Derby Hospitals NHS Foundation
Trust
Library and Knowledge Service

D1758642

WITHDRAWN

The Premenstrual Syndromes: PMS and PMDD

Edited by

PM SHAUGHN O'BRIEN MD FRCOG
Professor, Women and Children's Division
University Hospital of North Staffordshire
Keele University
Stoke-on-Trent
UK

ANDREA J RAPKIN MD
Professor, Department of Obstetrics and Gynecology
David Geffen School of Medicine at ULCA
Los Angeles, CA
USA

PETER J SCHMIDT MD FRCP(C)
National Institute of Mental Health
Bethesda, MD
USA

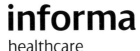

© 2007 Informa UK Ltd

First published in the United Kingdom in 2007 by Informa Healthcare, Telephone House, 69-77 Paul Street, London EC2A 4LQ. Informa Healthcare is a trading division of Informa UK Ltd. Registered Office: 37/41 Mortimer Street, London W1T 3JH. Registered in England and Wales number 1072954.

Tel: +44(0)20 7017 5000
Fax: +44 (0)20 7017 6699
Website: www.informahealthcare.com

All rights reserved. No part of this publication may be reproduced, stored in a retrieval system, or transmitted, in any form or by any means, electronic, mechanical, photocopying, recording, or otherwise, without the prior permission of the publisher or in accordance with the provisions of the Copyright, Designs and Patents Act 1988 or under the terms of any licence permitting limited copying issued by the Copyright Licensing Agency, 90 Tottenham Court Road, London W1P 0LP.

Although every effort has been made to ensure that all owners of copyright material have been acknowledged in this publication, we would be glad to acknowledge in subsequent reprints or editions any omissions brought to our attention.

Although every effort has been made to ensure that drug doses and other information are presented accurately in this publication, the ultimate responsibility rests with the prescribing physician. Neither the publishers nor the authors can be held responsible for errors or for any consequences arising from the use of information contained herein. For detailed prescribing information or instructions on the use of any product or procedure discussed herein, please consult the prescribing information or instructional material issued by the manufacturer.

A CIP record for this book is available from the British Library.
Library of Congress Cataloging-in-Publication Data

Data available on application

ISBN-10: 0 415 39974 2
ISBN-13: 978 0 415 39974 6

Distributed in North and South America by
Taylor & Francis
6000 Broken Sound Parkway, NW, (Suite 300)
Boca Raton, FL 33487, USA

Within Continental USA
Tel: 1 (800) 272 7737; Fax: 1 (800) 374 3401
Outside Continental USA
Tel: (561) 994 0555; Fax: (561) 361 6018
Email: orders@crcpress.com

Distributed in the rest of the world by
Thomson Publishing Services
Cheriton House
North Way
Andover, Hampshire SP10 5BE, UK
Tel: +44 (0)1264 332424
Email: tps.tandfsalesorder@thomson.com

Composition by Exeter Premedia Services Private Ltd., Chennai, India
Printed and bound in India by Replika Press Pvt Ltd

Contents

Contributors

Zenab Amin PhD
Department of Psychiatry
Yale University School of Medicine
New Haven, CT
USA

Lotta Andréen MD PhD
Umeå Neurosteroid Research Center
Department of Clinical Sciences
Norrland University Hospital
Umeå
Sweden

Torbjörn Bäckström MD PhD
Umeå Neurosteroid Research Center
Department of Clinical Sciences
Norrland University Hospital
Umeå
Sweden

Inger Björn MD PhD
Umeå Neurosteroid Research Center
Department of Clinical Sciences
Norrland University Hospital
Umeå
Sweden

Candace Brown MSN PharmD
Professor, Departments of Pharmacy
Obstetrics and Gynecology, and Psychiatry
University of Tennessee Health Science Center
Memphis TN
USA

Vandana Dhingra MBBS
University Hospital of North Staffordshire
Keele University
Stoke-on-Trent
UK

C Neill Epperson MD
Departments of Psychiatry, Obstetrics
Gynecology, and Reproductive Sciences
Yale University School of Medicine
New Haven, CT
USA

Elias Eriksson MD
Professor of Pharmacology
Institute of Neuroscience and Physiology
Sahlgrenska Academy
Göteborg University
Göteborg
Sweden

Edzard Ernst MD PhD FRCP FRCPEd
Complementary Medicine
Peninsula Medical School
Universities of Exeter and Plymouth
Exeter
UK

Ellen W Freeman PhD
Departments of Obstetrics/Gynecology
and Psychiatry
University of Pennsylvania
Philadelphia, PA
USA

Uriel Halbreich MD
Biobehavioral Program
State University of New York at Buffalo and WPA
Section on Interdisciplinary Collaboration
New York, NY
USA

Khaled MK Ismail MSc MD MRCOG
Academic Unit of Obstetrics and Gynecology
University Hospital of North Staffordshire
UK

Inga-Maj Johansson PhD
Umeå Neurosteroid Research Center
Department of Clinical Sciences
Norrland University Hospital
Umeå
Sweden

John Kuo MD
Department of Obstetrics and Gynecology
David Geffen School of Medicine at UCLA
Los Angeles, CA
USA

Frank W Ling MD
Department of Obstetrics and Gynecology
Vanderbilt University
Women's Health Specialists, PLLC
Germantown, TN
USA

Magnus Löfgren PhD-Student
Umeå Neurosteroid Research Center
Department of Clinical Sciences
Norrland University Hospital
Umeå
Sweden

Julia L Magnay MSc CSci FIBMS
Institute for Science and Technology in Medicine
Keele University
Stoke-on-Trent
UK

Graeme F Mason PhD
Departments of Psychiatry and Diagnostic Radiology
Yale University School of Medicine
New Haven, CT
USA

Kara Lynn McCunn MD
Assistant Professor of Psychiatry
Yale School of Medicine
New Haven, CT
USA

Judy Mikacich MD
Department of Obstetrics and Gynecology
David Geffen School of Medicine at UCLA
Los Angeles, CA
USA

PM Shaughn O'Brien MD FRCOG
Professor, Women & Children's Division
University Hospital of North Staffordshire
Keele University
Stoke-on-Trent
UK

Nick Panay BSc MD FRCOG
Consultant Gynaecologist
Queen Charlotte's and Chelsea and Chelsea and
Westminster Hospital
London
UK
and
Honorary Senior Lecturer
Imperial College
London
UK

Teri Pearlstein MD
Associate Professor of Psychiatry and Human
Behavior
Warren Alpert Medical School of Brown
University
Director, Women's Behavioral Health and
Infants' Hospital
Providence, RI
USA

Andrea J Rapkin MD
Professor of Obstetrics and Gynecology
David Geffen School of Medicine at ULCA
Los Angeles, CA
USA

Robert L Reid MD
Professor, Obstetrics and Gynecology, Physiology
Queen's University
Kingston, Ontario
Canada

David R Rubinow MD
Professor and Chairman
Department of Psychiatry
University of North Carolina at Chapel Hill
Chapel Hill, NC
USA

Peter J Schmidt MD
Section on Behavioral Endocrinology
National Institute of Mental Health
Bethesda, MD
USA

Claudio N Soares MD PhD
Associate Professor, Department of Psychiatry and
Behavioural Neurosciences, McMasters University
Director, Women's Health Concerns Clinic
St Joseph's Healthcare
Hamilton, ON
Canada

Meir Steiner MD PhD FRCPC
Professor of Psychiatry and Behavioural Neurosciences
and Obstetrics and Gynecology
McMaster University
Professor, Department of Psychiatry and Institute of
Medical Sciences
University of Toronto
Adjunct Sceintist, the Hospital for Sick Children,
Toronto
Founding Director, Women's Health Concerns Clinic
St Joseph's Healthcare
Hamilton, ON
Canada

John WW Studd DSc MRCOG MFFP
Professor of Gynaecology
Chelsea and Westminster Hospital
London
UK
and
The Lister Hospital
London
UK

Dean A Van Vugt PhD
Professor and Chair
Division of Reproductive Endocrinology and Infertility
Queen's University
Kingston, Ontario
Canada

Kimberly A Yonkers MD
Associate Professor of Psychiatry, Obstetrics and
Gynecology and Reproductive Sciences
Yale School of Medicine
New Haven, CT
USA

Preface

Somatic, affective, and behavioral symptoms can occur during the premenstrual phase of the menstrual cycle of nearly all ovulatory women. The nature and severity of these symptoms constitute a spectrum from minimal to disabling; however, the distinction between normal and pathological symptoms is one of the principal dilemmas in this area of research. The severity of interference with daily activities depends on various as yet poorly defined factors, but etiology probably includes genetic, neurochemical, and environmental factors. Are we really, in this era of high technology, limited to the use of simple paper-based rating scales to record the impact of symptoms on normal functioning, on school and work performance, and on ability to socialize? Yes, at present, this remains the most reliable way to distinguish between what is physiological and what constitutes a premenstrual disorder, premenstrual syndrome (PMS) or premenstrual dysphoric disorder (PMDD).

Awareness of such premenstrual problems amongst women, their partners, general practitioners, gynecologists, psychiatrists, other health professionals and, particularly, the media has increased dramatically over the past 30 years.

Even so, there are sceptics who say that premenstrual symptoms or disorders have been exaggerated and medicalized by the profession and the pharmaceutical industry, in order to 'peddle' their hormones (progestagens and estrogen) or antidepressants (notably selective serotonin reuptake inhibitors, SSRIs). Complementary and alternative practitioners have also offered a range of treatments: some ineffective; others, poorly studied, but possibly effective. Premenstrual symptoms, similar to many affective and behavioral symptoms, exhibit a very high response to placebo, and significant symptoms can occur in at least 20% of women. The lack of consensus on the nature of this condition creates a void

of knowledge, in which some women may unfortunately become targets for exploitation. However, it is of paramount importance that scientific research continues and that the medical community recognizes and cares for these disorders. It would be a great disservice to women and society if those in the medical community (who have insufficient knowledge and understanding) approach these problems with disdain.

Premenstrual syndrome is amongst a unique, small number of disorders where the patient frequently arrives at the specialist with their own diagnosis and it is the practitioner's role to exclude or confirm the diagnosis. The lack of an objective means of confirming the diagnosis and monitoring treatment is a great problem. This may be one of the reasons why the credibility of the diagnosis of PMS has been questioned. Although this is probably true for other psychological disorders, it is probably more so for PMS.

In the USA and in Australasia, PMS is recognized as a serious entity, but in the UK and continental Europe less so. The National Institute of Mental Health (NIMH) in Washington, DC, the American Psychiatric Association, and the American College of Obstetricians and Gynecologists (ACOG) respect the validity of these disorders in that research program grants, evidence-based clinician guidance, and patient information are well-established and widely disseminated. By contrast, in the UK, all PMS/PMDD research has been led by the pharmaceutical industry and only now, for the first time, is the Royal College of Obstetricians and Gynaecologists developing evidence-based guidance for treatment. The situation in the rest of Europe probably falls somewhere between these two extremes. A patient/consumer group in the UK, The National Association of Premenstrual Syndrome, has been the focus of activity in the field and has a relatively scientific view of most matters relating to PMS. In the UK and rest of Europe, the only licensed preparations for managing PMS are progesterone and various progestins, yet we will see in the following chapters that there is incontrovertible evidence that these are ineffective. Many other effective but unlicensed approaches are used in the UK and Europe: we have a situation where everything that is licensed is ineffective and everything that works is unlicensed! By contrast, in the USA, Canada, and Australasia, both the SSRI class of drugs as well as a novel oral contraceptive pill (for women who also want hormonal contraception), are licensed and prescribed extensively with guidelines for psychiatrists and gynecologists (ACOG) recommending either SSRIs or the newer drospirenone-containing oral contraceptive pill as first-line therapies for severe PMS or PMDD.

Clinical and basic science researchers in wide-ranging fields of study, including gynecology, psychology, psychiatry, endocrinology, genetics, brain imaging, and neurophysiology, have been interested in the exploration of this disorder for over 70 years, with an escalation of interest around the mid 1970s until today. This is the first multi-author textbook of its kind to focus solely on the premenstrual disorders of PMS and PMDD. Contributions have been received from individuals from most the units in Europe and the USA who have extensively researched and treated premenstrual tension, PMS, and PMDD.

The three editors have been involved in research into PMS for decades. They comprise a UK professor of obstetrics and gynecology from Keele University (PMSOB) who is currently also vice president of the Royal College of Obstetricians and Gynaecologists; a research and clinical psychiatrist from the NIMH in Washington, DC (PJS), and a well-established professor of obstetrics and gynecology from UCLA (AJR).

When setting about this book, we decided to choose authors who could represent virtually every major unit actively investigating aspects of PMS and PMDD in the UK, continental Europe, and the USA. It is hoped that no subject area has been left uncovered and no research group from these geographical areas overlooked.

Within the book there will be areas that are repeated or are contradictory, as views differ and it was felt inappropriate to edit out these views simply to be uniform. The reader will be able to appreciate ideological contrast and differing perceptions and experiences between psychiatrists and gynecologists, Europeans and Americans, clinicians and basic scientists, geneticists and endocrinologists. There is also, not surprisingly, agreement and disagreement within members of the same specialist areas. This adds to the richness of the debate and gives a fuller understanding of the current landscape. They are very much chapters written as the individuals see the issues, and often the emphasis will differ markedly. For instance, few authors from the USA contemplate giving estrogen, even though the evidence would support it. Few US authors would contemplate surgery. In the UK, there are strong advocates of ovulation suppression with transcutaneous estrogen therapy and, though only rarely and in severely affected patients, UK clinicians would be more willing to offer a surgical option – meaning, of course, the curative but very invasive decision to allow patients who request surgery to undergo hysterectomy and bilateral salpingo-oophorectomy. The research on this dramatic approach, however, has come from Canada and the USA as well as from the UK.

US psychiatrists, particularly, favor the use of the term PMDD and the use of SSRIs in management. The oral contraceptive pill is more readily advocated by US gynecologists, whereas the use of the levonorgestrel intrauterine system (LNG IUS, Mirena) is used extensively by UK gynecologists, not as a primary treatment method but to protect the endometrium from estrogen-induced hyperplasia during ovulation suppression using transcutaneous estrogen therapy. The use of psychotropic therapy and, more specifically, the SSRIs has been led by US and Canadian psychiatrists and Swedish researchers.

I think it is true to say that the study and publication of work on SSRI therapy predated any serious understanding of the neurobiology of PMS/PMDD, but this is now such a fascinating area that involves animal research, biochemical study, brain imaging with functional magnetic resonance imaging (fMRI) and positron emission tomography (PET) scanning, and finally genetics. This combination of research, which is all being currently undertaken, will give us the best chance of succeeding in reaching a valid explanation for the etiology and then the cure of the premenstrual disorders within the early part of the 21st century.

The science of the premenstrual disorders and, hopefully, this textbook should stimulate and whet the appetite of anyone who has not already embarked on the investigation of this area.

PMSO

1

History of the premenstrual disorders

PM Shaughn O'Brien and Khaled MK Ismail

INTRODUCTION

The study of premenstrual syndrome (PMS) appears to have been full of contradictions over many decades. However, progress in understanding the etiology and providing therapy for this condition has accelerated in recent years.

The easiest and most appropriate way to describe the history of the premenstrual disorders is to divide it into four eras based on the historical changes in terminology used in the literature. These four landmark stages parallel our understanding of the premenstrual disorders. The eras are:

- From the 'agitations' of Hippocrates (370 BC) to premenstrual tension (PMT);[1] in this period, the recognition and description of symptoms were first realized and the beginnings of an understanding of the problem began.
- From PMT to PMS;[2] in this period, the link between the ovarian hormone cycles and symptoms was recognized.
- From PMS to the American Psychiatric Association's definition of premenstrual dysphoric disorder (PMDD) (via late luteal phase dysphoric disorder [LLPDD]); in this period, a great deal of scientific energy was expended in an attempt to define and quantify premenstrual disorders and the theory of progesterone deficiency was explored and refuted.
- From PMDD to the present day; in this period there has been the realization that women are sensitive to *normal* levels of ovulatory progesterone, that this possibly has a neuroendocrine explanation, and that therapy can be achieved by altering neuroendocrine status with psychotropic drugs (notably selective serotonin reuptake inhibitors [SSRIs]) or by elimination of ovulation.

FROM HIPPOCRATES' 'AGITATIONS' TO FRANK'S PMT

Much is written in historical and religious texts regarding menstruation. There seems to be a strong need to claim that premenstrual symptoms were first described in the Torah, the Talmud, or the works of Hippocrates. Although there is extensive discussion and teaching related to menstruation in the two religious works, it is difficult to find anything that can be directly considered to describe premenstrual symptoms before the works attributed to Hippocrates. Much was written in myth related to menstruation and behavior, but one cannot clearly distinguish what does and what does not refer to the menstrual, pre-, or perimenstrual time phase associations with mood and behavior. What was written originally (often in Greek mythology) tended to be positive about menstruation, but as time progressed this became more negative. There are, however, several instances in Hippocrates' works where there are statements or aphorisms which clearly describe premenstrual symptoms:

> The blood of females is subject to intermittent 'agitations' and as a result the 'agitated blood' makes its way from the head to the uterus whence it is expelled.[3]

> Women experience a feeling of heaviness prior to menstruation.[4]

Beyond Hippocrates, many years passed before the literature identifies further reference to premenstrual symptoms. Halbreich[5] cites three important descriptions of severe premenstrual symptoms.

The first of these was by an 11th century female Italian scholar, Trotulo of Salerno, who wrote:

> There are young women who suffer in the same manner, who are relieved when their menses are called forth.

The second was also Italian; Giovani da Padua in the 16th century described fairly clearly a link between menstruation and depression.

Finally, Halbreich quotes the English physician James Cowles Prichard, who wrote:

> Some females at the period of the catamenia undergo a considerable degree of nervous excitement, morbid dispositions of mind are displayed by them at these times, a wayward and capricious temper, excitability in the feelings, moroseness in disposition, a proneness to quarrel with their dearest relatives and sometimes a dejection of mind approaching to melancholia.

What could be closer to this as a description of PMS, published in 1837?[6]

Ian Brockington's work on menstrual psychosis[7] is another valuable source of historical information. In it, he quotes the works of JE Hitzig, Briere de Boismont, and Richard von Krafft-Ebing.

In 1828, Hitzig described menstrual mood disorder in relation to an acquittal for filicide. Having been condemned to death for drowning her child, a mother confided in a fellow prisoner that she experienced inexplicable symptoms before and during her period. Following medical observation of this and various physical phenomena, she was acquitted.

Briere de Boismont described four cases of premenstrual psychosis and described the relationship between menstruation and *surexcitation* or overstimulation and agitation:

> Surexcitation: 8 synonymes: agitation, bouillonnement, délire, ébullition, échauffement, effervescence, exaltation, fièvre.

Brockington quotes frequently the seminal work of Richard von Krafft-Ebing,[8] in which he described 60 cases of menstrual psychosis.

FROM PMT TO DALTON'S PMS: PREMENSTRUAL TENSION

Robert Tilden Frank (1875–1949)[1] was a New York gynecologist who graduated from Harvard and subsequently worked in Columbia University and as chief of the gynecological service at Mount Sinai Hospital in New York. In 1931 he described for the first time the condition premenstrual tension in a paper read at the Academy of Medicine, New York:

> My attention has been increasingly directed to a large group of women who are handicapped by premenstrual disturbances of a manifold nature.

It is well known that normal women suffer varying degrees of discomfort preceding the onset of menstruation. Employers of labour take cognisance of this fact and make provision for the temporary increased fatigability, irritability, lack of concentration and attacks of pain. In another group of patients the symptoms complained of are of sufficient gravity to require rest in bed for one or two days. In this group particularly, pain plays a prominent role. There is still another class of patients in whom grave systemic disorders manifest themselves predominantly during the premenstrual period.

Frank suggested initially that an excess of ovarian estrogen (due to diminished excretion) was the underlying cause, and he went on to illustrate this with cases – some of which were treated by irradiation of the ovaries, presumably resulting in a radiation menopause. Jeliffe (1906) had hinted at this previously in a report in the New York State Journal of Medicine (cited in Halbreich),[5] but it was Frank who brought the subject and its probable link with the ovarian cycle to the attention of the medical world. Frank clearly was the first to describe premenstrual tension but, at the same time, Karen Horney, a German psychoanalyst who moved to the USA in the early 1930s, described (independently from Frank) 'Die pramenstruellen Verstimmungen' in 1931.[9] She highlighted the disappearance of symptoms with the onset of menstruation and its recurrent nature. She attributed the symptoms to estrogenic hormone from the ovary but recognized that this was related to the corpus luteum.

Between Frank's publication and the writings of Katherina Dalton in 1953, many theories were developed and proposed for the etiology, including antidiuretic hormone, hormone allergy, deficiency of various vitamins and minerals (including potassium, calcium, and magnesium), hypoglycemia/insulin excess, estrogen/progesterone imbalance, pelvic congestion, 'menotoxin', progesterone deficiency, and salt and water retention, and of course there were many purely psychological theories. It is not appropriate to discuss every one of these: those that are important are discussed in other chapters of this book, whereas those which are less important can be found in the editor's (P.M.S.O.) earlier textbook, Premenstrual Syndrome.[10]

FROM PMS TO THE AMERICAN PSYCHIATRIC ASSOCIATION'S PMDD

In 1950, Morton was first to advocate the (subsequently disproved) theory of progesterone deficiency and estrogen/progesterone imbalance. Dalton[2] took this theory, and the claim that 'pure' progesterone would provide treatment, to a high level of consciousness internationally in the medical, lay, and political world. She coined the new term premenstrual syndrome (PMS) and this is the term still largely used throughout the world by the majority of women and most physicians, general practitioners, gynecologists, and (with the exception of North America), most psychiatrists.

Dalton must be credited for bringing this syndrome to the attention of the medical world, as without her crusading intervention the problem of PMS may well have been ignored. Her blind support for progesterone therapy in the face of the evidence of its inefficacy was unscientific but of course she was practicing and her views did stem from the early 1950s.

Katherina Dalton was a charismatic general practitioner in London. As a medical student, she suffered severe menstrual migraine that disappeared during her four pregnancies. She put two and two together, and, with the endocrinologist Dr Raymond Greene,* embarked on a personal exploration of progesterone therapy. Katherina Dalton became free from premenstrual migraines by administration of daily injections of progesterone from ovulation to menstruation. Accordingly, and not surprisingly, her enthusiasm and dedication grew from here on and she went on in the 1950s and 1960s to report subsequently on a series of anecdotal cases of successful treatment of premenstrual asthma, eczema and migraines in her patients.

Between the time of Dalton's early descriptions of PMS and the era which led to more precise diagnosis and measurement, many theories were proposed and much research was undertaken. Many of these efforts led to today's research, but it must be admitted that much of what we know from that era was based on diagnostic criteria that were imprecise and thus limited lasting conclusions can be drawn from much of that work.

The dominant theories and work focused on several areas over the time span of 1953 to the late 1980s (Table 1.1). These areas were:

- etiology – ovarian endocrine: estrogen excess, progesterone deficiency, estrogen/progesterone imbalance
- etiology – other non-ovarian hormones
- therapy – anecdotal, uncontrolled trials and randomized controlled trials (RCTs)
- quantification techniques and definitions.

*Brother of Graham Greene, the English novelist and playwright, and Sir Hugh Greene, former director of the BBC.

Ovarian endocrine research dominated this era. Research focused on estrogen and, particularly, progesterone, arising from Dalton's progesterone deficiency crusade. By the end of this historical phase it became clear that research had produced studies demonstrating high, low, or no differences in progesterone or estrogen levels in PMS patients compared with controls. Researchers, and, more so, the pharmaceutical industry, selected those data that supported their case. The case for progesterone deficiency was more or less dispelled but this did not stop the continued prescription of, and indeed licensing of, progesterone by several routes and progestogens orally. It is of interest to note that in the UK these preparations continue to be the only preparations licensed for PMS and so they are widely prescribed in the face of overwhelming evidence that they are ineffective.

Although some studies did demonstrate differences to support these theories, it must be realized that few were replicated and probably what is more important is that the specific criteria and quantification techniques used now were not available. Reliance cannot be made on supportive or negative findings for most of these studies.

Where these findings are relevant to today's practice and research they will be addressed in the individual chapters which follow. More detailed reference can again be found in O'Brien's Premenstrual Syndrome (1987), which covers the available research up to that year.[91]

Table 1.1 Hormones, minerals, and vitamins considered as possible etiologic agents in this era

- Estrogen excess
- Progesterone deficiency
- Prolactin excess
- Sex hormone-binding globulin
- Testosterone
- Prostaglandins
- Pituitary hormone/gonadotropins
- Aldosterone–renin–angiotensin system
- Cortisol
- Thyroid hormones
- Antidiuretic hormone
- Atrial natriuretic peptide
- Magnesium, calcium, and vitamins (including vitamin B_6) deficiency

Table 1.2 Proposed or researched PMS treatments

Non-pharmacological treatments:
- Counseling
- Relaxation therapy
- Psychotherapy
- Cognitive behavioral therapy (CBT)
- Stress management
- Homeopathy
- Intravaginal electrical stimulation
- Rest
- Isolation
- Yoga
- Aromatherapy
- Exercise
- Music therapy
- Hypnosis
- Dietary manipulation
- Salt restriction
- Self-help groups
- Agnus castus
- Irradiation of ovaries

Non-hormonal pharmacological treatments:
- Tranquilizers
- Antidepressants
- Lithium
- SSRIs initial studies
- Vitamin B_6
- Beta-blockers
- Evening primrose oil
- Diuretics, spironolactone
- Magnesium, zinc, and calcium

Hormonal treatments:
- Progesterone (pessaries, injections, vaginal gel)
- Progestogens (norethisterone, dydrogesterone, medroxyprogesterone acetate, Depo-Provera)
- COC pill: cyclical/continuous
- Testosterone
- Bromocriptine
- Mifepristone, RU-486
- Cyproterone acetate
- Tibolone
- Danazol, gestrinone
- Estradiol (oral, patch, implant)
- GnRH agonist analogs
- Non-steroidal anti-inflammatory drugs

(Continued)

Table 1.2 (Continued)

Surgical treatments:
- Hysterectomy
- Hysterectomy and bilateral oophorectomy
- Endometrial ablation techniques

Therapy

In the era from 1950 to the late 1980s and early 1990s, treatment research moved from anecdotal reporting of cases through non-blind trials to well-controlled randomized double-blind trials. However, meta-analysis had not yet made any impact in this sphere of research. The area of these studies matched that of the studies of etiology to a large extent. The number of therapeutic studies conducted during that time period was huge, as the existence of PMS had reached public consciousness – everything available was being used to treat PMS. With such a large initial placebo response and the existence of many patients labeled as PMS who had much milder problems, the pharmaceutical industry and complementary and alternative therapy companies were having a field day.

Again, it is not appropriate to list every study: details will again be found in the individual chapters of this book or in O'Brien's book.[1]

Table 1.2 aims to summarize the different treatments which had been proposed or researched. The list is not intended to be exhaustive but gives a flavor of the range and number of therapies proposed during the era.

Quantification and definitions

Most early studies relied on the patient's perception of her symptoms or the clinician's diagnosis from history and observation alone. Through this time period, a great deal of work was conducted aiming to define PMS more precisely and to devise methods to measure symptoms.

The first method dedicated specifically to menstrual or premenstrual symptoms was the Moos, Menstrual Distress Questionnaire.[11] This was a rating scale which used a 47-symptom six-point rating scale. Subsequent new scales followed this template, which used different combinations of symptom types; scores which ranged from 0 to 3, 4, 5, 6, and 7. In the same era, the first use of a visual analog scale (VAS) was published (1979) and, much later, improvements led to VAS charts that adhered to the criteria required for PMDD.

Definitions and diagnostic criteria also evolved over this time period. Having begun with Frank's PMT and

Dalton's PMS, new, more precise terms were developed. In 1987, the terminology and criteria for late luteal phase dysphoric disorder (LLPDD) for the Diagnostic and Statistical Manual of Mental Disorders, third edition (DSM-III) of the American Psychiatric Association were published. This is only now of historical interest, as the later definition and criteria of premenstrual dysphoric disorder, which was defined in DSM-IV,[12] has replaced it. In 1990 the Daily Record of Severity of Problems (DRSP) provided a categorical rating (0–6) scale of all of the symptom components required for PMDD.[13,14]

This was an important milestone in the evolution of the science of premenstrual disorders. It provided clear-cut guidance and criteria, but unfortunately with some important limitations: e.g. the need for five symptom groups excludes many patients with a severe premenstrual disorder but with fewer symptoms. Additionally, it also confines the range of physical symptoms to a single category, virtually excluding the diagnosis of PMDD in a patient with predominantly physical symptoms. Cynics have been heard to say that this was intentional in order to exclude gynecology and to strengthen the case for psychotropic therapy – particularly the (then) newly emerging SSRIs.

FROM PMDD TO THE PRESENT DAY AND BEYOND

The key events following the introduction of the concept of PMDD represent the journey to our current understanding of all premenstrual disorders. This understanding will provide a real chance of determining a full explanation of the mechanisms of premenstrual disorders (and subsequently their treatment) in the early part of this century.

Developments in treatment approach over the past 20 years

Given that current treatment offers the ability either to suppress ovulation or to rectify an unknown neural biochemical derangement, we will again consider developments under these headings and with a causal theory/treatment modality pairing.

Therapeutic research

In this era, hormonal therapy, cognitive behavioral therapy, and psychotropic therapy became all-important: in particular, transdermal estrogen, new combined contraceptive pills with novel progestogens (such as drospirenone), and gonadotropin-releasing hormone (GnRH) analogues (with and without add-back) became serious contenders. The levonorgestrel IUS (intrauterine system) was also introduced, first as a contraceptive technique, then as a treatment for menorrhagia, and next as the progestogenic component of hormone replacement therapy (HRT). In the clinical arena, many were using it to protect the endometrium from hyperplasia during ovarian suppression with estrogen in the management of PMS – the rationale being, parallel with its use in HRT, that the endometrium would be protected while systemic levels remained low, thus avoiding restimulation of PMS symptoms. Meta-analysis was introduced as a new powerful method to analyze several trials that were relatively underpowered to draw conclusions from the single studies. Finally, a whole new research direction assessing psychotropic therapy, particularly the SSRIs, began.

Hormone therapy

Katherina Dalton's theory of progesterone deficiency and therapy using progesterone replacement was largely dismissed during this time. It is an irony that her views were the main stimulus to our interest in PMS in the third quarter of the 20th century. For the same reasons, the administration of oral progestogens was also considered valueless. This said, these two approaches remain the only drugs prescribable under license in the UK for PMS and, consequently, the most commonly prescribed therapy in UK general practice.[15]

In the mid 1980s there was a transient enthusiasm for theories related to prolactin excess and, thus, the use of dopamine agonists. This enthusiasm waned after finding that prolactin differences did not exist and that PMS did not respond to bromocriptine therapy. It should be mentioned that cyclical mastalgia does respond to bromocriptine. Side effects can be problematic. It is considered that late evening administration and luteal-phase only treatment may minimize this, but there is no confirmatory research. Bromocriptine therapy is thus limited to PMS patients suffering with premenstrual mastalgia.

Around the same time, similar views were being held for the use of the androgenic preparation, danazol. There was more evidence in favor of its positive benefit for PMS symptoms (compared with bromocriptine) but the doses required to suppress ovulation reliably were associated with the risk, or at least perceived risk, of side effects, particularly masculinizing side effects. Luteal phase administration of low-dose danazol was studied and published with slightly conflicting findings. Certainly, such a regimen was shown to be effective for cyclical mastalgia (with minimal side effects)[16] and one study showed a beneficial effect on most PMS symptoms.[17]

During the same era, there began an enthusiasm for the use of evening primrose oil containing γ-linolenic acid. This was largely driven by the manufacturer and based on quite spurious data. Again, though, breast symptoms appeared to be effectively relieved with minimal side effects. Until quite recently there was a UK pharmaceutical license for mastalgia and, despite the lack of supportive evidence of efficacy, relatively high doses were available in 'Premenstrual Packs' as over-the-counter preparations in the high street pharmacy.

In the UK, a small group of clinical researchers had always maintained a high degree of enthusiasm for estrogen therapy, believing that such therapy should be considered first line. John Studd, an eminent UK gynecologist, with his research group, had been as great an advocate and enthusiast for estrogen therapy as Katherina Dalton had been for progesterone. The difference, however, with Studd's work was that:

- the therapeutic approach was based on a realistic theory; i.e. suppression of ovulation was achievable using transdermal estrogen
- he published well-controlled research to support the efficacy of transdermal estrogen therapy.

Serotonin and SSRIs

Part of this historical research phase could reasonably be known as the 'serotonin phase' of the science of PMS. Research trials of SRIs/SSRIs (serotonin reuptake inhibitors/selective serotonin reuptake inhibitors) had begun as early as 1986 and had been reported soon after. Beneficial effects had been shown, particularly for fluoxetine, paroxetine, citalopram, sertraline, and venlafaxine. The Steiner et al[19] fluoxetine paper was pivotal in the approval of SSRIs by the US Food and Drug Administration (FDA) and the UK Committee in Safety of Medicines (CSM) licensing authorities, with long-acting fluoxetine being recognized subsequently. The UK and European license was lost when it was withdrawn by the European Medicines Agency (EMEA), the European licensing agency, thus depriving a whole continent of the benefits of such treatment regimens. Fluoxetine is used off-license extensively for PMS, but this advice is usually only given by the small number of medical practitioners with specialized knowledge in the area and, maybe, some well-informed general practitioners who choose to label the patients with this problem as a variant of depression in order to justify its prescription. It is probably true to say that SSRIs are now accepted as the first-line, non-hormonal therapy for PMS. Some doctors would now consider them *the* first choice in patients with severe PMS/PMDD. As a comment on European intransigence to the licensing, it should also be added that the acceptance of PMDD as an entity is far from widespread.

Soon after the acceptance of SSRIs as treatment, there began the realization that the actions of these drugs were probably different from the mechanism found in its antidepressant effect, to such an extent that luteal phase dosing began and was shown to be effective in appropriately conducted trials. As the following chapters will show, many researchers have been involved in the development and subsequent phases of this area of research, which includes most SSRI work (see Chapter 15).

Systematic reviews are useful in establishing consistencies and significant variations in healthcare effects. They are essential for the efficient integration of valid information, and hence provide a basis for rational decision-making.[19] The use of explicit, systematic methods in systematic reviews limits bias (systematic errors) and reduces chance effects, thus providing more robust results upon which to draw conclusions and make decisions.[20,21] Moreover, quality assessment of individual studies included in a systematic review helps to gain insight into potential comparisons and guides interpretation of findings. Factors that warrant assessment are those related to applicability of findings, validity of individual studies, and specific design characteristics that affect interpretation of results. 'Meta-analysis' is the term given to the process of using statistical methods to summarize data of included independent studies. This collective analysis can provide more precise estimates of the effects of health care than those derived from the individual studies included in a single review,[22–24] thus facilitating decisions that are based on the totality of the available evidence. With the widespread acceptance of this methodology as the gold standard for determining evidence-based management in medicine, a series of systematic reviews were conducted to evaluate the effectiveness of therapeutic interventions used in PMS/PMDD.[25–29] Meta-analysis is now well-established internationally and benefits from the visual presentation of collective data using Forest Plots. The Cochrane database and library were the forerunners of this approach. The strength of meta-analysis over uncontrolled trials, individual trials, unstructured reviews, and even structured reviews should be noted. The power of meta-analysis was realized, and analysis of many therapeutic modalities was carried out in this way for many medical areas, particularly for obstetrics and menstrual disorders. The Cochrane Collaboration led this approach to research.

For PMS/PMDD, meta-analyses were produced for vitamin B_6, progesterone, progestogens, GnRH analogues, GnRH analogues with add-back, and the SSRIs, luteal phase SSRIs, and antidepressants, with danazol and estrogen therapy to be published in the near future.

Many other therapeutic areas have been covered in systematic views but not meta-analysis, which, as we have said, represents the gold standard for clarity, power, and precision.

Research into etiology

Much new work on estrogen, progesterone levels, suppression of the ovarian and cycle, and the investigation of endocrine cycle paradigms became prominent (see Chapter 10) during this era, led by the NIMH (National Institute of Mental Health) group in Washington, DC, and two groups in Sweden, at the Universities of Gothenburg and Umea (see Chapters 3 and 13, respectively). This research was very much cause-driven, not leading to an immediate therapeutic modality. Landmark research was undertaken on hypotheses related to neuroanatomy, ovarian suppression with GnRH and re-stimulation paradigms, and neuronal biochemistry; this work was particularly directed at serotonin and γ-aminobutyric acid (GABA) and conducted from the mid 1990s onwards.

Although no excess or deficiency in estrogen or progesterone levels has ever been demonstrated, the possibility of differences in progesterone receptors or progesterone metabolites was considered by the UCLA (University of California at Los Angeles) group (see Chapter 9). Because of the affinity of allopregnanolone for the GABA receptor and the lower measured levels of allopregnanolone in PMS patients, it became a prominent recent theory of causation. It has not yet led to specific treatment recommendations.

As it became clear that ovulation is the trigger for premenstrual events rather than differences in hormone levels, attention became focused on the probability that neural factors permitted an increased sensitivity to ovarian steroids, particularly progesterone. Therapeutic research on the SSRIs very convincingly demonstrated a high level of efficacy, although it was realized that effective therapy does not automatically imply causality in PMS (i.e. headache is not due to aspirin deficiency!). Effective SSRI treatment does not prove serotonin deficiency.

It is not surprising that research thereafter led to the investigation of most neurotransmitters, including the genetics of serotonin (5-hydroxytryptamine, 5-HT), GABA, and PMS/PMDD. The editors of this book (and several other groups) are currently investigating the genetic basis of PMS and PMDD. Despite many differences being found in such disorders as depression, seasonal affective disorder (SAD), and anxiety, the exploration of polymorphisms in PMDD appeared initially unfruitful, although it now seems possible that differences in polymorphisms for the 5-HT1A receptor may be present compared with controls, and ultimately these may show a linkage to cause and/or therapeutic response (Vandana Dhingra, pers comm).

The inaccessibility of the brain makes the understanding of any psychological process or illness a major challenge. If we analyze what has been available to investigators, our research tools are found to be sadly lacking. Certainly, there is no objective test available to make a diagnosis: peripheral blood tests need not necessarily reflect central nervous system (CNS) levels or activity (e.g. platelet and blood serotonin, β-endorphin); no physical test has been identified; for measurements, we are limited to patient-completed questionnaires; and detailed psychiatric interviews have been available to only a small number of studies.

The challenge of the complex inter-relationships seen in neurological biochemistry and associated genetics is made even more exciting by developments in brain imaging. A greater understanding of this whole field is poised to be unfolded by the arrival of techniques (see Chapter 11) such as positron emission tomography (PET), single-photon emission computed tomography (SPET), and functional magnetic resonance imaging (fMRI). These techniques offer a real chance of investigating and understanding brain function and blood flow, which may link us to an understanding of premenstrual disorders.

CONCLUSION

It has taken more than 20 centuries to move from Hippocrates' observation that women appeared to have cerebral 'agitations' (which were released from the uterus at menstruation) to developing the ability to visualize these 'agitations' by modern brain imaging technology. There seems to be little doubt that the normal ovarian endocrine cycle provides the trigger in women with CNS sensitivity to these endocrine changes. We are in the process of explaining the reason for this sensitivity incrementally – the more we learn, the more an explanation points towards specific neurotransmitters in the CNS. A combination of molecular genetics, endocrinology, and brain imaging will certainly lead us to this goal. In the meantime, we have a plethora of therapeutic approaches to help us manage our patients until scientific study leads to a cure.

REFERENCES

1. Frank RT. The hormonal causes of premenstrual tension. Arch Neurol Psychiatry 1931; 26:1053.
2. Dalton Greene. The premenstrual syndrome. BMJ 1953; 1: 1016–17.
3. Farrington B. The Medical Works of Hippocrates by John Chadwick, W.N. Mann. J Hellen Stud 1952; 72:132–3.

4. Simon B. Mind and Madness in Ancient Greece: the Classical Roots of Modern Psychiatry. Ithaca: Cornell University Press; 1978.

5. Halbreich U. History and trajectory of PMS: towards a balanced adaptation and a biosocial homeostasis. J Reprod Infant Psychol 2006; 24(4):336–46.

6. Prichard J. Treatise on Insanity and Other Disorders Affecting the Mind. London: Sherwood, Gilbert and Piper; 1837.

7. Brockington I. Menstrual psychosis. World Psychiatry 2005; 4(1): 9–17.

8. Krafft-Ebing R. Psychosis Menstrualis. Stuttgart: Verlag von Ferdinand Enke; 1902.

9. Horney K. Die Pramenstruellen Verstimmungen. Zeitscher f psychoanalytische Padagogik 1931; 5:1–7.

10. O'Brien P. Premenstrual Syndrome. London: Blackwell Science; 1987.

11. Moos RH. The development of a menstrual distress questionnaire. Psychosom Med 1968; 30(6):853–67.

12. American Psychiatric Association. Diagnostic and Statistical Manual of Mental Health, 4th edn. Washington, DC: American Psychiatric Press; 1994.

13. Endicott J, Harrison W. Daily rating of severity of problems form. New York: Department of Research Assessment and Training, New York State Psychiatric Institute; 1990.

14. Endicott J, Nee J, Harrison W. Daily Record of Severity of Problems (DRSP): reliability and validity. Arch Womens Ment Health 2006; 9(1):41–9.

15. Wyatt KM, Dimmock PW, Frischer M, Jones PW, O'Brien SPM. Prescribing patterns in premenstrual syndrome. BMC Womens Health 2002; 2(1):4.

16. O'Brien PM, Abukhalil IE. Randomized controlled trial of the management of premenstrual syndrome and premenstrual mastalgia using luteal phase-only danazol. Am J Obstet Gynecol 1999; 180(1 Pt 1):18–23.

17. Sarno AP Jr, Miller EJ Jr, Lundblad EG. Premenstrual syndrome: beneficial effects of periodic, low-dose danazol. Obstet Gynecol 1987; 70(1):33–6.

18. Steiner M, Steinberg S, Stewart D et al. Fluoxetine in the treatment of premenstrual dysphoria. Canadian Fluoxetine/Premenstrual Dysphoria Collaborative Study Group. N Engl J Med 1995; 332(23):1529–34.

19. Mulrow CD. Rationale for systematic reviews. BMJ 1994; 309 (6954):597–9.

20. Antman EM, Lau J, Kupelnick B, Mosteller F, Chalmers TC. A comparison of results of meta-analyses of randomized control trials and recommendations of clinical experts. Treatments for myocardial infarction. JAMA 1992; 268(2):240–8.

21. Oxman AD, Guyatt GH. The science of reviewing research. Ann NY Acad Sci 1993; 703:125–33.

22. Cohen J. Statistical Power Analysis for the Behavioral Sciences. New Jersey: Lawrence Erlbaum Associates; 1988.

23. Sacks HS, Berrier J, Reitman D, Ancona-Berk VA, Chalmers TC. Meta-analyses of randomized controlled trials. N Engl J Med 1987; 316(8):450–5.

24. Thacker SB. Meta-analysis. A quantitative approach to research integration. JAMA 1988; 259(11):1685–9.

25. Wyatt K, Dimmock P, Jones P, Obhrai M, O'Brien S. Efficacy of progesterone and progestogens in management of premenstrual syndrome: systematic review. BMJ 2001; 323(7316):776–80.

26. Wyatt KM, Dimmock PW, Jones PW, Shaughn O'Brien PM. Efficacy of vitamin B-6 in the treatment of premenstrual syndrome: systematic review. BMJ 1999; 318(7195):1375–81.

27. Wyatt KM, Dimmock PW, O'Brien PM. Selective serotonin reuptake inhibitors for premenstrual syndrome. Cochrane Database Syst Rev 2002; (4):CD001396.

28. Wyatt KM, Dimmock PW, Ismail KM, Jones PW, O'Brien PM. The effectiveness of GnRHa with and without 'add-back' therapy in treating premenstrual syndrome: a meta analysis. BJOG 2004; 111(6):585–93.

29. Dimmock PW, Wyatt KM, Jones PW, O'Brien PM. Efficacy of selective serotonin-reuptake inhibitors in premenstrual syndrome: a systematic review. Lancet 2000; 356(9236):1131–6.

Derby Hospitals NHS Foundation Trust
Library and Knowledge Service

2

The diagnosis of PMS/PMDD – the current debate

Uriel Halbreich

INTRODUCTION

Despite several decades of research and progress in knowledge on premenstrual syndrome (PMS), acceptance by most laypeople in Western countries and the availability of reasonably effective treatment modalities, the definitions and diagnostic criteria for PMS remain controversial. We are still far from a biomedical and/or biopsychosocial model of a diagnostic entity based on etiology, pathophysiology, phenomena, time course, and treatment response. Even descriptive diagnoses are fragmented with at least two main pathways: gynecological and psychiatric. Furthermore, there is still a group that doubts the existence of PMS – mostly on political–psychosocial grounds.

Diagnostic criteria are important for the clinical relevance and treatment of PMS as well as for delineation of the public health impact. According to the criteria of the American Psychiatric Association (APA) Diagnostic and Statistical Manual, fourth edition (DSM-IV)[1] and DSM-IV – text revision (DSM-IV-TR)[2] for premenstrual dysphoric disorder (PMDD), the prevalence of that dysphoric premenstrual syndrome is widely cited as being 3–8% of women of reproductive age.[3–10] However, if the clinically relevant impairment, suffering, and distress are considered as important, as opposed to the arbitrary cut-off number of five symptoms, the 12 months prevalence of dysphoric PMS is closer to 20% of women of reproductive age. The impact of definitions on the reported prevalence is demonstrated in Table 2.1.

When viewed in relation to other mental disorders,[16] it is demonstrated[17] that PMS/PMDD should be viewed as a major problem for the individual and the public. According to the strict minimalist criteria, the impact of PMDD on quality of life and social adjustment is similar to that of dysthymic disorder and is comparable to the impact of major depressive disorder (MDD) on marital and parental social adjustment as well as housework and leisure functioning.[17,18] Clinically relevant amendments to the criteria would probably increase the documented prevalence of dysphoric PMS and its impact.

The public health impact of PMDD may be demonstrated by using the global burden of disease (GBD) model and calculating the number of years of healthy life lost to disability, or – in other words – the disability adjusted life years (DALYs).[19] Detailed conservative considerations and calculations have been previously published.[17] The calculated burden of PMDD for the USA as well as the European Union, using very strict criteria for PMDD, is summarized in Table 2.2.

The actual total DALYs are probably much higher, because the calculations in the table are limited to the estimate of 5% of women who would meet strict criteria for PMDD and do not take into account women with significant premenstrual impairment with only 3–4 symptoms, or who have only physical symptoms. If global DALYs for PMS were to be calculated, the number would be staggering.

Considering the clinical and public health impact of premenstrual syndromes, an interdisciplinary internationally accepted diagnosis is needed.

EARLY DIAGNOSTIC CONCEPTS OF PMS[21]

As early as 1906[22] catamenial migraine was identified as a menstrually related endocrinological disorder. Various descriptions of premenstrual catamenial disorders followed. In 1931, the American gynecologist Frank[23] coined the term PMT – premenstrual tension, which described mostly behavioral and mood symptoms and their timeframe, 7–10 days before menstruation. It is of interest that in the same year (1931) the prominent

Table 2.1 The reported prevalence of premenstrual dysphoric disorder and severe premenstrual symptoms depends on the definitions applied

Author (year)	Symptoms/criteria	N	Percent
Robinson and Swindle (2000)[11]	Comparison of three assessment measures: global self-report, DSM-IV PMDD, and 'summative symptom' severity	1022 (age: 18–49 years)	Global self-report: severe symptoms, 4.9%; PMDD, 11.3%; severe summative symptoms, 16.2%; 'stronger severe' impairment, 17.1%
Angst et al (2001)[3]	Perimenstrual symptoms, subjective distress and impairment measure. 15 years prospective cohort study	299 (age: 21–35 years)	Severe distress, 8.1%. Moderate distress, 13.6%
Steiner et al (2002)[12] (abstract)	Retrospective list of DSM-IV PMDD items	508 (age: 18–55 years)	PMDD, 5.1%. Impairment with ≤4 PMDD items (near threshold), 20.7%
Cohen et al (2002)[13]	Prospective DRSP	513 (age: 36–44 years)	PMDD, 6.4%
Chawla et al (2002)[14]	Modified prospective DRSP	1194 (age: 21–45 years)	OMDD, 4.7%. Subthreshold severe PMS, 12.6%
Wittchen et al (2002)[15]	Prevalence and 4-year incidence for symptoms and diagnosis of PMDD based on DSM-IV criteria	1091 (age: 14–24 years)	Strict 12-month prevalence, 5.3%. Cumulative lifetime incidence, 7.4%. Near threshold cases, 18.6%

Adapted from Halbreich et al.[17]

psychoanalyst Karen Horney[24] expressed a more interdisciplinary approach, describing Prämenstruallen Verstimmungen (premenstrual negative predispositions) as a variety of syndromes – physical and mental – affecting vulnerable women and triggered by changes in gonadal hormones.

Although several hormonal and psychological treatment modalities of PMT were suggested, the definition of PMT as a clinical entity was debated from time to time with no operational solution. Notably the problems were delineated by a distinguished interdisciplinary panel gathered in New York in 1953,[25] the same year that the term premenstrual tension syndrome, PMTS started to replace PMT. Later it was abbreviated to PMS. Still, the diagnosis of PMS (or PMTS or PMT)

was a practical individual art depending on the physician's specialty, awareness, philosophy, and skills. No specific criteria were suggested, established, or accepted.

This has not been changed even with the more official but vague inclusion of premenstrual tension syndrome (PMTS) in the ICD nomenclature.

CURRENT DIAGNOSTIC ENTITIES OF PMS

ICD-10

The World Health Organization (WHO)'s International Classification of Diseases, 10th edition (ICD-10),[26] includes premenstrual tension syndrome (PMTS) in its

Table 2.2 The burden of PMDD/PMS in the USA and the EU according to most conservative-strict definition: disability adjusted life years (DALY)[a] lost

• Severity weight of severe PMS	0.50 (Class 5)	
• Age of onset of PMS	14–17 years[b]	
• Prevalence in teenagers	5.3–7.8%	
• Duration of disease 14–51 years	37 years	
• Cycles affected 481–22 (2 pregnancies and postpartum)	459 cycles	
• Average days of severe PMS per cycle	6.1 days[c]	
• Total days/years of disorders	2800 days/7.671 years	
• DALY (7.671 × 0.5)	3.835 per woman	
	USA	**EU**
• Women ages 14–51 (USA); 15–49 (EU) 2000 census	75,580,000	91,445,000
• Women who would meet criteria for PMDD (>5%)	>3,779,000	>4,572,250
Total DALYs, lost years of healthy life	**>14,492,465**	**>17,534,579**
The number would be even higher if all women suffering from PMS with impairment are counted		

Data from [a]Murray and Lopez,[19] [b]Wittchen et al,[15] and [c]Hylan et al.[20]

section of gynecological disorders, as a disorder of the female genital organs. The significance of the ICD-10 diagnosis is that it focuses on the two main aspects of PMS:

• the association with the menstrual cycle
• cyclicity and timing.

It requires that symptoms occur exclusively during the premenstrual period and remit following menses. It de-emphasizes the nature of specific symptoms or phenomena. It only gives examples such as tension or migraine or any other molimen – any menstrually related symptoms. It does not specify any level of required severity or impairment, no degree of change from the non-symptomatic phase of the menstrual cycle, and no differential diagnosis or exclusion criteria (Table 2.3). The ICD-9 code for PMS is 625.4.

ACOG diagnostic criteria

Conceptually similar, but a step forward from the ICD-10 criteria are the American College of Obstetricians and Gynecologists (ACOG) diagnostic criteria for premenstrual syndrome (PMS)[27] (Table 2.3).

The ACOG diagnostic criteria require the reporting of at least any one of six affective or one of four somatic symptoms that should exist during the 5 days before the menses at each of three prior menstrual cycles and be relieved within 4 days of onset of menses. They should not exist until the periovulatory phase of the menstrual cycle, be present in the absence of any pharmacological therapy, be associated with impairment or dysfunction in social or economic performance, and be prospectively confirmed during two menstrual cycles.

The significance of the ACOG criteria is that they acknowledge the importance of dysfunction and impairment, specify the symptomatic and the asymptomatic periods, and require prospective confirmation of retrospective reports. In my opinion, the emphasis on timing, with vagueness of nature of symptoms and requirement for at least one symptom without a threshold of minimal number of symptoms, is a conceptual and practical strength of the ACOG criteria.

APA DSM-IV criteria

The most elaborate diagnostic criteria of a subtype of PMS are the APA DSM-IV criteria for premenstrual dysphoric disorder – PMDD.[1,2] This set of criteria requires an initial retrospective report that symptoms, their luteal–follicular cyclicity, luteal occurrences, and follicular absence have been presented for the majority of cycles during the previous year. At least five out of 11 listed symptoms must be present; at least one of them should be a major mood symptom – depression, anxiety, irritability, or affective lability. Symptoms should cause impairment and interfere with work, social activities,

	ICD-10	ACOG	DSM-IV
Table 2.3 Current diagnostic criteria for PMS/PMDD			
Diagnostic entity (and ICD-9 code)	PMTS (625.4)	PMS (625.4)	PMDD (311)
Category	Gynecology	Gynecology	Psychiatry
Temporal pattern	Occur premenstrually Remit following menses		
		Occur 5 days before menses Remit within 4 days of onset of menses No recurrence at least until day 13 of cycle	Occur during the last week before menses Remit within few days after onset of follicular phase
			At least five symptoms, with at least one of: depression, anxiety, or tension, anger or irritability, and monthly swings Other qualifying symptoms are: decreased interest, difficulty concentrating, lack of energy, changed sleep, overwhelmed, out of control, change in appetite Other physical symptoms such as breast tenderness, bloating headaches, pain Markedly interferes with work, social activities, relationships Most menstrual cycles during past year At least two consecutive cycles Not merely an exacerbation of another disorder Not associated with pharmacological, hormone, alcohol or drug use or abuse

and/or relationships, not be an exacerbation of another chronic disorder and be prospectively confirmed by daily ratings during at least two consecutive cycles. Because of differing opinions during the APA's DSM-IV process, PMDD is listed in the DSM-IV and DSM-IV-TR as one of the criteria sets and axes provided for further study, and is designated as 'Depressive Disorder not otherwise specified' – ICD-9 code 311.

The three main diagnostic criteria are summarized in Table 2.3.

UNSOLVED ISSUES WITH CURRENT DIAGNOSTIC CRITERIA

The main shortcomings of the current diagnostic criteria are lack of universal agreement on the nature of the PMS as well as lack of universal acceptance of the criteria per se. The closest to universal acceptance is the ICD-10 entity. However, the PMTS description is vague and does not provide specific diagnostic process and criteria: actually, it just acknowledges the existence of the entity.

Universal acceptance of a diagnostic entity is needed for unified coding and for regulatory purposes. It has financial ramifications for service delivery and reimbursement as well as for prescriptions and their reimbursements.

The lack of clear, acceptable definitions inhibits the development of drugs and other treatments. Regulatory agencies, like the US Food and Drug Administration (FDA) and the European Union's European Medicines Agency (EMEA) require clear clinical indication for pivotal clinical trials and clear projected outcome measures. In the USA, the indication of PMDD is acceptable mainly because it is included in the influential DSM-IV and follows its descriptive principles; PMS, though, is still not acceptable despite the weight of the ACOG.

The implied dichotomy between the physical symptoms of PMS and the mental symptoms of PMDD is arbitrary. The association between physical and mental symptoms is still unclear, especially when any of them is severe enough to cause dysfunction and/or distress. The repeated and widely presumed reference to PMDD as a severe form of PMS is not supported by data, either. It also assumes a continuum of basically the same manifestation of an entity along a severity gradation and attributes lesser severity to perception of physical and other non-dysphoric symptoms.

A major unsolved issue is the definition of PMDD as a diagnostic entity, independent of PMS. This may well be correct but so far data to the contrary are no less convincing. Most catamenial disorders (Table 2.4) are characterized as an episode whose phenomena and etiology are similar to generally occurring disorders, but the timing of the episode is entrained to the menstrual cycle – mostly due to hormonal fluctuations. Therefore, the menstrually related changes trigger the occurrence of the specific episode but do not influence the basic etiology and pathophysiology or the vulnerability to the parent disorder. Only a few physical symptoms of PMS or catamenial disorders (e.g. breast tenderness) may be attributed to the influence of estrogen or progesterone per se.

Review of the literature (for example, Refs 28–33) demonstrates that PMDD may be a catamenial disorder like any other catamenial disorder. The phenomena are similar to other depressions and anxiety disorders and there is a statistical association with them. In some cases treatment interventions and responses are similar.

A vulnerability–trigger conceptualization[33–35] of etiology and pathophysiology of PMS/PMDD suggests that some women are vulnerable to develop specific phenotypes of dysphoric disorders. Vulnerability implies a symptomatic threshold in response to hormonal or situational triggers. In many people symptoms appear even without a currently known trigger and the course of illness depends on currently unknown mechanisms.

Table 2.4 Is PMDD conceptually similar to the following catamenial episodes?	
• Epilepsy	• Genital herpes
• Migraine headache	• Asthma
• Other headaches	• Pneumothorax
• Meningioma symptoms	• Pulmonary endometriosis
• Kleine–Levin syndrome (hypersomnia)	• Rheumatoid arthritis
• Myoclonus	• Diabetes mellitus
• Neuralgia paresthetica	• Porphyria
• Paraparesis	• Platelets disorders
• Autoimmune diseases (SLE, MS)	• Cholelithiasis
• Suicidal behavior	• Urticaria and anaphylaxis
• Sleep disorders	• Glaucoma
	• Pain

Therefore, the main difference between DSM-IV affective and anxiety disorders and subtypes of PMS/PMDD would be the added vulnerability to menstrually related triggers and probably also an intact or strong normalization process that prevents the episode from extending for a long time beyond the expiration of the menstrually related transitory stimulus.

According to this conceptualization, the distinction between PMDD (or PMS) and premenstrual exacerbation (PME) of other mental or physical disorders may not be substantial, especially when the exacerbations are limited to or occur mostly during the premenstrual period. Biologically, PMS and PME may represent stages on a continuum of vulnerability–(threshold)–stimulus interactions.

Even if PMDD is viewed as a separate entity, it presents a plethora of unsolved issues.

Despite the acceptance of the PMDD entity by the US FDA and despite several FDA-approved medications for that indication, the definitions of PMDD are far from being perfect. The main weakness of that diagnostic entity is the requirement of endorsing five of the 11 listed symptoms. The reason for the choice of a specific numerical threshold is unclear and it is not necessarily clinically relevant. A significant proportion of women report severe impairment but of only three or four symptoms.[15] They seek and certainly warrant treatment no less than the 5% of women who report the highly specific and restrictive five symptoms. Even though a multitude of premenstrual dysphoric symptoms[29] have been reported, only 11 are listed. There is no latitude for accounting for other symptoms, even though for a specific individual they may be no less severe than the listed ones. The requirement of impairment of functioning does not consider the possibility of women who manage to continue reasonable day-to-day functioning despite having severe symptoms, but they do have severe *distress*.

As is the case with most DSM-IV clinical entities, the putatively quantitative measures are actually descriptive and are vaguely defined (e.g. 'most menstrual cycles', 'most of the time', 'within few days', 'markedly' interfere, 'marked' anxiety) and therefore are subject to additional subjective interpretations.

The contribution of inclusion of PMDD in the DSM-IV to recognition of the entity and to improving treatment of women suffering from PMS should not be underestimated. The media coverage of that disorder as well as industry promotion of FDA-approved medications certainly increased alertness of patients and clinicians as well as acceptance of the concept, but this does not negate the need to further improve and refine the diagnostic entity.

The ACOG criteria of PMS consider the individual diversity of symptoms and avoid the trap of a specific numerical symptom's threshold. They follow previous suggestions[33] (and Mortola, unpublished work) for the logic of PMS diagnosis but do not carry it to specificity and well-rounded inclusiveness.

THE DURATION OF THE PREMENSTRUAL PERIOD

The DSM-IV criteria require qualified symptoms to occur during the week before menses, and the ACOG criteria require them to occur within 5 days before menses. Both do not specify for how many days should the symptoms exist, nor does the DSM-IV specify how soon should symptoms remit ('within few days after the onset of follicular phase').

For clinical trials, inclusion criteria usually specify 'severe symptoms for at least 4 days' or 'average severity during 7 days'. When duration of premenstrual symptoms is reported[20] it is apparent that there is a large individual variability in the number of premenstrual symptomatic days. The mean has been reported to be 6.1 days. However, in the USA, UK, and France, 44%, 36%, and 19% of women, respectively, reported in retrospective telephone interviews that their PMS lasts no longer than 3 days. Up to 10% of women with PMS report duration of symptoms for the entire luteal phase and 1–2% report that their symptoms actually included

the periovulatory period; 12–18% report only 1–2 symptomatic days. My clinical experience is that some women may have extremely severe PMS symptoms for only 1–2 days, especially those with premenstrual manic or psychotic episodes.[36] The possibility that different lengths of the premenstrual phase of symptoms may be associated with different phenotypes and underlying mechanisms has not been fully elucidated yet, partially because women with a very short premenstrual period (PMP) do not meet criteria for current clinical trials, as is often the case for women with a very long symptomatic phase.

The time-related different patterns of PMP and their differentiation from chronic non-PMS pattern is demonstrated in Figure 2.1.

PROPOSED DEFINITION AND DIAGNOSTIC CRITERIA FOR PMS

If the diagnosis of PMS/PMDD is to be widely accepted, two complementary conceptual procedural operational steps should be taken. First, an international authoritative organization should take the lead in formulating and establishing the diagnosis and its criteria. Indeed the WHO should perform that task and update the ICD-10 definition and criteria of PMTS, as a component of the future ICD-11. The groundwork for such an update has recently been performed. An interdisciplinary panel of 16 experts from 13 countries in four continents recommended diagnostic criteria for PMS and their quantification for research.[37] The panel was convened by the World Psychiatric Association (WPA) Section on Interdisciplinary Collaboration, and its recommendations still need to be endorsed by diversified major professional organizations of the related disciplines. Secondly, it should be recognized that PMS is an interdisciplinary domain: it involves many aspects of endocrinology, gynecology, mental health, and clinical neurosciences, and several subdisciplines of internal medicine, as well as social and developmental sciences. It is the domain of all of these disciplines and none of them can claim it exclusively.

The main aspects of a proposed widely accepted definition of PMS have already been widely accepted:

- The entity is distinguished from other similar entities mostly by its timing: symptoms appear mostly cyclically during the luteal phase of the menstrual cycle and disappear shortly following the beginning of menses, and are temporally entrained to the menstrual cycle.
- To be considered a disorder, symptoms should cause impairment and/or dysfunction. I suggest to add 'and/or distress'.

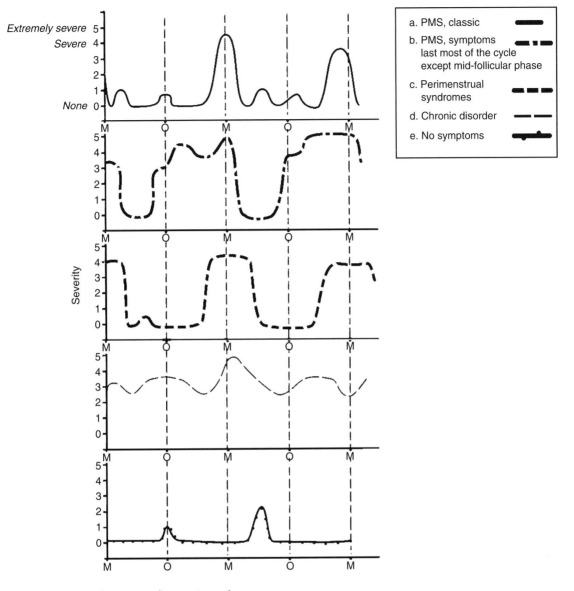

Figure 2.1 PMS and non-PMS fluctuations of symptoms.

It is also quite widely accepted that individual vulnerability is an important contributor to the development of PMS. It should be recognized that, as is increasingly suggested for affective disorders in general, there are probably diversified vulnerability traits to PMS.[31] The diversified vulnerabilities are probably associated with diversified genotypes,[36] pathophysiological processes (e.g. 5-hydroxytryptamine (5-HT), γ-aminobutyric acid (GABA)[35]), and ensuing phenotypes. Once the concept of multiple phenotypes or subtypes of PMS is accepted,

this is important not only for the diagnosis of PMS but also for phenotype-targeted treatment, which is the ultimate purpose of appropriate diagnosis.

The main arguments in support of diversified vulnerabilities to PMS are:

- Over 200 symptoms have been reported as appearing premenstrually; they involve many body systems and none of them is exclusively related to the menstrual cycle per se.[29,36–38]

- The nature and clusters of symptoms are quite consistent from cycle to cycle within individual women, although the severity may fluctuate.[39]
- Individual women may tend to present with similar symptoms at other times of physical, psychosocial, or hormonal stress.
- The rate of treatment response to any currently approved medication for PMDD (currently only selective serotonin reuptake inhibitors (SSRIs)) is barely 20% better than placebo.[40] One may suggest that only a subgroup of women with PMS respond to these medications. Subgroups with other vulnerabilities may respond to treatment modalities.[41]

The suggested diversified genotypes and phenotypes lead to a need to de-emphasize the descriptive approach to PMS and to replace it with a generalized approach that has already been partly adopted by ACOG. Accordingly, the following diagnostic criteria for PMS have been proposed,[33,42] but they are not widely accepted:

- *Any* mood, behavioral or physical symptom(s), or cluster(s) of symptoms that occur recurrently and cyclically during the luteal phase of the menstrual cycle.
- The symptom(s) remit(s) shortly following the beginning of menses and consistently do not exist for at least 1 week of the follicular phase of most menstrual cycles.
- The symptom(s) cause emotional or physical distress and/or suffering and/or impairment in daily functioning, and/or impairment in relationships.
- The recurrence, cyclicity, and timing of the cycle, and severity of the symptoms as well as existence of a menstrually related symptom-free period are documented by daily monitoring and/or reports.

Whether or not exclusively premenstrually repeated episodes of any disorder may be considered as PMS or a catamenial disorder is a matter of definition. This may be addressed as part of the differential diagnosis of PMS (see Table 2.5).

Indeed, as is the case with many mental or physical entities, there is a debate between 'splitters' (those who are searching for specific phenotypes or subgroups of patients with very specific and narrow clinical and etiological common denominators and similarities) and 'lumpers' (those who prefer a broader clinical approach and are convinced that the differences between the various subgroups and phenotypes are overpowered by the similarities within the larger group). Although I believe that there are multiple premenstrual syndromes with different vulnerabilities and phenotypes but a common trigger, this debate has not been resolved yet.

Similarly, there is no consensus on the role of catamenial episodes (see Table 2.4) as menstrually related disorders (MRDs) and their relation with PMS. If the definition of PMS is based mostly on timing and not on descriptive phenomena, and if genotypes and dynamically evolving vulnerability[35,42,43] contribute to specific phenotypes of PMS, then one may argue that catamenial episodes appearing during the premenstrual period are subtypes of PMS (as long as they do not appear during other times during the cycle). If the catamenial episodes consistently appear at other times (non-premenstrual phase of the menstrual cycle, e.g. periovulatory), then they are a part of the broader definition of MRD.

As is the case with subtypes or phenotypes of PMS, this is not just a heuristic discussion. It has direct clinical treatment implications. In the case of catamenial episodes, treatment should involve the disorder-specific intervention *as well as* suppression of hormonal cyclicity. This may also be the case with specific phenotypes of PMS.

The diagnostic concept of multiple premenstrual syndromes, as opposed to a single PMS, was not accepted by about half of the members of the international interdisciplinary consensus panel[44] (consensus was considered when at least 14/16 participants agreed).

The panel agreed that a PMS ICD diagnostic code should be incorporated in a new 'Interdisciplinary diagnoses' section and the title should be PMS – Premenstrual Syndrome (different patterns of symptoms or clusters of symptoms may appear as part of the syndrome).

The panel achieved a consensus on the pivotal role of timing as a crucial criterion of PMS and settled on '2 weeks before menses in most menstrual cycles', as well as 'remit following onset of menses'. Prospective documentation of cyclicity is required, by clinician and/or daily monitoring by the patient.

The panel required that the symptoms are not just an exacerbation or worsening of another mental or physical chronic disorder, and recommended issues for field trials that are quite similar to the ones that will be described later. These field trails require quantification of the diagnostic criteria that were also recommended by the panel.

RESEARCH DIAGNOSTIC CRITERIA FOR PMS/PMDD

Owing to the vagueness on severity and other definitions of the DSM-IV PMDD, quantitative replicable definitions and procedures for diagnosis and outcome measures had to be developed – to be translated into inclusion and exclusion criteria for enrollment of patients in clinical trials.

Table 2.5 Differential diagnosis of PMS	
Mental disorders (may be with premenstrual exacerbations)	**General medical conditions** (with menstrually related worsening or exacerbations)
• Major depressive episodes • Dysthymia • Chronic major depression • Bipolar disorder • Generalized anxiety disorder • Panic disorder • Seasonal affective disorder • Somatoform disorder • Personality disorders • Substance abuse • Repeated stress • ADHD	• Dysmenorrhea • Endometriosis • Polycystic ovaries • Adverse effects of hormonal contraceptives • Perimenopausal symptoms • Seizure disorders • Autoimmune diseases (e.g. MS, SLE) • Hypothyroidism • Hyperglycemia • Anemia • Allergies

The research procedures are for quantification of PMDD criteria of severity (quantify 'marked'), duration of symptomatic period, duration of non-symptomatic period, and degree of impairment, as well as non-existence of other diagnostic entities.

In addition, degree of change from non-symptomatic to symptomatic periods and cyclicity are sometimes measured.

The most acceptable research method to establish the severity of symptoms, their entrainment to the menstrual cycle, and their fluctuation and cyclicity is by daily rating forms (DRFs).

Most widely applied DRFs provide a range of severity for each item, from non-existent to extremely severe. There are some anchor definitions for each level of severity. For research purposes, a cut-off point is introduced, mostly between mild and moderately severe. However, that distinction is subjective and varies from individual to individual. If there was an objective measure of severity (at present, there is none) it would be subjectively described by some women as not severe and by some others as very severe – according to their tolerance, coping style, ability, personality, perception, and subjective definition of 'what is severe'.

The difference between 'mild' and 'moderate' may determine a woman's eligibility or ineligibility for enrollment in a clinical trial, especially if it is a symptom that would make the fifth required symptom of PMDD or is a crucial perception of impairment.

Since the symptoms should be absent in the week post menses, the same cut-off (though as an upper ceiling) applies to the mid-follicular period as well. Here another issue is pertinent. Since women are humans, there may be external stressful situations during the mid-follicular phase, and therefore women subjects may rate some of the symptoms higher than 'mild' and thus would be disqualified if clinical judgment was not exercised. An average severity across 5 days may control for incidental stressful days, but even then a more flexible-realistic schedule (e.g. allowing for several external stress-related items above 'mild' severity) may reflect a representative patient group.

Since the duration of PMS varies among patients, a reasonable required duration of the severe symptoms may be at least 2 days, with lesser severity during the rest of the PMP.

Some DRFs provide an overall daily score for the questionnaire, which may be averaged for the entire designated PMP (usually 7 days) as well as for the mid-follicular phase – allowing for calculation of total change from mid-follicular to late-luteal phase, and hence a measure of overall fluctuation and cyclicity. At least two issues may be considered in this regard. First, a total score does not reflect severity of PMS in a woman who complains of only a few but very severe premenstrual symptoms. This would also be the case with the determination of percentage change from mid-follicular to late-luteal periods. Secondly, the percentage change assumes a linear continuous score from non-existent to extremely severe that is identical for all individuals. This is not necessarily the case with the highly subjective description at focus here. Furthermore, a combined requirement of a minimal late-luteal total score and a minimal percentage increase from mid-follicular to late-luteal phase may be too strict for some women and very permissive for others (who may have many mild symptoms which do not exist at mid-follicular phase).

The same considerations apply also to the impairment items. However, there are women who do not have actual premenstrual impairment of their performance but maintain their function with a *high level of distress*. This should be considered as a measure of severity no lesser than impairment in function.

For research purposes, regular menstrual cycles are obligatory: usually 21–35 days are considered to be 'regular'. However, currently there is no requirement for the limit of individual cycle-to-cycle duration stability within this wide range.

FUTURE DIRECTIONS FOR RESEARCH ON THE DIAGNOSIS OF PMS/PMDD

The main *diagnostic issues* that, to my opinion, are still unsolved are:

1. Are there multiple diversified premenstrual syndromes that also include diversified premenstrual dysphoric phenotypes? This issue is also of crucial importance for the understanding of the pathophysiology of PMS and effective treatment (beyond the current efficacy ceiling of 60%).
2. If there are diversified phenotypes, can we move beyond the DSM-IV-style descriptive arbitrary cut-off points towards a diagnosis based on the pattern(s) of symptoms, past history and time course, biological changes (etiology and pathobiology), and treatment outcome? Once phenotypes are established, are they specifically associated with specific genotypes?
3. If our present understanding of PMS involves the concept of vulnerability and menstrually related trigger(s) of symptoms, then is it justified to distinguish between premenstrual syndromes and PMEs or catamenial disorders? The difference may be the degree of the threshold and the magnitude of the trigger needed to cause expression of symptoms, but not necessarily a fundamental difference between premenstrual syndromes and PMEs. If the vulnerability level changes over time, and may increase or decrease according to life events and their perception, as well as repeated assaults (kindling and dynamically evolving vulnerability), then there may be a continuum between at least some premenstrual syndromes, PMEs, and more chronic major disorders – this notion deserves investigation.
4. What is a clinically relevant PMS (or PMDD)? When do women warrant and benefit from treatment?

5. Can we develop clinically relevant diagnostic procedures that would not require prospective monitoring of symptoms for two consecutive menstrual cycles (which are too much of a burden for many women and their primary care physicians)?

There are many more unsolved diagnostic issues of PMS/PMDD, even before we tackle issues of underlying mechanisms that may vary from phenotype to phenotype.

REFERENCES

1. American Psychiatric Association. Diagnostic and Statistical Manual of Mental Disorders, 4th edn. Washington, DC: American Psychiatric Press; 1994.
2. American Psychiatric Association. Diagnostic and Statistical Manual of Mental Disorders, 4th edn, text revision (DSM-IV-TR). Washington, DC: American Psychiatric Press; 2000: 771–4.
3. Angst J, Sellaro R, Merikangas KR et al. The epidemiology of perimenstrual psychological symptoms. Acta Psychiatr Scand 2001; 104(2):110–16.
4. Johnson SR. The epidemiology and social impact of premenstrual symptoms. Clin Obstet Gynecol 1987; 30(2):367–76.
5. Merikangas KR, Foeldenyi M, Angst J. The Zurich Study. XIX. Patterns of menstrual disturbances in the community: results of the Zurich Cohort Study. Eur Arch Psychiatry Clin Neurosci 1993; 243:23–32.
6. Ramcharan S, Love EJ, Fick GH et al. The epidemiology of premenstrual symptoms in a population-based sample of 2650 urban women: attributable risk and risk factors. J Clin Epidemiol 1992; 45(4):377–92.
7. Rivera-Tovar AD, Frank E. Late luteal phase dysphoric disorder in young women. Am J Psychiatry 1990; 147(12):1634–6.
8. Sveindottir H, Backstrom T. Prevalence of menstrual cycle symptom cyclicity and premenstrual dysphoric disorder in a random sample of women using and not using oral contraceptives. Acta Obstet Gynecol Scand 2000; 79(5):405–13.
9. Wittchen HU, Hoyer J. Generalized anxiety disorder: nature and course. J Clin Psychiatr 2001; 62(Suppl 11):15–19; discussion 20–1.
10. Woods NF, Most A, Dery GK. Prevalence of perimenstrual symptoms. Am J Public Health 1982; 72(11):1257–64.
11. Robinson RL, Swindle RW. Premenstrual symptom severity: impact on social functioning and treatment-seeking behaviors. J Womens Health Gend Based Med 2000; 9(7):757–68.
12. Steiner M, Brown E, McDougall M. The burden of illness of premenstrual symptoms. J Womens Health Gend Based Med 2002; 11:324.
13. Cohen LS, Soares CN, Otto MW et al. Prevalence and predictors of premenstrual dysphoric disorder (PMDD) in older premenopausal women. The Harvard Study of Moods and Cycles. J Affect Disord 2002; 70(2):125–32.
14. Chawla A, Swindle R, Long S, Kennedy S, Sternfeld B. Premenstrual dysphoric disorder: is there an economic burden of illness? Med Care 2002; 40(11):1101–12.
15. Wittchen HU, Becker E, Lieb R, Krause P. Prevalence, incidence and stability of premenstrual dysphoric disorder in the community. Psychol Med 2002; 32(1):119–32.
16. Narrow WE, Rae DS, Robins LN, Regier DA. Revised prevalence estimates of mental disorders in the United States: using a clinical significance criterion to reconcile 2 surveys' estimates. Arch Gen Psychiatry 2002; 59(2):115–23.

17. Halbreich U, Borenstein J, Pearlstein T, Kahn LS. The prevalence, impairment, impact, and burden of premenstrual dysphoric disorder (PMS/PMDD). Psychoneuroendocrinology 2003; 28: 1–23.

18. Pearlstein TB, Halbreich U, Batzar ED et al. Psychosocial functioning in women with premenstrual dysphoric disorder before and after treatment with sertraline or placebo. J Clin Psychiatry 2000; 61(2):101–9.

19. Murray CJL, Lopez AD, eds. The Global Burden of Disease: a Comprehensive Assessment of Mortality and Disability from Diseases, Injuries, and Risk Factors in 1990 and Projected to 2020. Boston: The Harvard School of Public Health, on behalf of the World Health Organization and the World Bank; 1996.

20. Hylan TR, Sundell K, Judge R. The impact of premenstrual symptomatology on functioning and treatment-seeking behavior: experience from the United States, United Kingdom, and France. J Womens Health Gend Based Med 1999; 8(8):1043–52.

21. Halbreich U. History and trajectory of PMS: towards a balanced adaptation and a biosocial homeostasis. J Reprod Infant Psychol 2006; 24(4):1–11.

22. Jeliffe. New York State J Med (Report) 1906.

23. Frank RT. The hormonal causes of premenstrual tension. Arch Neurol Psychiatry 1931; 26:1053.

24. Horney K. Die prämenstruellen Verstimmungen. Zeitschrift für psychonal Padagogiei 1931; 5:1–7.

25. Morton JH. Symposium on premenstrual tension. Int Record Med 1953; 166: 463–510.

26. WHO. International Classification of Diseases, 10th rev. Geneva: World Health Organization; 1996.

27. American College of Obstetricians and Gynecologists (ACOG). Premenstrual Syndrome. Washington, DC: ACOG; 2000.

28. Halbreich U, Endicott J. Relationship of dysphoric premenstrual changes to depressive disorders. Acta Psychiatr Scand 1985; 71(4):331–8.

29. Halbreich U, Endicott J, Schacht S, Nee J. The diversity of premenstrual changes as reflected in the Premenstrual Assessment Form. Acta Psychiatr Scand 1982; 65(1):46–65.

30. Halbreich U. Menstrually related disorders: what we do know, what we only believe that we know, and what we know that we do not know. Crit Rev Neurobiol 1995; 9(2–3):163–75.

31. Halbreich U. Premenstrual dysphoric disorders: a diversified cluster of vulnerability traits to depression. Acta Psychiatr Scand 1997; 95(3):169–76.

32. Halbreich U. Premenstrual syndromes. Ballière's Clinical Psychiatry: International Practice and Research: London: Ballière & Tindall; 1996; 2:667–86.

33. Halbreich U. Menstrually related changes and disorders: conceptualization and diagnostic considerations. Neuropsychopharmacology 1993; 9(1):25–9.

34. Halbreich U, Alt IH, Paul L. Premenstrual changes. Impaired hormonal homeostasis. Neurol Clin 1988; 6(1):173–94.

35. Halbreich U. The etiology, biology and evolving pathology of premenstrual syndromes. Psychoneuroendocrinology 2003; 28: 55–99.

36. Halbreich U, Endicott J, Nee J. Premenstrual depressive changes. Value of differentiation. Arch Gen Psychiatry 1983; 40(5): 535–42.

37. Halbreich U. The diagnosis of premenstrual syndromes and premenstrual dysphoric disorder – clinical procedures and research perspectives. Gynecol Endocrinol 2004; 19:320–34.

38. Halbreich U, Endicott J. Methodological issues in studies of premenstrual changes. Psychoneuroendocrinology 1985; 10(1):15–32.

39. Bloch M, Schmidt PJ, Rubinow DR. Premenstrual syndrome: evidence for symptom stability across cycles. Am J Psychiatry 1997; 154(12):1741–6.

40. Halbreich U, Marshall-Hobika D, Garde J. Response rates to selective serotonin reuptake inhibitors for treatment of premenstrual dysphoric disorder. Proceedings of 2nd World Congress of Women's Mental Health, March 17–20. Washington, DC, 2004.

41. Halbreich U. Premenstrual syndromes: closing the 20th century chapters. Curr Opin Obstet Gynecol 1999; 11:265–70.

42. Halbreich U. Menstrually related disorders – towards interdisciplinary international diagnostic criteria. Cephalalgia 1997; 20(Suppl 17):1–4.

43. Halbreich U. Future directions for studies of women's mental health. Psychopharmacol Bull 1998; 34(3):327–31.

44. Halbreich U, Backstrom T, Eriksson E et al. Clinical diagnostic criteria for PMS and guidelines for their quantification for research studies. Gynecol Endocrinol 2007; 23(3): 123–30.

3

Premenstrual syndrome: a case of serotonergic dysfunction?

Elias Eriksson

SHOULD PMS BE REGARDED AN ENDOCRINE CONDITION OR AS A BRAIN DISORDER?

Triggered by sex steroids produced by the ovaries, premenstrual syndrome (PMS) and premenstrual dysphoric disorder (PMDD) may be, and have often been, regarded primarily as endocrine conditions. Attempts to explain, in terms of differences with respect to hormone levels, why certain women are afflicted by premenstrual symptoms, while other women are spared from such complaints, however, have consistently failed. Therefore, it is nowadays generally agreed that women with premenstrual complaints differ from controls *not* with respect to ovarian function, but with respect to how responsive the target organs are to the influence of gonadal steroids. Supporting this view, administration of exogenous sexual hormones following the suppression of the endogenous gonadal steroid production elicits PMS-like complaints in women with PMS but not in controls.[1]

One important target organ for sex steroids is the central nervous system. Receptors for sex hormones are thus abundant in many brain regions including the amygdala and the hypothalamus. Since mood and behavioral symptoms are key features of PMS, the brain obviously is where underlying processes at least partly must be sought. Consequently, a better understanding of the mechanisms underlying PMS clearly requires insight into the neurochemical basis of the influence of sex steroids in relation to mood and behavior and why certain individuals are particularly sensitive to this influence. Hence, studies of PMS have to deal with the same difficulties, and apply the same methodological approaches, as research on the pathophysiology of other psychiatric disorders.

Two factors render studies on the mechanisms underlying psychiatric illness more difficult than other fields of medical research. First, the brain is much more complex than any other organ; hence, our knowledge of how it operates to produce consciousness, thoughts, memories, executive functioning, and emotions is as yet very limited. And secondly, it is – as compared to many other organs – relatively inaccessible for exploration. Because of these difficulties, it is as yet impossible to measure to what extent a certain individual is characterized – for example – by shortage or excess of a certain brain transmitter.

Notwithstanding these problems, over the past 50 years, very reasonable hypotheses concerning the involvement of specific brain transmitters in conditions such as depression, anxiety, schizophrenia, and attention deficit hyperactivity disorder have been formulated. These hypotheses have, without exception, been based primarily on pharmacological observations: whereas certain drugs have been found, accidentally, to reduce the symptoms of the condition in question, other compounds have been found to aggravate them. And by then analyzing how these different compounds influence brain neurotransmitters, using animal experiments, researchers have been able to draw tentative conclusions regarding the pathophysiology underlying the studied condition.[2] Subsequently, usually decades later, it has often been possible to obtain at least partial confirmation of these theories by means of other methodological approaches, such as brain imaging[3,4] or genotyping.[5] But the foundation of theories linking brain neurotransmitters to psychiatric disorders has always been the presumed mechanism of action of drugs.

With respect to the brain mechanisms underlying PMS, one particular neurotransmitter, serotonin, has been proposed to play a key role. As is the case for other theories implicating specific transmitters in specific conditions, also this hypothesis is first and foremost based on pharmacological data: whereas drugs facilitating brain serotonergic transmission effectively reduce the symptoms of PMS, treatments counteracting serotonergic activity may aggravate them. In addition to these findings, there are however also reports, though difficult to interpret, suggesting that women with PMS differ from controls with respect to serotonergic activity. In this chapter, the different arguments supporting an involvement of serotonin in PMS will be presented and discussed.

HOW IS HUMAN BEHAVIOR INFLUENCED BY SEROTONIN?

Serotonin is a monoamine, formed from the essential amino acid tryptophan, with 5-hydroxytryptophan as intermediate.[6] Whereas the cell bodies of the neurons using serotonin as transmitter are all localized to the brainstem, serotonergic nerve terminals are found in most parts of the brain. The effects of this transmitter on adjacent neurons are mediated by at least 15 receptor subtypes, the different functions of which are as yet poorly understood.

Serotonin has long since been assumed to be of importance for the regulation of mood and behavior, partly because of observations made in preclinical studies, and partly because of the antidepressant and anxiety-reducing effect exerted by serotonin-facilitating drugs, such as the serotonin reuptake inhibitors (SRIs) (see below). Recently, the importance of serotonin for depression and anxiety has been reinforced by studies applying brain imaging[4] and/or molecular genetics.[5,7,8]

Although serotonin has been implicated in psychiatric conditions as disparate as depression, obsessive compulsive disorder, and panic disorder, little is known regarding the normal, physiological role of this transmitter. Interestingly, however, the most clear-cut changes in the behavior of rodents exposed to serotonin depletion is an increase in aggression and sexual activity,[6] i.e. those aspects of behavior that are most clearly sex steroid-driven. These findings may suggest that a major physiological task for serotonin in rats and mice is to modulate or dampen sex steroid-driven behavior. That this may be the case not only in rodents but also in humans gains support from the fact that reduced libido is probably the most common side effect of long-term treatment with SRIs.[9]

Studies showing sex steroids to influence serotonin transmission in rodents[10–14] and non-human primates[15,16] suggest that the effects of gonadal hormones on behavior may be mediated in part by an influence on serotonergic pathways. However, an alternative scenario would be that sex steroids influence neuronal circuits regulating mood and behavior, which do not constitute serotonergic neurons per se, but are under the dampening influence of serotonergic terminals. Reinforcing the notion that interactions between sex steroids and serotonin may be of clinical importance, almost all indications for SRIs – including depression, dysthymia, social phobia, panic disorder, generalized anxiety disorder, and eating disorders – display a marked gender difference in prevalence, being considerably more common in women than in men.

If it is true that a major role for serotonin is to dampen the influence of sex steroids on behavior, the theory that serotonin is of importance for PMS, one of the most obvious examples of sex steroids influencing behavior, is not farfetched, and even less so given the fact that enhanced irritability is a cardinal symptom of PMS, and, at the same time, one of the most characteristic features of serotonin-depleted animals. Given what we know from animal studies regarding the neurochemical regulation of aggression, for any condition in which irritability and anger are prominent symptoms, an involvement of serotonin should in fact be suspected.

SEROTONIN REUPTAKE INHIBITORS IN PMS

The most well-established way of facilitating brain serotonergic neurotransmission is to block the serotonin transporter, i.e. the protein inactivating serotonin by transporting this molecule from the synaptic cleft back into the presynaptic neuron. Such an effect may be achieved by SRIs, some of which selectively inhibit the reuptake of serotonin only (selective SRIs = SSRIs), and some of which inhibit the reuptake of both serotonin and norepinephrine (tricyclic antidepressants and serotonin/norepinephrine reuptake inhibitors = SNRIs).

To a large extent, the notion that serotonergic neurons are part of – or capable of influencing – the neuronal networks that generate premenstrual changes in mood and behavior stems from the observation that SRIs very effectively reduce such symptoms. This has now been shown with the tricyclic antidepressant clomipramine, the selective SRIs citalopram, escitalopram, fluoxetine, paroxetine, and sertraline, and the SNRI venlafaxine.[17–19]

In addition to reducing the symptoms of PMS, the SRIs are also antidepressants. Whereas studies aiming to reveal an effect of these treatments in depression however sometimes fail to show a difference between active drug and placebo, due to insufficient statistical power, the superiority of SRIs over placebo in PMS/PMDD has been robustly replicated in a large number of consecutive studies, one small early trial being the sole exception.[17–19] In PMS patients with irritability or depressed mood as the most prominent symptoms, the response rate to an

SRI may be around 90%, and the effect size – which is a measure of the difference between active drug and placebo – for the most responsive symptoms, such as irritability, as high as 1.4, which is much higher than what is usually found in studies on the effect of SRIs in other conditions.[20] It may hence be argued that premenstrual irritability is an extraordinarily SRI-responsive condition, more so than, e.g. depression.

For the treatment of depression, reuptake inhibitors selectively or primarily influencing serotonin appear to be neither more nor less effective than reuptake inhibitors primarily influencing norepinephrine. For the treatment of PMS, on the other hand, only reuptake inhibitors with a marked effect on serotonin, such as those listed above, seem to be effective.[21–23] These findings suggest that the effect of SRIs in PMS is not equivalent to the antidepressant effect of these drugs, and underline the importance of serotonin, rather than norepinephrine, for the influence of antidepressants in PMS.

Animal studies have revealed an immediate increase in synaptic serotonin concentrations following SRI administration,[24] and there are also reasons to assume that SRIs are capable of exerting an almost immediate facilitation of serotonin activity in humans. Endocrine responses to these drugs,[25] as well as some of the side effects (including nausea[26]) and influence on sexual function[27], hence appear shortly after drug intake. In spite of this, the beneficial effect of SRIs in depression and several anxiety disorders usually requires several weeks of treatment. Interestingly, such a delay in onset is not seen when these drugs are used for the treatment of PMS; SRIs are thus capable of reducing premenstrual irritability within a few days after treatment has started. As first shown for clomipramine[28] and later confirmed for citalopram, escitalopram, fluoxetine, paroxetine, and sertraline,[19] this short onset of action renders intermittent administration of SRIs, during luteal phases only, a feasible alternative to continuous administration.

The difference between PMS and other indications with respect to the onset of action of SRIs has prompted some authors to suggest that the effect of these drugs in PMS must be unrelated to serotonin. Such a conclusion is however unjustified, since SRIs do exert a prompt effect on serotonergic transmission; the speed of onset of the clinical response hence does not at all argue against the effect being mediated by serotonin. Yet the difference between PMS on the one hand, and depression and other indications on the other, with respect to the onset of action of SRIs, reinforces the assumption that the effect in PMS is not equivalent to the antidepressant and antianxiety effects of these drugs, but probably mediated by other serotonergic pathways. Of considerable interest in this context are studies suggesting that

symptoms such as anger and affect lability, i.e. two cardinal symptoms of PMS, respond within a very short onset of action to SRIs also when being the consequence of conditions such as dementia, stroke or brain injury.[29–32] Moreover, SRIs have been shown to reduce estrous cycle-related aggression without delay in a rodent model of PMS.[33]

EFFECTS OF OTHER MEANS OF MODULATING SEROTONERGIC TRANSMISSION

If the assumption that SRIs reduce premenstrual symptoms by facilitating serotonergic transmission is correct, then other treatments enhancing serotonin activity would be expected to reduce premenstrual complaints. Conversely, manipulations reducing serotonergic activity would be expected to aggravate or trigger symptoms and/or to reverse the symptom-reducing effect of SRIs. Indeed, a large number of observations indicate this to be the case:

1. mCPP and fenfluramine – two compounds known to release serotonin into the synaptic cleft by interacting with the transporter, but in a different way as compared with the SRIs[34] – have both been reported to reduce premenstrual symptoms.[35,36]
2. The serotonin precursor tryptophan, which should be expected to cause at least a moderate increase in serotonin formation, has also been shown to be superior to placebo for this condition.[37]
3. Pyridoxine, which is a cofactor for an enzyme of critical importance for serotonin formation, also appears to exert some (though modest) beneficial effect.[38]
4. Buspirone, which is a partial agonist at the serotonergic 5HT1A receptor, has been shown to be superior to placebo in reducing at least one important premenstrual symptom, i.e. irritability.[39]
5. Depletion of tryptophan from the diet, leading to a reduction in serotonergic transmission, has been shown to aggravate premenstrual irritability.[40]
6. The symptom-reducing effect of SRIs in PMS is at least partly counteracted by administration of a serotonin receptor antagonist, metergoline.[41]

Taken together, these observations speak very strongly in favor of the hypothesis that premenstrual dysphoria may indeed be dampened by serotonergic neurons. Given this body of evidence, the notion sometimes put forward that the effect of some of the SRIs in PMS is in fact independent of serotonin, and instead mediated by other mechanisms,[42] seems somewhat unlikely.

IS PMS DUE TO SEROTONERGIC DYSFUNCTION?

Needless to say, the fact that enhancing or reducing serotonergic activity may alleviate or aggravate PMS does not necessarily mean that the symptoms are the result of serotonergic dysfunction. As discussed below, many studies however do lend support to the notion that women with PMS/PMDD differ from controls with respect to various indices of serotonergic activity, indicating that serotonin in fact may play a significant part in the pathophysiology of this condition.

One tentative way of assessing serotonergic activity in living humans is to utilize the fact that certain serotonin-related proteins, including the serotonin transporter and the serotonin-metabolizing enzyme monoamine oxidase (MAO), are expressed not only by serotonergic neurons in the brain but also by platelets. Several studies comparing PMS subjects and controls with respect to serotonin uptake into thrombocytes, platelet serotonin transporter density, and platelet MAO activity, do suggest a difference either throughout the menstrual cycle or at a certain phase of the cycle.[43,44] Although it remains unclear to what extent these peripheral markers reflect brain serotonin activity, and how the observed differences should be interpreted in terms of function, these findings provide some evidence for the notion that PMS may be associated with aberrations in serotonergic activity.

Hypothalamic serotonergic neurons exert a stimulatory influence on the release of prolactin from the pituitary. One tentative way of addressing the function of brain serotonergic neurons and/or the responsiveness of central postsynaptic serotonin receptors is to assess the prolactin response to indirect or direct serotonin receptor agonists. Several studies indicate that women with PMS differ from controls also with respect to this parameter.[45-47] However, how this measure corresponds to the activity of those serotonergic neurons that are involved in the regulation of mood and behavior remains to be clarified.

Another crude way of assessing brain serotonergic transmission is to measure levels of the serotonin metabolite 5-hydroxyindoleacetic acid (5-HIAA) in the cerebrospinal fluid. One study has reported reduced levels of the ratio between the dopamine metabolite homovanillic acid and 5-HIAA in women with PMS.[48] This finding is of some interest since a similar aberration has previously been reported in subjects with depression, but it cannot be easily interpreted in terms of function.

A more sophisticated strategy to assess brain serotonergic transmission in humans than those mentioned above is the use of brain imaging techniques, such as positron emission tomography. Although research on PMS using this method are as yet sparse, there are two recent pilot studies suggesting that symptomatic women differ from non-symptomatic controls with respect to uptake of a serotonin precursor and density of serotonergic 5HT1A receptors, respectively.[49,50] Both these studies are small, and should be interpreted with caution until replicated, but they do lend further support to the notion that PMS may be associated with abnormal serotonin activity.

It should be emphasized that all of the different techniques mentioned above yield results that are difficult to interpret, and that they provide, at best, an indirect and/or very limited insight into the status of the different serotonergic pathways in the brain. Moreover, most of the studies that have been published in this field are small, and should for this reason be regarded as preliminary until replicated. Notwithstanding these caveats, the fact that such a large number of studies indicate that PMS women and controls differ significantly with respect to various serotonin-related indices supports the notion that PMS is indeed associated with serotonergic dysfunction. In this context, the possible influence of publication bias, i.e. the tendency for studies finding a difference to get published more often than studies not finding a difference, should however not be ignored.

If certain variants of serotonin-related genes were found to increase the susceptibility to PMS, this would provide a reasonable explanation both to the symptoms characterizing this condition and to the many positive findings regarding serotonin-related biological markers, including peripheral indices of serotonergic function, that have been published. However, association studies showing a relationship between serotonin-related genes and PMS have yet to be published. In one study, women with PMS were found to display reduced platelet density of the serotonin transporter, but this difference could not be linked to any of the more well-known polymorphisms in the serotonin transporter gene.[43]

To conclude, the hypothesis that the enhanced responsiveness to sex steroids in women with PMS is at least partly due to a dysfunction in brain serotonergic neurons is not far-fetched and gains some support from the available literature, but remains to be confirmed. Brain imaging studies and extensive studies of serotonin-related genes in large and well-characterized cohorts should shed further light on this issue.

THE POSSIBLE ROLE OF SEROTONIN IN THE PATHOPHYSIOLOGY OF SOMATIC SYMPTOMS

One issue that has for long been debated, but remains unresolved, is if premenstrual somatic symptoms–such as breast tenderness, bloating, joint and muscle pain, and headache–are due to the influence of sex steroids in the brain, modulating the subject's awareness of minor bodily changes, or to direct effects of sex steroids in hormone-responsive tissues in the periphery.

Supporting the former notion, several studies have failed to confirm fluid retention or breast enlargement by objective means in women reporting these symptoms.[51] Moreover, many studies have demonstrated that SRIs reduce not only mood and behavioral symptoms but also somatic complaints. Worth considering in this context is the fact that SRIs have been reported to influence the sensitivity to pain also in other conditions.[52]

On the other hand, it should be emphasized that the SRIs exert a more robust effect on premenstrual mood and behavioral symptoms than on somatic symptoms, a difference that is particularly evident when the treatment is given intermittently[20]. Moreover for one common premenstrual symptom, headache, no superiority of SRIs over placebo has been reported. Hence, the suggestion put forward in this chapter that serotonin is critically involved in the pathophysiology of PMS is probably more relevant for the mood and behavioral aspects of this syndrome than for the somatic complaints.

UNRESOLVED ISSUES

To conclude, there is strong evidence to support the notion that sex steroids and serotonergic neurons interact, and that an important task for the serotonergic pathways is to dampen sex steroid-driven behavior, such as aggression and sexual activity. In all likelihood, the rapid and very impressive effect of SRIs on many of the cardinal symptoms of PMS, such as irritability and affect lability, should be regarded as a manifestation of this interaction, and of the well-established inhibitory influence of serotonin on anger and irritability. Although there are reasons to believe that the amygdala and the hypothalamus are brain areas of particular importance in this context, much more work is required to map the pathways involved, and to clarify how and where sex steroids and serotonergic neurons interact. It is also important to elucidate which of the many different serotonin receptors that mediate these effects of serotonin, and with which other transmitters serotonin interacts in this context. In particular, the interplay between serotonin and another transmitter, dopamine, that is known to exert effects opposite to those of serotonin on aggression, warrants further study.

Although the efficacy of SRIs in PMS is well established, it remains to be clarified if women with premenstrual symptoms differ from controls with respect to serotonin activity, or if the mechanisms making certain women particularly responsive to the influence of sex steroids reside elsewhere. Studies of serotonin-related genes, assessment of brain serotonergic activity using brain imaging techniques, and projects combining these strategies are likely to shed further light on this issue.

REFERENCES

1. Schmidt PJ, Nieman LK, Danaceau MA et al. Differential behavioral effects of gonadal steroids in women with and in those without premenstrual syndrome. N Engl J Med 1998; 338:209–16.
2. Carlsson A. A paradigm shift in brain research. Science 2001; 294:1021–4.
3. Abi-Dargham A, Rodenhiser J, Printz D et al. Increased baseline occupancy of D_2 receptors by dopamine in schizophrenia. Proc Natl Acad Sci 2000; 97:8104–9.
4. Parsey RV, Hastings RS, Oquendo MA et al. Lower serotonin transporter binding potential in the human brain during major depressive episodes. Am J Psychiatry 2006; 163:52–8.
5. Kendler KS, Kuhn JW, Vittum J, Prescott CA, Riley B. The interaction of stressful life events and a serotonin transporter polymorphism in the prediction of episodes of major depression: a replication. Arch Gen Psychiatry 2005; 62:529–35.
6. Eriksson E, Humble M. Serotonin in psychiatric pathophysiology. A review of data from experimental and clinical research. In: Pohl R, Gershon S, eds. The Biological Basis of Psychiatric Treatment. Prog Basic Clin Pharmacol. Basel: Karger; 1990:66–119.
7. Lesch KP, Bengel D, Heils A et al. Association of anxiety-related traits with a polymorphism in the serotonin transporter gene regulatory region. Science 1996; 274:1527–31.
8. Hariri AR, Mattay VS, Tessitore A et al. Serotonin transporter genetic variation and the response of the human amygdala. Science 2002; 297:400–3.
9. Rosen RC, Lane RM, Menza M. Effects of SSRIs on sexual function: a critical review. Clin Psychopharmacol 1999; 19:67–85.
10. Sundblad C, Eriksson E. Reduced extracellular levels of serotonin in the amygdala of androgenized female rats. Eur Neuropsychopharmacol 1997; 7:253–9.
11. Rubinow DR, Schmidt PJ, Roca CA. Estrogen–serotonin interactions: implications for affective regulation. Biol Psychiatry 1998; 44:839–50.
12. Zhang L, Ma W, Barker JL, Rubinow DR. Sex differences in expression of serotonin receptors (subtypes 1A and 2A) in rat brain: a possible role of testosterone. Neuroscience 1999; 94:251–9.
13. Robichaud M, Debonnel G. Oestrogen and testosterone modulate the firing activity of dorsal raphe nucleus serotonergic neurones in both male and female rats. J Neuroendocrinol 2005; 17:179–85.
14. Hiroi R, McDevitt RA, Neumaier JF. Estrogen selectively increases tryptophan hydroxylase-2 mRNA expression in distinct subregions of rat midbrain raphe nucleus: association between gene expression and anxiety behavior in the open field. Biol Psychiatry 2006; 1:288–95.
15. Bethea CL, Lu NZ, Gundlah C, Streicher JM. Diverse actions of ovarian steroids in the serotonin neural system. Front Neuroendocrinol 2002; 23:41–100.
16. Barrett GM, Bardi M, Guillen AK, Mori A, Shimizu K. Regulation of sexual behavior in male macaques by sex steroid modulation of the serotonergic system. Exp Physiol 2006; 91:445–56.
17. Wyatt KM, Dimmock PW, O'Brien PM. Selective serotonin reuptake inhibitors for premenstrual syndrome. Cochrane Database Syst Rev 2002; CD001396.

18. Steiner M, Pearlstein T, Cohen LS et al. Expert guidelines for the treatment of severe PMS, PMDD, and comorbidities: the role of SSRIs. J Womens Health 2006; 15:57–69.

19. Eriksson E, Andersch B, Ho HP, Landén M, Sundblad C. Diagnosis and treatment of premenstrual dysphoria. J Clin Psychiatry 2002; 63:16–23.

20. Landén M, Nissbrandt H, Allgulander C et al. Placebo-controlled trial comparing intermittent and continuous paroxetine in premenstrual dysphoric disorder. Neuropsychopharmacology 2007; 32: 153–61

21. Eriksson E, Hedberg MA, Andersch B, Sundblad C. The serotonin reuptake inhibitor paroxetin is superior to the norepinephrine reuptake inhibitor maprotiline in the treatment of premenstrual syndrome. Neuropsychopharmacology 1995; 12:167–76.

22. Pearlstein TB, Stone AB, Lund SA et al. Comparison of fluoxetine, bupropion, and placebo in the treatment of premenstrual dysphoric disorder. J Clin Psychopharmacol 1997; 17:261–6.

23. Freeman EW, Rickels K, Sondheimer SJ, Polansky M. Differential response to antidepressants in women with premenstrual syndrome/premenstrual dysphoric disorder: a randomized controlled trial. Arch Gen Psychiatry 1999; 56:932–9.

24. Rutter JJ, Auerbach SB. Acute uptake inhibition increases extracellular serotonin in the rat forebrain. J Pharmacol Exp Ther 1993; 265:1319–24.

25. Golden RN, Hsiao J, Lane E et al. The effects of intravenous clomipramine on neurohormones in normal subjects. J Clin Endocrinol Metab 1989; 68(3):632–7.

26. Coupland NJ, Bailey JE, Potokar JP, Nutt DJ. 5-HT3 receptors, nausea, and serotonin reuptake inhibition. J Clin Psychopharmacol 1997; 17:142–3.

27. Waldinger MD, Zwinderman AH, Olivier B. On-demand treatment of premature ejaculation with clomipramine and paroxetine: a randomized, double-blind fixed-dose study with stopwatch assessment. Eur Urol 2004; 46:510–15.

28. Sundblad C, Hedberg MA, Eriksson E. Clomipramine administered during the luteal phase reduces the symptoms of premenstrual syndrome: a placebo-controlled trial. Neuropsychopharmacol 1993; 9:133–45.

29. Muller U, Murai T, Bauer-Wittmund T, von Cramon DY. Paroxetine versus citalopram treatment of pathological crying after brain injury. Brain Inj 1999; 13:805–11.

30. Sloan RL, Brown KW, Pentland B. Fluoxetine as a treatment for emotional lability after brain injury. Brain Inj 1992; 6:315–19.

31. Nahas Z, Arlinghaus KA, Kotrla KJ, Clearman RR, George MS. Rapid response of emotional incontinence to selective serotonin reuptake inhibitors. J Neuropsychiatry Clin Neurosci 1998; 10: 453–5.

32. Burns A, Russell E, Stratton-Powell H et al. Sertraline in stroke-associated lability of mood. Int J Geriatr Psychiatry 1999; 14:681–5.

33. Ho HP, Olsson M, Westberg L et al. The serotonin reuptake inhibitor fluoxetine reduces sex steroid-related aggression in female rats: an animal model of premenstrual irritability? Neuropsychopharmacology 2001; 24:502–10.

34. Rothman RB, Baumann MH. Serotonin releasing agents. Neurochemical, therapeutic and adverse effects. Pharmacol Biochem Behav 2002; 71:825–36.

35. Su TP, Schmidt PJ, Danaceau M, Murphy DL, Rubinow DR. Effect of menstrual cycle phase on neuroendocrine and behavioral responses to the serotonin agonist m-chlorophenylalanine in women with premenstrual syndrome and controls. J Clin Endocrin Metab 1997; 82:1220–8.

36. Brzezinski AA, Wurtman JJ, Wurtman RJ et al. d-Fenfluramine suppresses the increased calorie and carbohydrate intakes and improves the mood of women with premenstrual depression. Obstet Gynecol 1990; 76:296–301.

37. Steinberg S, Annable L, Young SN, Liyanage N. A placebo-controlled clinical trial of L-tryptophan in premenstrual dysphoria. Biol Psychiatry 1999; 45:313–20.

38. Macdougall M. Poor-quality studies suggest that vitamin B_6 use is beneficial in premenstrual syndrome. West J Med 2000; 172:245.

39. Landén M, Eriksson O, Sundblad C et al. Compounds with affinity for serotonergic receptors in the treatment of premenstrual dysphoria: a comparison of buspirone, nefazodone and placebo. Psychopharmacology 2001; 155:292–8.

40. Menkes DB, Taghavi E, Mason PA, Spears GF, Howard RC. Fluoxetine treatment of severe premenstrual syndrome. BMJ 1992; 305:346–7.

41. Roca CA, Schmidt PJ, Smith MJ et al. Effects of metergoline on symptoms in women with premenstrual dysphoric disorder. Am J Psychiatry 2002; 159:1876–81.

42. Pinna G, Costa E, Guidotti A. Fluoxetine and norfluoxetine stereospecifically and selectively increase brain neurosteroid content at doses that are inactive on 5-HT reuptake. Psychopharmacology 2006; 24:1–11.

43. Melke J, Westberg L, Landén M et al. Serotonin transporter gene polymorphisms and platelet [^{3}H] paroxetine binding in premenstrual dysphoria. Psychoneuroendocrinology 2003; 28:446–58.

44. Ashby CR Jr, Carr LA, Cook CL, Steptoe MM, Franks DD. Alteration of platelet serotonergic mechanisms and monoamine oxidase activity in premenstrual syndrome. Biol Psychiatry 1988; 24:225–33.

45. Steiner M, Yatham LN, Coote M, Wilkins A, Lepage P. Serotonergic dysfunction in women with pure premenstrual dysphoric disorder: is the fenfluramine challenge test still relevant? Psychiatry Res 1999; 87:107–15.

46. Yatham LN. Is 5HT1A receptor subsensitivity a trait marker for late luteal phase dysphoric disorder? A pilot study. Can J Psychiatry 1993; 38:662–4.

47. Halbreich U, Tworek H. Altered serotonergic activity in women with dysphoric premenstrual syndromes. Int J Psychiatry Med 1993; 23:1–27.

48. Eriksson E, Alling C, Andersch B, Andersson K, Berggren U. Cerebrospinal fluid levels of monoamine metabolites. A preliminary study of their relation to menstrual cycle phase, sex steroids, and pituitary hormones in healthy women and in women with premenstrual syndrome. Neuropsychopharmacology 1994; 11:201–13.

49. Eriksson O, Wall A, Marteinsdottir I et al. Mood changes correlate to changes in brain serotonin precursor trapping in women with premenstrual dysphoria. Psychiatry Res 2006; 146:107–16.

50. Jovanovic H, Cerin Å, Karlsson P et al. A PET study of 5HT1A-receptors at different phases of the menstrual cycle in women with premenstrual dysphoria. Psychiatry Res 2006; 148:185–93.

51. Faratian B, Gaspar A, O'Brien PM et al. Premenstrual syndrome: weight, abdominal swelling, and perceived body image. Am J Obstet Gynecol 1984; 150:200–4.

52. Arnold LM, Hess EV, Hudson JI et al. A randomized, placebo-controlled, double-blind, flexible-dose study of fluoxetine in the treatment of women with fibromyalgia. Am J Med 2002; 112:191–7.

4

Quantification of premenstrual syndrome and premenstrual dysphoric disorder

Vandana Dhingra and PM Shaughn O'Brien

INTRODUCTION

Gynecological practice is almost always informed by an objective test or visual information on which to base diagnosis and provide treatment. No such objective tests are available for quantification for premenstrual syndrome/premenstrual dysphoric disorder (PMS/PMDD), and this may be a challenge for gynecologists treating patients or undertaking research.

Psychiatrists are used to this problem in the diagnosis, management, and documentation of most psychiatric disorders and, while they are well acquainted with disorders that are periodic in nature, it is rare that prospective assessment and the wait for repeated menstrual cycles impacts on their practice regularly. Similarly, they are less well acquainted with the vagaries of the menstrual cycle, its endocrinology and its other symptoms.

As we know, PMS and even PMDD are commonly encountered amongst women of reproductive age, and these can have a major impact. (see Chapter 6). Literally hundreds of symptoms have been described, spanning a spectrum of mood and physical disturbance, and so it is not surprising that symptomatology overlaps with many other medical problems. We will see in several of the following chapters that the exclusion of both psychiatric and organic medical/gynecological disorders is of critical importance: gynecological disorders that may be confused include pelvic pain syndrome, endometriosis, dysmenorrhea, and the perimenopause. Psychological disorders to be distinguished, amongst many others, include subtypes of depression, personality disorder, anxiety disorders, and seasonal affective disorder. Investigators lack agreement regarding the particular symptoms that define PMS and the specific methodology to diagnose this condition. Whether the method of assessment needs to be different for clinical purposes and research is also a matter for debate.

There is currently no objective means of assessing PMS, and clinical diagnosis relies predominantly on the subjective self-reporting of symptomatology. If we look again at the criteria required for the diagnosis of PMS and PMDD, it is clear that several factors must be quantified.

Any technique needs to provide an easily completed means of assessing *individual symptoms* on a prospective daily basis. To ensure compliance, this must be simple and not time consuming for the patient. The symptoms should be easily converted into numerical data and so free text should be avoided. The first aim is to demonstrate that symptoms occur in the luteal phase and, perhaps most importantly, to show that they resolve by the end of menstruation. Secondly, the *severity* of symptoms needs to be quantified in a numerical format. Thirdly, a means of assessing whether or not there is an *underlying psychiatric disorder* and how this is to be quantified needs consideration; psychiatric interview, rating scales, or questionnaires for psychological illness are all possibilities. At its most simple, given that there is considerable overlap between symptoms of PMS/PMDD and those of other psychological disorders, the absence of symptoms in the follicular phase on PMS/PMDD scales may well suffice for clinical practice for the exclusion of depression but probably not for disorders such as obsessive compulsive disorder (OCD) and post-traumatic stress disorder (PTSD) which require structured psychiatric interview. Finally, an important factor which we must measure, and in fact the key factor which enables us to distinguish between physiological premenstrual symptoms, PMS, and PMDD, is the determination of the *impact* on normal functioning, well-being, and interpersonal relationships.

METHODS OF MEASUREMENT REPORTED TO DATE

Early research projects attempted to use rating scales that were essentially established and designed to quantify other psychiatric and psychological conditions. Examples of this are the use of the Hamilton Rating Scale for Depression[1] and the Beck Depression Inventory.[2] The lack of specificity of these techniques to quantify PMS led to the development of new 'bespoke' techniques.

The earliest published measure specific to premenstrual symptoms was the Moos' Menstrual Distress Questionnaire (MDQ),[3] which used a 47-item 0–6 rating scale. The first use of visual analog scales (VAS) was published as the Premenstrual Mood Index, which was used for the first time within the context of a randomized clinical trial of spironolactone at the University of Nottingham, UK.[4] We will look at the use of VAS first.

Visual analog scales

VAS techniques demonstrate admirably the character and cyclicity of symptoms. It is likely that visual analog scales (VAS) are the most sensitive measure of PMS/PMDD, as they allow a continuous rating. When first used back in 1976, each score had to be measured by hand, and this was tedious and onerous. The VAS can be used to look at individual scores and their response to therapy or a global score. Visual analog scales have been found to be an effective tool in measuring the change in premenstrual symptoms over time, and their validity and reliability have since been well documented.[4–6] Bipolar visual analog scales, which record mood changes, differ in one important respect from the more usual unipolar ratings; the 100 mm line has both positive and negative mood adjectives, with the midline being 'a normal day'; they are thus rated either side of 50 mm scores. Bipolar visual analog scales are more difficult to handle in a statistical sense.

Unipolar VAS consists again of a 100 mm horizontal line with vertical line anchors at each end. The anchors are 0 = 'not at all' (i.e. the way you normally feel when you don't have premenstrual symptoms) and 100 = 'extreme symptoms' (i.e. the way you feel when your premenstrual symptoms are at their worst). Data collected from more recent trials of women with severe premenstrual symptoms indicate that the use of the revised VAS, which better reflects the current DSM-IV (Diagnosis and Statistical Manual of Mental Disorders, fourth edition) definition of PMDD, provides a reliable measure of premenstrual symptoms when evaluated against the well-validated Premenstrual Tension

Syndrome – Observer (PMTS-O). It is more user friendly and also improves compliance. However, the relentless measuring of the 100 mm lines of the scales was at the time a disincentive to further development of the method.[7] Later on, the ability to optically read the scores and to provide a measuring technique on touch-sensitive PDA screens showed the promise of greater simplicity and utility (Figure 4.1). This is discussed in detail later.

OTHER RATING SCALES

The original Moos MDQ had significant limitations, mainly related to the specificity of the symptoms. Even so, this is the model on which most other PMS rating techniques were based. It used a 46-item 0–6 rating scale; the various newer techniques rate from 0 to 3, 4, 5, 6, or 7, using categorical rating scales. The cynic might observe that there are about the same number of scales as there are research groups. Early scales included the Clinical Global Impression Scale (CGIS), the Global Assessment Scale (GAS),[8] the Steiner Self-Rating Scale,[9] while later the more widely used scales included Premenstrual Assessment Form (PAF),[10] Prospective Record of the Impact and Severity of Menstrual Symptoms (PRISM),[11] and the Calendar of Premenstrual Experiences (COPE).[12] These and many other tools used over the past 30 years are summarized in Table 4.1.

The Daily Record of Severity of Problems

During the evolution of these various methods, the DSM-III and DSM-IV criteria[23] were developed for late luteal phase dysphoric disorder (LLPDD), and then PMDD. In line with that, in 1990, Endicott and Harrison[20] published the somewhat simple tool named Daily Record of Severity of Problems (DRSP). DRSP was developed to help individual women and their therapist assess the nature, severity, and timing of onset and offset of problems which may develop during specific phases of the menstrual cycle. The feelings and behaviors which are to be rated each day are those which make up the diagnostic criteria for PMDD. Completion of such rating is essential to determine the nature of the problem being experienced.[20]

Daily ratings made for several menstrual cycles help to establish when specific symptoms first appear or become more severe, how severe they become, how much impairment in functioning they cause, and when they go away or become less severe. The pattern of change in the symptoms helps the woman and her therapist to determine which of the following conditions are

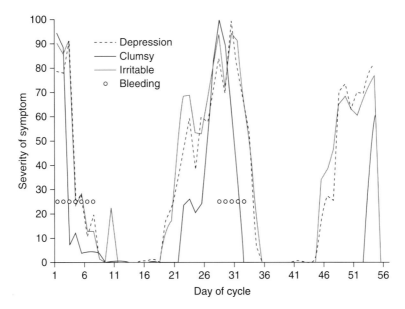

Figure 4.1 Daily visual analog scale scores for psychological symptoms derived from electronic data capture of VAS measurement on PDA.[30]

most likely to be present (J Endicott, unpublished data):

1. Premenstrual worsening of her ongoing condition, which is present throughout her cycle.
2. PMDD with patterns of changes that clearly meet criteria.
3. PMS that is clearly present but does not meet the severity or impairment criteria for PMDD.
4. Symptoms and impairment that show no evidence of being linked to phases of the menstrual cycle.

The reason such a diagnostic evaluation is important is that it will identify the diagnosis and guide the treatment of the condition (Figure 4.2)

The Premenstrual Symptoms Screening Tool

The Premenstrual Symptoms Screening Tool (PSST) is a simple user-friendly screening tool devised by Steiner et al[22] to identify women who suffer from severe PMS/PMDD and who are likely to benefit from treatment. The PSST reflects and translates categorical DSM-IV criteria into a rating scale with degrees of severity and impact of premenstrual symptoms. It is less time consuming and more practical than two cycles of prospective charting and, hence, is an important starting point for further assessment. Following screening, the clinician still must rule out other psychiatric

and medical conditions and, if in doubt, more comprehensive assessment measures including prospective charting should be initiated (Figure 4.3).

This chart has the potential to provide a simple easy-to-used chart for clinical purposes but probably not for research. Even for clinical purposes, most clinicians believe it still needs to be validated against the DRSP.

When using any chart for either research or clinical purposes, ideally, symptoms should be rated prospectively in order to avoid the inaccuracies inherent in retrospective rating, including the incorrect recall of symptom timing and exaggeration of symptom severity. Symptoms recorded over several cycles will illustrate any inter-cycle variability in the nature and severity of symptoms. Statistical measures have to be used to establish if a cyclical change exists or not.

Quantifying severity with VAS and other techniques poses problems. In 1983 the National Institute of Mental Health workshop on PMS/PMDD stated that premenstrual changes should show at least 30% increase from the intensity of symptoms measured in the follicular phase (i.e. on days 5–10 of the menstrual cycle), compared with those measured in the premenstrual phase (on the 6 days before menstruation). Many of those involved in that workshop consider the 30% change in the ratings of symptoms has been shown to be too liberal and a poor discriminator when comparing women with self-reported severe PMS, women using contraceptives whose natural cyclicity has been

Table 4.1 Techniques used to quantify premenstrual syndrome

Reference	Method	Comment
[a]Hamilton 1960[13]	Hamilton Rating Scale for Depression (HAM-D)	Observer-rated instrument to assess 17/21 items in premenstrual mood disturbance
[a]Beck et al 1961[2]	Beck Depression Inventory (BDI)	21-item self-report questionnaire; symptoms rated 0–3 to give an overall depression score
Moos 1968[3]	Moos Menstrual Distress Questionnaire (MDQ)	47 symptoms rated on a six-point scale
[a]McNair et al 1971[14]	Profile of Mood States (POMS)	65 symptoms rated on 0–4 scale combined to give summary scores for five dimensions
[a]Weissman and Bothwel 1976[15]	Social Adjustment Scale (SAS)	Self-report instrument containing 56 questions in seven different sections
Endicott et al 1976[8]	Global Assessment Scale (GAS)	Has not been used extensively
[a]Guy 1976[16]	Clinical Global Impression Scale (CGIS)	Seven-point observer/patient-rated global scale
[a]Derogatis and Cleary 1977[17]	Symptom Checklist-90 (SCL-90)	General index of psychological and physical symptoms plus additional nine subscales
O'Brien et al 1979[4]	Visual analog scale (VAS): Premenstrual Mood Index	100 mm line at either end of which are opposing adjectives representing the symptoms
Steiner et al 1980[9]	Self-Rating Scale for Premenstrual Syndrome	A 36-item yes/no rating scale
Steiner et al 1980[9]	Premenstrual Tension Syndrome – Observer (PMTS-O) and Self-Rating (PMTS-SR)	Assess symptoms in 10 different domains. 36 symptoms with severity ranging from 0 to 4
Halbreich et al 1982[10]	Premenstrual Assessment Form (PAF)	Retrospective questionnaire based on psychological and behavioral symptoms
Reid 1985[11]	Prospective Record of the Impact and Severity of Menstrual Symptoms (PRISM)	Daily chart records a large number of symptoms rated 1–3
Rubinow et al 1984[6]	Visual analog scale (VAS)	100 mm line at either end of which are opposing adjectives representing the symptoms
Magos et al 1986[18]	Modified Moos Menstrual Distress Questionnaire (MDQ)	Ten items derived from MDQ, usually subjected to Trigg's trend analysis
Casper and Powell 1986[5]	Visual analog scale (VAS)	100 mm line at either end of which are opposing adjectives representing the symptoms
Magos and Studd 1988[19]	Premenstrual Tension-Cator (PMT-Cator)	Five symptoms rated 0–3S

(Continued)

Table 4.1 (Continued)		
Reference	**Method**	**Comment**
Mortola et al 1990[12]	Calendar of Premenstrual Experiences (COPE)	
Endicott and Harrison 1990[20]	Daily Record of Severity of Problems (DRSP)	22-item rated 0–6 specifically for symptoms of PMDD
[a]Rivera-Tovar and Frank 1990[21]	Daily Assessment Form (DAF)	33-item symptom checklist rated from 0 (none) to 6 (extreme)
Steiner et al 2003[22]	Premenstrual Screening Tool (PSST)	Retrospective 0–3 scale. Retrospective for PMDD

[a]Methods originally designed for diagnoses other than PMS or PMDD.

suppressed, and women with normal cyclicity who report no premenstrual symptoms.[24,25] They now believe that if a 30% increase is to be used, it must relate to the symptom score *range* rather than *baseline*. Additionally, Gallant et al emphasized that what may be more clinically relevant is women's perceptions of variations in social and occupational functioning and 'the way in which having PMS is meaningful in a woman's life'. The authors' concern is that ever more stringent criteria might result in the exclusion from studies or treatment of significantly troubled individuals.

As early as 1986, Magos et al had applied Trigg's trend analysis[18] to evaluating severity and cyclicity and produced quite a useful tool for this purpose. Ekholm et al[26] compared four different methods to assess the cyclicity and severity, based on the daily prospective symptoms rating. The methods compared were:

- the non-parametric Mann–Whitney U-test,
- effect size
- run-test
- a 30% of change in symptom degree between the follicular and the luteal phases.

They concluded that three of the methods used seemed to correctly identify the same patients as having or not having cyclical changes. However, some differences in the outcome of validity testing and the 30% change methods seemed less valid than the other three methods.

DIAGNOSIS AND STATISTICAL MANUAL OF MENTAL DISORDERS (DSM-IV)

The diagnosis of PMS was operationalized with the introduction of the term 'late luteal phase dysphoric disorder' (LLPDD) into DSM-III-R (American Psychiatric Association, 1987) under the section headed 'Proposed diagnostic categories needing further study'. Subsequently a work group on LLPDD reported to the Diagnosis and Statistical Manual of Mental Disorders (DSM) IV task force, culminating in its inclusion in DSM-IV[23] as 'Premenstrual dysphoric disorder' in the section 'Mood disorders not otherwise specified', with its clinical criteria laid out in Appendix B – 'For further study' (Table 4.2). PMDD criteria require the presence of both certain types or number of symptoms (five of 11 symptoms present premenstrually, at least one being one of four mood symptoms – depression, anxiety, irritability, and affective lability) and certain phenomenal characteristics (present premenstrually and absent postmenstrually). Symptoms should cause impairment and interference with work/school/social activity and/or relationships premenstrually, not be an exacerbation of another chronic disorder, and be prospectively confirmed by daily ratings during at least two consecutive cycles. A change in symptoms from the follicular to the luteal phase of at least 50% is suggested for the diagnosis of PMDD.

There is little question that the creation of diagnostic criteria has improved the generalizability of findings in psychiatric research by assuring greater cross-study sample homogeneity. While this has certainly been true for PMS, questions can be legitimately raised about the stringency of the criteria and the means of their operationalization.

Unfortunately, the DSM-IV does not specify for how many days the symptoms should exist, nor does it specify how soon the symptoms should remit: additionally, it fails to pay much attention to the importance of physical symptoms. For clinical trials, inclusion criteria usually specify 'severe symptoms for at least 4 days' or

DAILY RECORD OF SEVERITY OF PROBLEMS

Name or Initials--------------------------------------Month/Year--

Each evening note the degree to which you experienced each of the problems listed below. Put an "x" in the box which corresponds to the severity: 1 - not at all, 2 - minimal, 3 - mild, 4 - moderate, 5 - severe, 6 - extreme.

BLEEDING																			
Cycle Day	1	2	3	4	5	6	7	8	9	10	11	12	13	14	15	16	17	18	40
Felt depressed, sad, "down", or "blue"																			
Felt hopeless																			
Felt worthless or guilty																			
Felt anxious, tense, "keyed up" or "on edge"																			
Had mood swings (eg suddenly felt sad or tearful)																			
Was more sensitive to rejection or my feelings were easily hurt																			
Felt angry, irritable																			
Had conflicts or problems with people																			
Had less interest in usual activities																			
Had difficulty concentrating																			
Felt lethargic, tired, fatigued, or had a lack of energy																			
Had increased appetite or overate																			
Had cravings for specific foods																			
Slept more, took naps, found it hard to get up when intended																			
Had trouble getting to sleep or staying asleep																			
Felt overwhelmed or that I could not cope																			
Felt out of control																			
Had breast tenderness																			
Had breast swelling, felt "bloated", or had weight gain																			
Had headache																			
Had joint or muscle pain																			
Impairment as demonstrated by interference with normal work, school or home activities or interference with usual social activities and relationships with others																			
At work, at school, at home, or in daily routine, at least one of the problems noted above caused reduction or productivity or inefficiency																			
At least one of the problems noted above interfered with hobbies, or social activities (eg avoid or do less)																			
At least one of the problems noted above interfered with relationships with others																			

Figure 4.2 Daily Record of Severity of Problems.

**Do you experience some or any of the following premenstrual symptoms which
start _before_ your period and _stop_ within a few days of bleeding?**
(please print and mark an "X" in the appropriate box)

SYMPTOMS	NOT AT ALL	MILD	MODERATE	SEVERE
1. Anger/irritability				
2. Anxiety/tension				
3. Tearful/Increased sensitivity to rejection				
4. Depressed mood/hopelessness				
5. Decreased interest in work activities				
6. Decreased interest in home activities				
7. Decreased interest in social activities				
8. Difficulty concentrating				
9. Fatigue/lack of energy				
10. Overeating/food cravings				
11. Insomnia				
12. Hypersomnia (needing more sleep)				
13. Feeling overwhelmed or out of control				
14. Physical symptoms: breast tenderness, headaches, joint/muscle pain, bloating weight gain				

Have your symptoms, as listed above, interfered with:

	NOT AT ALL	MILD	MODERATE	SEVERE
A. Your work efficiency or productivity				
B. Your relationships with co-workers				
C. Your relationships with your family				
D. Your social life activities				
E. Your home responsibilities				

Scoring

> The following criteria must be present for a diagnosis of **PMDD**
> 1.   at least one of #1, #2, #3, #4 is severe
> 2.   in addition at least four of #1-#1 4 are moderate to severe
> 3.   at least one of A, B, C, D, E is severe
>
> The following criteria must be present for a diagnosis of **moderate to severe PMS**
> 1.   at least one of #1, #2, #3, #4 is moderate to severe
> 2.   in addition at least four of #1-#14 are moderate to severe
> 3.   at least one of A, B, C, D, E is moderate to severe

Figure 4.3 Premenstrual Symptoms Screening Tool.

average severity during 7 days.[27] The possibility that different lengths of premenstrual period may be associated with different phenotypes and underlying mechanisms has not been fully elucidated.

DSM-IV allows the diagnosis of PMDD to be made alongside other disorders, but offers no guidance on differentiating between the two. The two disorders may coexist or indeed be intricately related to one another.

Table 4.2 Diagnosis and Statistical Manual of Mental Disorders IV Criteria

a. In most menstrual cycles during the past year, five (or more) of the following symptoms were present for most of the time during the last week of the luteal phase, began to remit within a few days after the onset of the follicular phase, and were absent in the week postmenses, with at least one of the symptoms being either (1), (2), (3), or (4):

   1. markedly depressed mood, feelings of hopelessness, or self-depreciating thoughts
   2. marked anxiety, tension, feeling of being 'keyed up' or 'on edge'
   3. marked affective lability (e.g. feeling suddenly sad or tearful or increased sensitivity to rejection)
   4. persistent and marked anger or irritability or increased interpersonal conflicts
   5. subjective sense of difficulty in concentrating
   6. lethargy, easy fatigability, or marked lack of energy
   7. marked change in appetite, overeating, or specific food cravings
   8. hypersomnia or insomnia
   9. a subjective sense of being overwhelmed or out of control
   10. other physical symptoms, such as breast tenderness or swelling, headaches, joint or muscle pain, a sensation of 'bloating', weight gain.

   Note: in menstruating females, the luteal phase corresponds to the period between ovulation and the onset of menses, and the follicular phase begins with menses. In non-menstruating females (e.g. those who have had a hysterectomy), the timing of luteal and follicular phase may require measurement of circulating reproductive hormones.

b. The disturbance markedly interferes with work or school or with usual social activities and relationships with others (e.g. avoidance of social activities, decreased productivity and efficiency at work or school).

c. The disturbance is not merely an exacerbation of the symptoms of another disorder, such as major depressive disorder, panic disorder, dysthymic disorder, or a personality disorder (although it may be superimposed on any of these disorders).

d. Criteria a, b, and c must be confirmed by prospective daily ratings during at least two consecutive symptomatic cycles. (The diagnosis may be made provisionally prior to this confirmation.)

Many of the scales listed in Table 4.1 have been used to make this distinction, in particular the Beck Depression Inventory,[2] Profile Of Mood States,[14] and Hamilton Depression Scale.[1] Other scales which can be administered to assess the woman's underlying psychiatric morbidity include the Hospital Anxiety and Depression Scale,[28] General Health Questionnaire,[29] Self-Reporting Questionnaire, and the Structured Clinical Interview for DSM-IV (SCID).[23]

Finally, it is important to reiterate that DSM-IV PMDD criteria fail to recognize the importance of physical symptoms, which is unfortunate as most women will complain of physical symptoms and for many this will be the most distressing feature. As an example, a woman with debilitating breast tenderness, bloatedness, and premenstrual headache with severe mood swings could be excluded from a diagnosis of PMDD if she had no other symptoms. More detailed and precise rating techniques must be devised and the authors of this chapter have proposed the concept of *Premenstrual Somatic Disorder (PMSD)*, for which specific rating scales have been devised but not yet evaluated or validated.

MENSTRUAL SYMPTOMETRICS

Various researchers have attempted to address the simplification of data collection. One of the simplest was the Premenstrual Tension-Cator (PMT-Cator), which was a gadget like an obstetric wheel calculator – although novel, it was never validated nor used in any further research. There have been several attempts at data acquisition, documentation, and transfer into a database by electronic means. The MiniDoc method has had limited use; it uses electronic data collection, but has not been published as a technique. At least one research study (within a clinical trial) using this technique was terminated prematurely because of difficulties with the system; the authors have been unable to locate other publications using the technique.

North Staffordshire Hospital/Keele University and Nottingham University investigated the menstrual symptometrics device, which was developed and validated against paper-based techniques. This method used a very early PDA (Amstrad PenPad, which is now obsolete). Visual analog scales were used to record scores for symptoms of PMS, dysmenorrhea, and perception of blood loss by means of a 'pen' on the touch-sensitive screen. It also incorporated the menstrual pictogram, a previously published pictorial method of measuring menstrual blood loss volume – hence, all symptoms related specifically to disorders of the menstrual cycle could be measured.[30]

Menstrual symptometrics was a simple 'palmtop' personal computer system programed to collect the daily menstrual cycle symptoms of PMS, blood loss, and pain, it was also programmed to include questionnaires to assess the woman's general health quality of life using an SF-36 (see next section for description) and a simple measure of underlying psychological pathology (General Health Questionnaire, GHQ) were also documented with other questionnaires incorporated into the system. It avoided the need to measure by hand the VAS, as the touch-sensitive screen allowed the instant measuring and storage of scores from VAS. It had a high level of patient acceptability and could provide instant pictorial feedback on symptoms for patients and clinicians.

This method is now obsolete, because of advances in PDA technology, and the menstrual pictogram is no longer valid because the blood absorbancy of those menstrual sanitary products acceptable to most women has changed dramatically.

MEASURES OF IMPAIRMENT

The measurement of impact or luteal phase impairment is critical in research and clinical practice if we are to distinguish PMS/PMDD from what are essentially normal or physiological symptoms of ovulatory menstrual cycles.

The diagnosis of PMDD also requires the confirmation of luteal phase impairment of social and/or work functioning. Commonly utilized ratings of role functioning and quality of life reported in prevalence and treatment studies include the Quality of Life Enjoyment

and Satisfaction Questionnaire (Q-LES-Q), the Sheehan Disability Scale (SDS), the Short Form of the Medical Outcomes Study functioning scale (SF-36), and the Social Adjustment Scale (SAS). The DRSP monitors three functioning items daily that assess impairment at work, school or home; interference with hobbies or social activities; and interference with relationships with others. Most researchers consider that to be adequate for most clinical trials.

CONCLUSION

The definitions and diagnosis of PMDD are still fragmented, not widely accepted, and, if accepted, not always applied in day-to-day clinical practice. We are still far from a biomedical and/or biopsychological model of a diagnostic entity based on etiology, pathophysiology, phenomena, time course, and treatment response.

Methods which use bipolar scores, optimize the thresholds separating PMS+ from PMS− cycles, and are based on known PMS symptom patterns are likely to be satisfactory whatever their level of sophistication.

The vast amount of paperwork involved in recording a woman's premenstrual symptoms daily over several months has meant that the data collection, measurement, and analysis of such data is time-consuming and labor-intensive, requiring many hours of data acquisition. A personal computer system for data collection and symptom measurement provides a simplified means of collecting large amounts of data on a daily basis, such as measurement of VAS, categorical scores, menstrual icons, and documentation of questionnaires. The ability to provide a graphic display provides an instant cyclic image of all the woman's menstrual cycle symptoms, making diagnosis and appropriate management of any disorder more accurate and straightforward.

Further studies are needed to validate the possibility of circumventing the need for prospective daily charting in establishing the diagnosis of PMS or PMDD possibly by validation of the PSST against the DRSP.

Until an objective means (genetic or magnetic resonance imaging [MRI]) of diagnosing PMS/PMDD is achieved, diagnosis is likely to rely on daily questionnaires such as the DRSP which most closely relates to the symptom factors within DSM-IV PMDD, unless of course the PSST can be shown to be valid. The concept of PMSD is a new one and, together with new rating tools, it warrants further exploration.

If such large numbers of data points continue to be required, electronic methods will increasingly be necessary and are really the only practical way forward. To consider PMS/PMDD management without reference to other gynecological and psychological comorbidities is inappropriate. This will need to be taken into account when these electronic methods are devised.

This chapter gives a summary of techniques and approaches used over the past 30 years and how we arrived at where we are today and where PMS/PMDD/PMSD research may take us in the future. The milestones are recorded, although it is not comprehensive and is likely to have some omissions. In Chapter 5, Pearlstein gives further insight into this area of research, particularly the valuable information that can be derived from many of the above techniques in relation to investigation, prevalence, and the impact of the disorder.

REFERENCES

1. Hamilton M. A rating scale for depression. J Neurol Neurosurg Psychiatry 1960; 23:56–62.
2. Beck AT, Ward CH, Mendelson M, Mock J, Eebaugh J. An inventory for measuring depression. Arch Gen Psychiatry 1961; 35:773–81.
3. Moos RH. The development of a menstrual distress questionnaire. Psychosom Med 1968; 30(6):853–67.
4. O'Brien PM, Craven D, Selby C, Symonds EM. Treatment of premenstrual syndrome by spironolactone. Br J Obstet Gynaecol 1979; 86(2):142–7.
5. Casper RF, Powell AM. Premenstrual syndrome: documentation by a linear analogue scale compared with two descriptive scales. Am J Obstet Gynecol 1986; 155(4):862–7.
6. Rubinow DR, Roy-Byrne P, Hoban MC, Gold PW, Post RM. Prospective assessment of menstrually related mood disorders. Am J Psychiatry 1984; 141(5):684–6.
7. Steiner M, Streiner DL. Validation of a revised visual analogue scale for premenstrual mood symptoms: results from prospective and retrospective trials. Can J Psychiatry 2005; 50(6):327–32.
8. Endicott J, Spitzer RL, Fleiss JL, Cohen J. The global assessment scale. A procedure for measuring overall severity of psychiatric disturbance. Arch Gen Psychiatry 1976; 33(6):766–71.
9. Steiner M, Haskett RF, Carroll BJ. Premenstrual tension syndrome: the development of research diagnostic criteria and new rating scales. Acta Psychiatr Scand 1980; 62(2):177–90.
10. Halbreich U, Endicott J, Schacht S, Nee J. The diversity of premenstrual changes as reflected in the Premenstrual Assessment Form. Acta Psychiatr Scand 1982; 65(1):46–65.
11. Reid RL. Premenstrual syndrome. Curr Probl Obstet Gynecol Fertil 1985; 8:1–57.
12. Mortola JF, Girton L, Beck L, Yen SS. Diagnosis of premenstrual syndrome by a simple, prospective, and reliable instrument: the calendar of premenstrual experiences. Obstet Gynecol 1990; 76(2):302–7.
13. Hamilton M. A rating scale for depression. J Neurol Neurosurg Psychiatry 1960; 23:56–62.
14. McNair DM, Lorr M, Droppleman LF. Profile of Mood States. San Diego: Educational and Industrial Telling Service; 1971.
15. Weissman MM, Bothwell S. Assessment of social adjustment by patient self-report. Arch Gen Psychiatry 1976; 33(9):1111–15.
16. Guy W. ECDEU. In: US Department of Health and Welfare, ed. Assessment Manual of Psychopharmacology. Washington, DC: National Institute of Mental Health, 1976:217–22.
17. Derogatis LR, Cleary PA. Factorial invariance across gender for the primary symptom dimensions of the SCL-90. Br J Soc Clin Psychol 1977; 16(4):347–56.
18. Magos AL, Brincat M, Studd JW. Trend analysis of the symptoms of 150 women with a history of the premenstrual syndrome. Am J Obstet Gynecol 1986; 155(2):277–82.
19. Magos AL, Studd JW. A simple method for the diagnosis of premenstrual syndrome by use of a self-assessment disk. Am J Obstet Gynecol 1988; 158(5):1024–8.
20. Endicott J, Harrison W. Daily rating of severity of problems form. New York: Department of Research Assessment and Training. New York State Psychiatric Institute, 1990.
21. Rivera-Tovar AD, Frank E. Late luteal phase dysphoric disorder in young women. Am J Psychiatry 1990; 147(12):1634–6.
22. Steiner M, Macdougall M, Brown E. The premenstrual symptoms screening tool (PSST) for clinicians. Arch Womens Ment Health 2003; 6(3):203–9.
23. American Psychiatric Association. Diagnostic and Statistical Manual of Mental Disorders, 4th edn. Washington, DC: American Psychiatric Press, 1994.
24. Gallant SJ, Popiel DA, Hoffman DM, Chakraborty PK, Hamilton JA. Using daily ratings to confirm premenstrual syndrome/late luteal phase dysphoric disorder. Part I. Effects of demand characteristics and expectations. Psychosom Med 1992; 54(2):149–66.
25. Gallant SJ, Popiel DA, Hoffman DM, Chakraborty PK, Hamilton JA. Using daily ratings to confirm premenstrual syndrome/late luteal phase dysphoric disorder. Part II. What makes a 'real' difference? Psychosom Med 1992; 54(2):167–81.
26. Ekholm UB, Ekholm NO, Backstrom T. Premenstrual syndrome: comparison between different methods to diagnose cyclicity using daily symptom ratings. Acta Obstet Gynecol Scand 1998; 77(5):551–7.
27. Halbreich U. The diagnosis of premenstrual syndromes and premenstrual dysphoric disorder – clinical procedures and research perspectives. Gynecol Endocrinol 2004; 19(6):320–34.
28. Zigmond AS, Snaith RP. The hospital anxiety and depression scale. Acta Psychiatr Scand 1983; 67(6):361–70.
29. Harding TW, de Arango MV, Baltazar J et al. Mental disorders in primary health care: a study of their frequency and diagnosis in four developing countries. Psychol Med 1980; 10(2):231–41.
30. Wyatt KM, Dimmock PW, Hayes-Gill B, Crowe J, O'Brien PM. Menstrual symptometrics: a simple computer-aided method to quantify menstrual cycle disorders. Fertil Steril 2002; 78(1):96–101.

5

Prevalence, impact on morbidity, and disease burden

Teri Pearlstein

PREVALENCE OF PREMENSTRUAL DYSPHORIC DISORDER

Many studies have examined the prevalence rates of premenstrual symptoms and premenstrual syndrome (PMS) in cross-sectional population cohorts and self-presenting clinical samples. Earlier studies included retrospective reports of PMS, either a 'Do you suffer from PMS, yes or no' or a one-time administered rating scale of premenstrual emotional, behavioral, and physical symptoms. The Premenstrual Assessment Form (PAF)[1] is one retrospective questionnaire that has been utilized in some studies. Several studies have suggested that retrospective reporting amplifies the frequency and severity of premenstrual symptoms. The reasons for the possible amplification of symptoms are unclear. Symptom severity peaks on or just before the first day of menses,[2–4] and the reporting of premenstrual symptoms may be influenced by menstrual cycle phase when questioned, wording of questions, expectations, and cultural issues.[2]

Since the introduction of research diagnostic criteria for premenstrual dysphoric disorder (PMDD) in the Diagnostic and Statistical Manual of Mental Disorders, fourth edition (DSM-IV),[5] women should prospectively rate their symptoms daily for two menstrual cycles to confirm the diagnosis. The prospective charting is designed to confirm the cyclical nature, timing, and magnitude of the symptoms. Commonly used daily rating forms reported in prevalence and treatment studies include the Daily Record of Severity of Problems (DRSP),[6] the Penn Daily Symptom Report (DSR),[7] the visual analog scale (VAS),[8] and the Moos Menstrual Distress Questionnaire (MDQ).[9] Determination of PMDD diagnosis, and thus, prevalence rates, can vary, depending on the scoring method applied to daily ratings. One study reported a PMDD prevalence rate range of 1–7% in 117 women, depending on the scoring method used,[10]

and another study reported a range of 14–45% in 670 women, depending on the scoring method used.[11]

The diagnosis of PMDD also requires the confirmation of luteal phase impairment of social and/or work functioning. Commonly utilized ratings of role functioning and quality of life reported in prevalence and treatment studies include the Quality of Life Enjoyment and Satisfaction Questionnaire (Q-LES-Q),[12] the Sheehan Disability Scale (SDS),[13] the Short Form of the Medical Outcomes Study functioning scale (SF-36),[14] and the Social Adjustment Scale (SAS).[15] In addition, the DRSP monitors three functioning items daily that assess impairment at work, school, or home; interference with hobbies or social activities; and interference with relationships with others.

Overall, studies utilizing prospective confirmation of PMDD, or retrospective assessment of PMDD criteria suggest PMDD prevalence rates of 3–8% in women of reproductive age. Recent studies also suggest that 15–20% of women meet criteria for 'subthreshold PMDD' or severe PMS with significant functional impairment. Irritability is consistently reported to be the most common and severe premenstrual symptom. One study noted that anxiety, irritability, and mood lability were the most stable symptoms over several cycles in women with PMDD, and were the symptoms associated with functional impairment.[16]

Prevalence studies using prospectively confirmed PMDD criteria

Three published studies have examined the prevalence of PMDD with prospective ratings and have reported very similar prevalence rates. Rivera-Tovar and Frank conducted a study in which 217 female college students (mean age 18.5 ± 1.8 years old) in Pittsburgh, Pennsylvania rated emotional and physical symptoms prospectively for 90 days.[17] Ten women (4.6%) met criteria for late luteal phase dysphoric disorder, now called PMDD. Cohen and colleagues reported on the prevalence of PMDD in 513 women (aged 36–44 years old) participating in the Boston area community Harvard Study of Moods and Cycles who rated their symptoms prospectively using the DRSP for one menstrual cycle.[18] The diagnosis of PMDD was confirmed in 33 (6.4%) of 513 women and was associated with previous major depressive disorder (MDD), lower education, and current cigarette smoking. Sternfeld and colleagues reported on the prevalence of premenstrual symptoms in 1194 women (aged 21–45 years old) enrolled in a California health maintenance organization who prospectively rated their symptoms for two cycles using the DRSP.[4] Fifty-six (4.7%) met criteria for PMDD and 151 (12.6%) women met criteria for severe PMS (defined as meeting PMDD criteria for one cycle with at least one symptom rated a 5 or 6 in the other cycle). The prevalence rates in this study may have been low due to the exclusion of women with known PMDD or psychotropic medication use. The number and severity of emotional premenstrual symptoms were inversely related to age and oral contraceptive use, and directly related to having a medical comorbidity and being Hispanic relative to being white.

Prevalence studies using PMDD criteria without prospective confirmation

Wittchen and colleagues published a study that has made a significant contribution to knowledge about prevalence and comorbidity data in an adolescent community sample.[19] These authors reported the 12-month prevalence and 4-year incidence rates of provisional PMDD in 1488 women aged 14–24 years old in a community cohort from Munich, Germany. Although women did not complete prospective ratings, subjects completed questions corresponding to the DSM-IV PMDD criteria relating to the past 12 months, with additional questions about impairment, psychosocial interference, and the absence of symptoms in the postmenses week. In addition, comorbid axis I disorders over the previous year were systematically assessed. At baseline, women aged 14–24 years old were enrolled, with 14–15 year olds sampled at twice the probability of 16–21 year olds, and 22–24 year olds sampled at half this probability. Follow-up assessments were conducted at approximately 2 and 4 years following enrollment; the age range of the sample at final follow-up was 18–29 years old.

At least one premenstrual symptom was endorsed by 79.8% of the total sample, with the five most common premenstrual symptoms being physical symptoms, affect lability, fatigability, depressed mood, and appetite/craving. The estimated 12-month prevalence of PMDD at baseline was 5.8% and the total overall cumulative incidence up to age 29 years old was 7.4%. When comorbid MDD and dysthymia were excluded, the baseline rate dropped to 5.3% and the cumulative incidence rate to 6.7%. PMDD was stable across the 4 years, with remission occurring in only 4.9%. The five most common PMDD symptoms were depressed mood (90.5%), affect lability (89.7%), irritability/anger (81.5%), fatigability (78.6%), and physical complaints (78.1%). Subthreshold PMDD was found in 18.6% of the total sample at baseline, defined as meeting most, but not all, of the PMDD criteria. The most frequent reason for not meeting full PMDD criteria was failure to meet the persistent impairment criterion. The rank order of premenstrual symptoms was similar for women with subthreshold PMDD but at lower frequencies compared to women with PMDD.

Both PMDD and subthreshold PMDD groups were significantly more likely to have a 12-month comorbidity of affective disorder, anxiety disorder, and nicotine dependence. Unusual findings from this study included the finding of suicide attempts having occurred in 15.8% of women with threshold PMDD, and significantly elevated 12-month rates of bipolar I, bipolar II post-traumatic stress disorder (PTSD), social phobia, and somatoform disorder compared with women without PMDD. Further analyses of this data have suggested that previous trauma or an anxiety disorder is associated with the development of PMDD, while having PMDD is associated with future episodes of depression.[19–21]

Steiner and colleagues developed a Premenstrual Symptoms Screening Tool (PSST) that assesses each of the PMDD criteria and five questions related to functioning and relationships rated as 'not at all', 'mild', 'moderate', or 'severe'.[22] The PSST was administered to 508 women attending a primary care clinic in Ontario, Canada. Although prospective ratings and evaluation of comorbid disorders were not obtained, the PSST directly inquired about symptoms that started before the period and stopped soon after menses. Results indicated that 26 (5.1%) women met criteria for PMDD and 105 (20.7%) women met criteria for moderate–severe PMS, similar to the results of the Wittchen study suggesting that approximately 1 in 5 women meet criteria for subthreshold PMDD.

In a cross-sectional telephone survey of 1045 women in the USA, UK, and France, Hylan and colleagues evaluated premenstrual symptoms based on the DSM-IV criteria by retrospective report, the extent to which the symptoms interfered with their home, school, work, or social life, and treatment-seeking behavior.[23] Between 23% and 31% of women were classified as having severe PMS. The most common symptoms occurring in about 80% of women in each country were irritability/anger, physical swelling/bloating, and fatigue. Robinson and Swindle conducted a cross-sectional survey of 1022 respondents from a nationally representative random sample of US women, evaluating premenstrual symptoms, social and occupational interference, healthcare beliefs, and treatment-seeking behavior. The results reported 11% meeting criteria for PMDD based on the DSM-IV criteria, and 63% of women having moderate–severe PMS.[24]

Prevalence studies in adolescent women with prospective charting of symptoms have not yet been conducted. Studies utilizing retrospective reporting of PMS have reported elevated and a wider range of prevalence rates of PMS compared with adult women. Two recent studies that retrospectively assessed the PMDD criteria in adolescent women reported prevalence rates of 31%[24a] and 13.4%.[24b]

Prevalence studies using retrospective PMS criteria

Reviews exist of older published studies of prevalence rates of PMS.[25,26] Some of the studies that were conducted in population cohorts will be mentioned, even though the studies utilized retrospective assessment of premenstrual symptoms. Two studies examined the prevalence of perimenstrual symptoms in a community cohort of women in Switzerland evaluated five times over 14 years.[27,28] Out of 299 women, 8.1% met criteria for severe, and 13.6% met criteria for moderate, perimenstrual emotional and somatic symptoms.[27] A study of 894 women in Virginia who were assessed over the telephone with the MDQ yielded 8.3% having PMS.[29] Severe premenstrual symptoms were endorsed by 2–3% of 1083 women in Sweden by mail survey.[30] Severe PMS with work impairment was reported in 3.2% of 730 nursing students in Iowa utilizing the PAF.[31] Between 2 and 7% of 2650 Canadian women in a population cohort met criteria for severe PMS by the MDQ.[32] In addition, 3–12% of 191 women in a Seattle area population cohort reported strong/disabling premenstrual symptoms by the MDQ.[33]

Prevalence studies in non-US countries

Several studies have examined the prevalence of premenstrual symptoms, PMS, and PMDD in non-US samples. Studies utilizing prospective confirmation of premenstrual symptoms over one or two menstrual cycles have reported prevalence rates of severe PMS or PMDD in 18.2% of 384 college students in Pakistan,[34] 6.4% of

52 volunteer women in India,[35] 12% of 150 women in a PMS clinic in Taiwan,[36] and 2.4% in 83 women in a population cohort in India.[37] Studies with retrospective reporting of premenstrual symptoms have also been conducted in Australia, Brazil, China, Egypt, Finland, France, Great Britain, Hong Kong, India, Japan, Mexico, Morocco, Nigeria, Spain, Taiwan, and Zimbabwe. Cross-cultural comparisons have suggested a predominance of somatic symptoms relative to emotional symptoms in several ethnic cultures. Caucasian women endorsed more emotional premenstrual symptoms compared with Afro-Caribbean and Asian subgroups in Great Britain,[38] and Australian and Italian women endorsed more emotional than somatic symptoms compared with Turkish, Vietnamese, and Greek subgroups in Australia.[39]

IMPACT OF PMDD ON FUNCTIONING, QUALITY OF LIFE, AND HEALTHCARE UTILIZATION

The morbidity of PMDD results from the severity of the symptoms, the chronic nature of the disorder, and the resulting impairment in work, relationships, and activities.[40] Halbreich et al estimated that women with PMDD endure 3.8 years of disability over their reproductive years based on the global burden of disease model, similar in magnitude to other major medical and psychiatric disorders.[25] The assessment of functioning and quality of life is difficult since it incorporates subjective views as well as measurable ratings of mental and physical health, work functioning, interpersonal functioning, and a sense of well-being.[41] In general, studies of role functioning in women with PMS and PMDD report greater subjective distress with the effect of premenstrual symptoms on interpersonal relationships compared to work performance.

In addition to the morbidity and functional impairment from PMDD, healthcare utilization also contributes to the disease burden. The assessment of healthcare utilization due to PMDD is difficult. Many studies assessing treatment utilization were conducted prior to the Food and Drug Administration (FDA) approval of selective serotonin reuptake inhibitors (SSRIs) for PMDD in 2000. Even though SSRIs are frequently used for PMDD currently, the diagnosis code attached to the SSRI prescription (as well as to the visit to the healthcare practitioner) is rarely the code for PMDD; it is more often a code for depression, anxiety disorder, or a medical condition. Thus, it is likely that prescription rates for medications for severe PMS and PMDD are largely underreported. The following summary of studies examines the effect of PMS and PMDD on interpersonal functioning, work functioning, and healthcare utilization.

Studies with PMS determined by a single-item question

Outpatient female veterans who endorsed PMS by a single (yes–no) item ($N = 445$) reported significantly lower SF-36 scores across all domains except energy/vitality compared with 574 women without any menstrual problems.[42] Compared with 26 women who claimed that they did not have PMS, 26 women who endorsed PMS had significantly more marital and family relationship dissatisfaction.[43] Another study reported a lack of absenteeism and objective work impairment in a group of women who reported having PMS.[44]

A random survey study of 220 women who stated that they had PMS reported that these women felt that the majority of physicians were not adequately informed to diagnose and treat them.[45] Even though satisfaction with antidepressants was high, only 15% of women had tried them. Many women had used vitamin/mineral supplements, exercise, natural progesterone, and diet changes in the past year. Phone assessment of a random national sample of 1052 women resulted in 41% of the women endorsing PMS.[46] Of these women, 42% took over-the-counter regimens for PMS, primarily analgesics, and only 3% took prescription medications. This study identified exercise and alternative and homeopathic treatments as also being tried.

Studies with PMS diagnosed by retrospective survey

Compared with women without PMS, women with PMS as defined by the PAF demonstrated marital dysfunction in the luteal phase.[47] In a population cohort from Sweden, 10% of 1083 women were unable to work at least once during the preceding 6 months due to PMS, and the inability to work was associated with the severity of emotional and physical symptoms.[30,48] In a survey of 658 women in Britain who stated that they had PMS after completing a questionnaire derived from the MDQ, 55% stated that PMS had a major effect on their relationship with their spouse, 43% stated an effect with their children, and 33% stated an effect on their work.[49] Almost half of this sample had visited their general practitioner specifically for PMS over the past year, and over the previous month 46% had taken analgesics, 9% had taken vitamins, and 11% had taken psychotropic medication.

Between 11% and 32% of 310 women were considered to have severe PMS as evaluated by the PAF on a cross-sectional retrospective survey of 310 women in general medicine practices in Australia.[50] Interpersonal relationship problems were more frequent than a negative impact on work attendance. Approximately half of the women had sought help for premenstrual symptoms and 85% had tried a prescription or over-the-counter medication. At least one-third of the women had tried analgesics, rest, exercise, drinking more fluids, vitamins, and oral contraceptives.

Studies with PMDD diagnosed by retrospective survey

In the study by Wittchen and colleagues described above, women with PMDD and subthreshold PMDD both reported significantly more acute impairment in their professional and everyday activities over the preious 4 weeks compared to women without PMDD.[19] Both PMDD groups also utilized medical and mental health practitioners significantly more than women without PMDD. However, the groups did not differ in use of psychotropic medication or over-the-counter preparations for premenstrual symptoms. The results of this study underscored that significant premenstrual symptoms, functional impairment, and healthcare utilization occurred in almost 25% of women aged 14–24 years old (combining the provisional PMDD and subthreshold PMDD groups) in a sizeable population cohort.

In the study by Steiner and colleagues described above, involving 508 women visiting a primary care clinic, the administration of the PSST confirmed decreased interest in work, home, and social activities in 57.7%, 69.2%, and 65.4%, respectively, of women meeting criteria for PMDD.[22] Decreased interest in work, home, and social activities was endorsed by 54.1%, 51.0%, and 48.5%, respectively, of women meeting criteria for moderate–severe PMS. These results lend further documentation of the substantial functional impairment in the 21% of women with severe PMS who do not meet the full severity criteria of PMDD.[22]

In the cross-sectional study of 1045 women conducted in the USA, UK, and France described above, functional impairment was highest at home; however, 8–16% of the sample reported missing work in the previous year due to premenstrual symptoms.[23] Approximately 25% of the women across the three nations had sought medical help for PMS, non-prescription medication use occurred in 20–47% of the sample, and prescription medication use occurred in 3–11% of the sample. Again, SSRIs had not yet been approved by regulatory authorities for PMDD at the time of this study.

Symptom severity was associated with impairment in work functioning and treatment-seeking. The cross-sectional study described above of 1022 women randomly assessed in the USA, reported that women who met criteria for PMDD had interference with all life domains assessed, particularly relationships, husband, and children.[24] Seeking treatment was associated with being older, greater severity and frequency of symptoms, and more positive attitudes toward PMS.

Studies with prospectively confirmed PMDD

A few studies with small samples of women with prospectively confirmed PMS or PMDD have examined work and family functioning. A study reported increased distress and increased functional impairment, as measured by the SDS, and reduced quality of life, as measured by the Q-LES-Q, in 15 women with PMDD vs 15 control women.[51] Another study compared impairment ratings in 31 women with late luteal phase dysphoric disorder (now PMDD) vs 34 control women.[52] Women with PMDD reported more negative interpersonal interactions at work, but not more family or work performance problems, compared with women without PMDD. Family functioning was assessed in 73 women with PMS and 50 women without premenstrual symptoms.[53] Women with PMS reported a higher amount of conflict in family relationships and more stress in their work environments compared with non-PMS controls. A group of 15 women with PMS and their husbands confirmed a negative effect of PMS on the marital relationship in another small study.[54]

Chawla and colleagues conducted further analyses on the data from 1194 women (aged 21–45 years old) enrolled in a California health maintenance organization who prospectively rated their symptoms with the DRSP.[55] As mentioned above, 56 (4.7%) met criteria for PMDD and 151 (12.6%) women met criteria for severe premenstrual syndrome, defined as meeting PMDD criteria for one cycle with at least one symptom rated a 5 or 6 in the other cycle.[4] Again, results from this study reflect women not seeking treatment for premenstrual symptoms, since women with known PMDD or psychotropic medication use were excluded. This study assessed work functioning and productivity with the Endicott Work Productivity Scale (EWPS),[56] the role-emotional subscale from the SF-36, and questions about time missed from work or decreased effectiveness in the past week. In addition, subjects were asked questions about utilization of medical services, and psychiatric services, and over-the-counter and prescription medications over the previous week.

As premenstrual symptom severity increased, the likelihood of emergency room visit, visit with a mental health clinician, or alternative medicine provider visit increased. There were no significant differences in healthcare expenditures across the mild, moderate, severe PMS and PMDD groups in terms of hospitalization rates or prescription drug utilization. Compared with the women with minimal PMS, women with PMDD had significantly more productivity impairment and role limitation during the luteal phase based on the EWPS score ($p < 0.01$), and the role-emotional score of the SF-36 ($p < 0.01$) and had less effectiveness ($p < 0.01$). Although full-day absenteeism from work was not significantly increased, women with PMDD and severe PMS reported significantly more hours missed from work than women with minimal PMS ($p < 0.01$).

Borenstein and colleagues examined data from a non-selected cohort of 436 women aged 18–45 years old enrolled in a medical group with capitated health insurance in Southern California who returned 2 months of DRSPs.[57,58] Approximately 30% of the women met criteria for a diagnosis of PMS in either one or both of the prospectively measured cycles. Measures of symptoms, functioning, healthcare utilization, work productivity, and absenteeism were compared between women with PMS and women without PMS. However, symptoms ratings may have been confounded by comorbid psychiatric or medical conditions, and psychotropic medication use, both of which were not systematically evaluated.

After analysis of the DRSP ratings, 47 women met criteria for PMS on both cycles, 78 women met criteria for PMS on one cycle, and 311 women who did not meet criteria for PMS were considered controls.[57,58] Women with one cycle of PMS had statistically significantly lower quality of life as measured by the physical components summary ($p < 0.0001$) and the mental components ($p < 0.0001$) summary measures of the SF-36 compared with controls.[57] Women who met PMS criteria for both cycles had significantly lower SF-36 summary scores than women who met PMS criteria for one cycle as well as controls. The magnitude of the reduction in mental health summary scores for the women with two cycles of confirmed PMS were comparable or exceeded the magnitude of reductions noted in studies of patients with depression and chronic medical illnesses.[57] Another study reported on the DRSP functioning items.[58] Women with PMS for both cycles showed significantly greater impairment than women with PMS for one cycle and women not meeting PMS criteria on work, school, and household activities ($p < 0.0001$), social activities and hobbies ($p < 0.0001$), and relationships with others ($p < 0.0001$).[58]

Women who met criteria for PMS for one or both cycles of PMS had significantly increased work absenteeism, decreased work productivity, and increased health provider visits than controls.[57] Further analysis demonstrated that women with PMS were 2–3 times more likely to miss at least 2 days of work per month and were 4–6 times more likely to report at least a 50% reduction in work productivity compared with women without PMS.[58] Women with PMS in both cycles showed significantly greater decrease in work productivity compared to women with one cycle of PMS and women not meeting PMS criteria. Women who met criteria for PMS in one or both cycles were significantly more likely to use calcium, vitamins, and other non-prescription medications ($p = 0.02$), and to use antidepressants, antianxiety medications, and other prescription medications ($p = 0.03$) for premenstrual symptoms than controls.[58]

The largest data available describing the functioning and quality of life in women with prospectively confirmed PMDD comes from women presenting for multisite clinical trials. Although women with PMDD seeking treatment may not be the same as women with PMDD in the community who do not seek treatment, the baseline evaluation of women seeking treatment in these studies has been systematic and comprehensive. In addition to baseline assessments, recent treatment trials have also examined the effect of treatment on functioning and quality of life as secondary outcome measures.

Fluoxetine trials

The largest multisite fluoxetine trial assessed the diagnosis of late luteal phase dysphoric disorder (now PMDD) with VAS in 313 women.[59] In later analyses, 8 items from the Premenstrual Tension Syndrome – Self Report[60] corresponding to work functioning were examined in 304 women.[61] At baseline, each of the 8 items were endorsed by a significantly larger percent of women during the luteal phase than in the follicular phase (each $p < 0.001$). Both fluoxetine 20 mg daily and 60 mg daily for 6 months were significantly better than placebo in improving the 8-item summed score, and the improvement occurred during the first cycle of treatment.

A multisite study compared luteal-phase fluoxetine 20 mg, fluoxetine 10 mg, and placebo in 260 women with PMDD diagnosed with the DRSP.[62] Both 20 mg ($p = 0.033$) and 10 mg ($p = 0.021$) fluoxetine for three cycles were significantly superior to placebo in improving the three DRSP functioning items. Another multisite study compared fluoxetine 90 mg administered 14 and 7 days before expected menses, placebo 14 days before, and fluoxetine 90 mg 7 days before expected menses, and placebo both 14 and 7 days before expected menses in 257 women with PMDD diagnosed with the DRSP.[63] The work, social life, and family life subscales of the SDS at luteal baseline were 4.8–5.2, 5.2–5.5, and

5.5–6.0, respectively, in the three treatment groups. The administration of fluoxetine 90 mg twice weekly before expected menses, but not once before expected menses, was significantly superior to placebo on improving the work ($p < 0.001$), social life ($p = 0.037$), and family life ($p = 0.005$) scores of the SDS and the sum of the three DRSP functioning items ($p = 0.035$). A cross-over study of flexible-dose fluoxetine and placebo, each administered for three cycles, in 20 women with PMDD reported superiority of fluoxetine over placebo for a composite social isolation and work efficiency score.[64]

Sertraline trials

A recent study[41] reported on a post-hoc analysis of the pretreatment Q-LES-Q scores of 437 women with prospectively confirmed PMDD by DRSP ratings who had participated in clinical trials of sertraline treatment.[65,66] The sum of items 1–14 correlated with the overall satisfaction and contentment item 16 ($r = 0.78$, $p < 0.0001$), suggesting that the broad set of functioning domains assessed by the Q-LES-Q individual items are related to the overall sense of quality of life. Thirty-one percent of women with PMDD were considered to have severe quality of life impairment, defined as two or more standard deviations below the community norm. Illness-specific symptom measures accounted for 26% of the variance in quality of life for women with PMDD, suggesting that quality of life assessment should be part of the diagnostic evaluation and treatment plan for women with PMDD in addition to specific premenstrual symptoms.[41]

Three studies have reported on the effect of sertraline and placebo on the functioning and quality of life in 243 women with PMDD who participated in a multisite trial of daily flexible-dose sertraline for three cycles.[65] Functioning was assessed by the SAS and the three DRSP items during the follicular and luteal phases at baseline and during the luteal phase of each treatment cycle. Quality of life was assessed with the Q-LES-Q at baseline and during each treatment cycle. The initial study reported that sertraline was significantly superior to placebo in improving functioning as measured by the three DRSP functioning items and the SAS scores.[65] Pearlstein and colleagues further examined the data.[67] Significant luteal phase impairment was evident compared with the follicular phase during the baseline cycle on the total and factor SAS scores, and on items 1–14 and the overall assessment score of the Q-LES-Q (all $p < 0.001$). Overall, the luteal impairment noted with SAS total and factor scores was similar to cohorts of women with dysthymia, but milder than women with MDD. Significant improvement with sertraline compared with placebo was evident by the second randomized treatment cycle on four of seven SAS factors, the Q-LES-Q and the three DRSP functioning items. Functional improvement as measured by the SAS and Q-LES-Q measures correlated with emotional and physical symptom improvement. Women who remitted (a Clinical Global Impressions-Improvement score of 1 after three cycles of sertraline treatment) had significantly higher premenstrual functioning at baseline compared with non-remitters as evidenced by the SAS total and factor scores, the Q-LES-Q scores, and the three DRSP functioning items (all $p < 0.001$).[67]

Halbreich and colleagues further compared baseline luteal SAS and Q-LES-Q scores of this same group of 243 women with PMDD participating in the sertraline trial[65] with baseline measures of women who participated in dysthymia ($N = 175$) and chronic MDD (MDD without remission or MDD and dysthymia, $N = 124$) sertraline trials.[25] Again, the pretreatment SAS and Q-LES-Q scores of women with PMDD and dysthymia did not significantly differ, except for significantly worse scores on the parental SAS factor in women with PMDD. Functional impairment in women with PMDD was not as severe as women with chronic MDD, overall, although the parental and social/leisure SAS factors demonstrated non-significant increased impairment with PMDD.

Halbreich and colleagues reported on a multisite trial of flexible-dose sertraline or placebo administered in the luteal phase over three menstrual cycles in 229 women with PMDD.[66] Functioning was assessed by the SAS and the three DRSP items during the follicular and luteal phases at baseline and during the luteal phase of each of three treatment cycles. Quality of life was assessed with the Q-LES-Q at baseline and during each treatment cycle. Significant improvement with sertraline compared with placebo was evident on the total and on four of seven SAS factor scores, the Q-LES-Q, and the three DRSP functioning items. The social/leisure and family unit SAS factor scores significantly improved with sertraline in both the daily dosing and luteal phase dosing studies.

A study in 167 women compared full-cycle sertraline, luteal phase sertraline, and placebo for 3 months.[68] This study utilized the DSR for prospective confirmation of premenstrual symptoms; 60% of the 167 women met strict criteria for PMDD and 40% met criteria for severe PMS. Global Ratings of Functioning assessed family life, work, and social activity functioning with ratings from 0 to 4, with 4 signifying 'severe disruption'. The Global Ratings of Functioning scores at baseline ranged from 2.1 to 2.7 in the 167 women. Results demonstrated that both dosing regimens of sertraline were significantly superior to placebo in improving

family relationships and social activities, but not work functioning.[68] An earlier study by this research group had utilized the DSR, Global Ratings of Functioning, and the Q-LES-Q in a study comparing full-cycle sertraline, desipramine, and placebo for three cycles.[69] In this study, 74% of 167 women met criteria for PMDD and 26% met criteria for severe PMS. At baseline, the Global Ratings of Functioning scores ranged from 2.37 to 2.81, and the Q-LES-Q averaged 45. Sertraline was more effective than both desipramine and placebo in improving family life, work, and social activity functioning. Sertraline was also more effective than placebo in improving quality of life as measured by the Q-LES-Q.

Paroxetine trials

Two multisite studies have been published reporting on the comparison of daily dosing of paroxetine controlled release (CR) 25 mg, paroxetine CR 12.5 mg, and placebo in women with PMDD.[70,71] In both studies the diagnosis of PMDD was determined by VAS ratings, and functioning was assessed with the SDS. In the first study, baseline values of the work, social/leisure, and family life SDS item scores for the sample of 313 women with PMDD at baseline were not provided. After three cycles of treatment, paroxetine CR 25 mg daily was significantly superior to placebo in each SDS domain, whereas 12.5 mg daily was superior to placebo in the improvement of social/leisure and family life functioning only.[70] In the second study, the ranges of SDS item scores at baseline in 371 women with PMDD were work (4.9–5.4), social life (5.7–6.0), and family life (6.5–6.9). Paroxetine CR 25 mg daily was significantly superior to placebo in each SDS domain, whereas 12.5 mg daily was superior to placebo in the improvement of family life functioning only.[71]

A multisite study of the luteal phase administration of paroxetine CR 25 mg, paroxetine 12.5 mg, and placebo was conducted in 366 women with PMDD.[72] Diagnosis of PMDD was determined by VAS ratings, and functioning was assessed with the SDS. The total SDS score ranged from 16.8 to 17.6 in the 366 women at baseline. Both doses of paroxetine CR were significantly superior to placebo after three cycles of treatment in improving functioning as reflected by reductions in the total SDS score.

Escitalopram trial

A recent small trial compared luteal phase dosing of escitalopram with symptom-onset dosing of escitalopram over three cycles in 27 women with PMDD.[73] There was no placebo condition. Diagnosis of PMDD was determined by the DSR, and functioning was assessed by the SDS. The average overall SDS score for both groups at baseline was 7.25–7.29. The overall SDS score significantly improved at endpoint compared to baseline with both escitalopram dosing regimens; there was no significant difference between the two dosing regimens.

Oral contraceptive trials

Two recently published studies with a new oral contraceptive containing drospirenone 3 mg and ethinyl estradiol 20 μg administered for three cycles have reported superior efficacy compared to placebo for premenstrual symptoms, functioning, and quality of life in women with PMDD.[74,75] In both studies, PMDD was determined by prospective DRSP ratings. One of the two studies was a parallel design study in 449 women. The DRSP functioning items averaged 3.7–4.2 (out of maximum possible score of 6) at baseline, and the sum of Q-LES-Q items 1–14 averaged 57.1–57.9 and overall life satisfaction score averaged 3.[74] The oral contraceptive was superior to placebo for the DRSP items of improved productivity, enhanced enjoyment in social activities, better quality of relationships, and items 1–14 of the Q-LES-Q. The second study was a crossover design study in 64 women. The sum of Q-LES-Q items 1–14 averaged 56.6–59.0 at baseline. The oral contraceptive was superior to placebo for the three DRSP functioning items (each $p < 0.001$), items 1–14, and the overall life satisfaction item of the Q-LES-Q (each $p = 0.04$).[75] Previous studies reported that a similar oral contraceptive with ethinyl estradiol 30 μg improved premenstrual sense of well-being[76] and improved the ability to perform usual activities as well as well-being premenstrually in women.[77] However, neither of these two latter studies included a formal assessment of PMS or PMDD in the samples.

A few small and older treatment studies deserve mention. An open study of fluvoxamine in 10 women with PMDD demonstrated a 20% improvement in Q-LES-Q scores after two cycles of treatment, but this was not statistically significant.[78] A small study comparing 12 sessions of individual cognitive therapy with waitlist in 23 women with prospectively confirmed PMS reported improvement in total and three SAS factor scores with cognitive therapy.[79] Cognitive therapy did not improve marital function compared with the waitlist condition, as measured by a marital questionnaire. A crossover study comparing luteal phase alprazolam to placebo in 30 women with late luteal phase dysphoric disorder (now PMDD) reported social dysfunction in 93% and vocational functioning in 59% of women at baseline.[80] A significant improvement in premenstrual social functioning was reported with alprazolam compared with placebo.

PMDD AND ECONOMIC COST OF DISEASE BURDEN

Borenstein and colleagues attempted to quantify the direct and indirect costs associated with PMS in the non-selected cohort of women enrolled in a medical group who returned DRSPs described above.[57,58,81] In addition to daily ratings of symptoms and functioning items, women were requested to answer three additional questions daily:

- How many hours did you plan to work today?
- How many hours of work did you miss today due to health reasons?
- Please rate your level of productivity at work today.

Direct costs can be assessed by the monetary costs for clinical visits, hospital care, prescription medications, laboratory tests, and radiological tests. Indirect costs can be assessed by work absenteeism and lost productivity at work, or 'presenteeism', such as employee errors, reduced quality, and reduced quantity of work.[81]

The most recent study from this research group assessed direct costs by medical claims and indirect costs by self-reported days of work missed, number of hours of intended work on a given day, number of intended work hours missed, and percentage of the total possible productivity level for the time worked.[81] From data available for 374 women, when women with PMS were compared to those without PMS, having PMS resulted, on average, in an additional $59 per patient per year in direct costs and an increase of $4333 in indirect costs per patient per year based on a 13.7% absenteeism rate and a 15% reduction in productivity. Similar to the economic burden with some chronic medical disorders, the potential economic impact of PMS was greater from work productivity losses than direct medical costs.[81]

Chawla and colleagues estimated that the cost of reported lost productivity for 56 women with prospectively confirmed PMDD was $890 per month in the studies described above.[4,55] The authors concluded that the economic burden associated with premenstrual symptoms was related more to self-reported decreased productivity than to direct healthcare costs.

CONCLUSION

Studies of prevalence rates of PMDD suggest 3–8% of menstruating women meet criteria for PMDD and 15–20% of menstruating women meet criteria for subthreshold PMDD or severe PMS. Several studies suggest that severity of premenstrual symptoms is associated with impairment in functioning, interference with relationships and activities, and decreased work productivity. From the subjective view of women with PMDD, interpersonal relationship interference is more problematic than work interference. Impaired functioning significantly affects the group of women with subthreshold PMDD/severe PMS as well as women with PMDD, expanding the burden of illness to approximately 1 in 5 women of reproductive age. The economic impact seems to be more severe for the employer than the health insurer, although prescription rates for PMS or PMDD are likely to be underreported. The pronounced negative impact of PMS and PMDD on quality of life, interpersonal functioning, and work productivity emphasizes the need for research inquiry into treatments for this burdensome disorder.

REFERENCES

1. Halbreich U, Endicott J, Schacht S et al. The diversity of premenstrual changes as reflected in the Premenstrual Assessment Form. Acta Psychiatr Scand 1982; 65:46–65.
2. Meaden PM, Hartlage SA, Cook-Karr J. Timing and severity of symptoms associated with the menstrual cycle in a community-based sample in the Midwestern United States. Psychiatry Res 2005; 134:27–36.
3. Pearlstein T, Yonkers KA, Fayyad R et al. Pretreatment pattern of symptom expression in premenstrual dysphoric disorder. J Affect Disord 2005; 85:275–82.
4. Sternfeld B, Swindle R, Chawla A et al. Severity of premenstrual symptoms in a health maintenance organization population. Obstet Gynecol 2002; 99:1014–24.
5. Premenstrual dysphoric disorder. In: Diagnostic and Statistical Manual of Mental Disorders, 4th edn, text revision. Washington, DC: American Psychiatric Press; 2000:771–4.
6. Endicott J, Nee J, Harrison W. Daily Record of Severity of Problems (DRSP): reliability and validity. Arch Womens Ment Health 2006; 9:41–9.
7. Freeman EW, DeRubeis RJ, Rickels K. Reliability and validity of a daily diary for premenstrual syndrome. Psychiatry Res 1996; 65:97–106.
8. Steiner M, Streiner DL, Steinberg S et al. The measurement of premenstrual mood symptoms. J Affect Disord 1999; 53:269–73.
9. Moos RH. The development of a menstrual distress questionnaire. Psychosom Med 1968; 30:853–67.
10. Gehlert S, Hartlage S. A design for studying the DSM-IV research criteria of premenstrual dysphoric disorder. J Psychosom Obstet Gynaecol 1997; 18:36–44.
11. Hurt SW, Schnurr PP, Severino SK et al. Late luteal phase dysphoric disorder in 670 women evaluated for premenstrual complaints. Am J Psychiatry 1992; 149:525–30.
12. Endicott J, Nee J, Harrison W et al. Quality of Life Enjoyment and Satisfaction Questionnaire: a new measure. Psychopharmacol Bull 1993; 29:321–6.
13. Sheehan DV, Harnett-Sheehan K, Raj BA. The measurement of disability. Int Clin Psychopharmacol 1996; 11 (Suppl 3):89–95.
14. Ware JE, Kosinski M, Bayliss MS et al. Comparison of methods for the scoring and statistical analysis of SF-36 health profile and summary measures: summary of results from the Medical Outcomes Study. Med Care 1995; 33:AS264–79.

15. Weissman MM, Bothwell S. Assessment of social adjustment by patient self-report. Arch Gen Psychiatry 1976; 33:1111–15.
16. Bloch M, Schmidt PJ, Rubinow DR. Premenstrual syndrome: evidence for symptom stability across cycles. Am J Psychiatry 1997; 154:1741–6.
17. Rivera-Tovar AD, Frank E. Late luteal phase dysphoric disorder in young women. Am J Psychiatry 1990; 147:1634–6.
18. Cohen LS, Soares CN, Otto MW et al. Prevalence and predictors of premenstrual dysphoric disorder (PMDD) in older premenopausal women. The Harvard Study of Moods and Cycles. J Affect Disord 2002; 70:125–32.
19. Wittchen HU, Becker E, Lieb R et al. Prevalence, incidence and stability of premenstrual dysphoric disorder in the community. Psychol Med 2002; 32:119–32.
20. Perkonigg A, Yonkers KA, Pfister H et al. Risk factors for premenstrual dysphoric disorder in a community sample of young women: the role of traumatic events and posttraumatic stress disorder. J Clin Psychiatry 2004; 65:1314–22.
21. Wittchen HU, Perkonigg A, Pfister H. Trauma and PTSD – an overlooked pathogenic pathway for premenstrual dysphoric disorder? Arch Womens Ment Health 2003; 6:293–7.
22. Steiner M, Macdougall M, Brown E. The premenstrual symptoms screening tool (PSST) for clinicians. Arch Womens Ment Health 2003; 6:203–9.
23. Hylan TR, Sundell K, Judge R. The impact of premenstrual symptomatology on functioning and treatment-seeking behavior: experience from the United States, United Kingdom, and France. J Womens Health Gend Based Med 1999; 8:1043–52.
24. Robinson RL, Swindle RW. Premenstrual symptom severity: impact on social functioning and treatment-seeking behaviors. J Womens Health Gend Based Med 2000; 9:757–68.
24a. Vichnin M, Freeman EW, Lin H et al. Premenstrual syndrome (PMS) in adolescents: severity and impairment. J Pediatr Adolesc Gynecol 2006; 19:397–402.
24b. Derman O, Kanbur NO, Tokur TE et al. Premenstrual syndrome and associated symptoms in adolescent girls. Eur J Obstet Gynecol Reprod Biol 2004; 116:201–6.
25. Halbreich U, Borenstein J, Pearlstein T et al. The prevalence, impairment, impact, and burden of premenstrual dysphoric disorder (PMS/PMDD). Psychoneuroendocrinology 2003; 28:1–23.
26. Logue CM, Moos RH. Perimenstrual symptoms: prevalence and risk factors. Psychosom Med 1986; 48:388–414.
27. Angst J, Sellaro R, Stolar M et al. The epidemiology of perimenstrual psychological symptoms. Acta Psychiatr Scand 2001; 104:110–16.
28. Merikangas KR, Foeldenyi M, Angst J. The Zurich Study. XIX. Patterns of menstrual disturbances in the community: results of the Zurich Cohort Study. Eur Arch Psychiatry Clin Neurosci 1993; 243:23–32.
29. Deuster PA, Adera T, South-Paul J. Biological, social, and behavioral factors associated with premenstrual syndrome. Arch Fam Med 1999; 8:122–8.
30. Andersch B, Wendestam C, Hahn L et al. Premenstrual complaints. I. Prevalence of premenstrual symptoms in a Swedish urban population. J Psychosom Obstet Gynaecol 1986; 5:39–49.
31. Johnson SR, McChesney C, Bean JA. Epidemiology of premenstrual symptoms in a nonclinical sample. I. Prevalence, natural history and help-seeking behavior. J Reprod Med 1988; 33:340–6.
32. Ramcharan S, Love EJ, Fick GH et al. The epidemiology of premenstrual symptoms in a population-based sample of 2650 urban women: attributable risk and risk factors. J Clin Epidemiol 1992; 45:377–92.
33. Woods NF, Most A, Dery GK. Prevalence of perimenstrual symptoms. Am J Public Health 1982; 72:1257–64.
34. Tabassum S, Afridi B, Aman Z et al. Premenstrual syndrome: frequency and severity in young college girls. J Pak Med Assoc 2005; 55:546–9.

35. Banerjee N, Roy KK, Takkar D. Premenstrual dysphoric disorder – a study from India. Int J Fertil Womens Med 2000; 45:342–4.

36. Hsiao MC, Liu CY, Chen KC et al. Characteristics of women seeking treatment for premenstrual syndrome in Taiwan. Acta Psychiatr Scand 2002; 106:150–5.

37. Sveindottir H. Prospective assessment of menstrual and premenstrual experiences of Icelandic women. Health Care Women Int 1998; 19:71–82.

38. van den Akker OB, Eves FF, Service S et al. Menstrual cycle symptom reporting in three British ethnic groups. Soc Sci Med 1995; 40:1417–23.

39. Hasin M, Dennerstein L, Gotts G. Menstrual cycle related complaints: a cross-cultural study. J Psychosom Obstet Gynaecol 1988; 9:35–42.

40. Freeman EW. Effects of antidepressants on quality of life in women with premenstrual dysphoric disorder. Pharmacoeconomics 2005; 23:433–44.

41. Rapaport MH, Clary C, Fayyad R et al. Quality-of-life impairment in depressive and anxiety disorders. Am J Psychiatry 2005; 162:1171–8.

42. Barnard K, Frayne SM, Skinner KM et al. Health status among women with menstrual symptoms. J Womens Health 2003; 12:911–19.

43. Winter EJ, Ashton DJ, Moore DL. Dispelling myths: a study of PMS and relationship satisfaction. Nurse Pract 1991; 16:34, 7–40,45.

44. Hardie EA. PMS in the workplace: dispelling the myth of cyclic dysfunction. J Occup Organiz Psychol 1997; 70:97–102.

45. Kraemer GR, Kraemer RR. Premenstrual syndrome: diagnosis and treatment experiences. J Womens Health 1998; 7:893–907.

46. Singh BB, Berman BM, Simpson RL et al. Incidence of premenstrual syndrome and remedy usage: a national probability sample study. Altern Ther Health Med 1998; 4:75–9.

47. Ryser R, Feinauer LL. Premenstrual syndrome and the marital relationship. Am J Fam Ther 1992; 20:179–90.

48. Hallman J, Georgiev N. The premenstrual syndrome and absence from work due to illness. J Psychosom Obstet Gynaecol 1987; 6:111–19.

49. Corney RH, Stanton R. A survey of 658 women who report symptoms of premenstrual syndrome. J Psychosom Res 1991; 35:471–82.

50. Campbell EM, Peterkin D, O'Grady K et al. Premenstrual symptoms in general practice patients. Prevalence and treatment. J Reprod Med 1997; 42:637–46.

51. Kuan AJ, Carter DM, Ott FJ. Distress levels in patients with premenstrual dysphoric disorder. Can J Psychiatry 2002; 47:888–9.

52. Gallant SJ, Popiel DA, Hoffman DM et al. Using daily ratings to confirm premenstrual syndrome/late luteal phase dysphoric disorder. Part II. What makes a "real" difference? Psychosom Med 1992; 54:167–81.

53. Kuczmierczyk AR, Labrum AH, Johnson CC. Perception of family and work environments in women with premenstrual syndrome. J Psychosom Res 1992; 36:787–95.

54. Frank B, Dixon DN, Grosz HJ. Conjoint monitoring of symptoms of premenstrual syndrome: impact on marital satisfaction. J Couns Psychol 1993; 40:109–14.

55. Chawla A, Swindle R, Long S et al. Premenstrual dysphoric disorder: is there an economic burden of illness? Med Care 2002; 40:1101–12.

56. Endicott J, Nee J. Endicott Work Productivity Scale (EWPS): a new measure to assess treatment effects. Psychopharmacol Bull 1997; 33:13–16.

57. Borenstein JE, Dean BB, Endicott J et al. Health and economic impact of the premenstrual syndrome. J Reprod Med 2003; 48:515–24.

58. Dean BB, Borenstein JE. A prospective assessment investigating the relationship between work productivity and impairment with premenstrual syndrome. J Occup Environ Med 2004; 46:649–56.

59. Steiner M, Steinberg S, Stewart D et al. Fluoxetine in the treatment of premenstrual dysphoria. Canadian Fluoxetine/Premenstrual Dysphoria Collaborative Study Group. N Engl J Med 1995; 332:1529–34.

60. Steiner M, Haskett RF, Carroll BJ. Premenstrual tension syndrome: the development of research diagnostic criteria and new rating scales. Acta Psychiatr Scand 1980; 62:177–90.

61. Steiner M, Brown E, Trzepacz P et al. Fluoxetine improves functional work capacity in women with premenstrual dysphoric disorder. Arch Womens Ment Health 2003; 6:71–7.

62. Cohen LS, Miner C, Brown EW et al. Premenstrual daily fluoxetine for premenstrual dysphoric disorder: a placebo-controlled, clinical trial using computerized diaries. Obstet Gynecol 2002; 100:435–44.

63. Miner C, Brown E, McCray S et al. Weekly luteal-phase dosing with enteric-coated fluoxetine 90 mg in premenstrual dysphoric disorder: a randomized, double-blind, placebo-controlled clinical trial. Clin Ther 2002; 24:417–33.

64. Su TP, Schmidt PJ, Danaceau MA et al. Fluoxetine in the treatment of premenstrual dysphoria. Neuropsychopharmacology 1997; 16:346–56.

65. Yonkers KA, Halbreich U, Freeman E et al. Symptomatic improvement of premenstrual dysphoric disorder with sertraline treatment. A randomized controlled trial. Sertraline Premenstrual Dysphoric Collaborative Study Group. JAMA 1997; 278:983–8.

66. Halbreich U, Bergeron R, Yonkers KA et al. Efficacy of intermittent, luteal phase sertraline treatment of premenstrual dysphoric disorder. Obstet Gynecol 2002; 100:1219–29.

67. Pearlstein TB, Halbreich U, Batzar ED et al. Psychosocial functioning in women with premenstrual dysphoric disorder before and after treatment with sertraline or placebo. J Clin Psychiatry 2000; 61:101–9.

68. Freeman EW, Rickels K, Sondheimer SJ et al. Continuous or intermittent dosing with sertraline for patients with severe premenstrual syndrome or premenstrual dysphoric disorder. Am J Psychiatry 2004; 161:343–51.

69. Freeman EW, Rickels K, Sondheimer SJ et al. Differential response to antidepressants in women with premenstrual syndrome/premenstrual dysphoric disorder: a randomized controlled trial. Arch Gen Psychiatry 1999; 56:932–9.

70. Cohen LS, Soares CN, Yonkers KA et al. Paroxetine controlled release for premenstrual dysphoric disorder: a double-blind, placebo-controlled trial. Psychosom Med 2004; 66:707–13.

71. Pearlstein TB, Bellew KM, Endicott J et al. Paroxetine controlled release for premenstrual dysphoric disorder: remission analysis following a randomized, double-blind, placebo-controlled trial. Prim Care Companion J Clin Psychiatry 2005; 7:53–60.

72. Steiner M, Hirschberg AL, Bergeron R et al. Luteal phase dosing with paroxetine controlled release (CR) in the treatment of premenstrual dysphoric disorder. Am J Obstet Gynecol 2005; 193:352–60.

73. Freeman EW, Sondheimer SJ, Sammel MD et al. A preliminary study of luteal phase versus symptom-onset dosing with escitalopram for premenstrual dysphoric disorder. J Clin Psychiatry 2005; 66:769–73.

74. Yonkers KA, Brown C, Pearlstein TB et al. Efficacy of a new low-dose oral contraceptive with drospirenone in premenstrual dysphoric disorder. Obstet Gynecol 2005; 106:492–501.

75. Pearlstein TB, Bachmann GA, Zacur HA et al. Treatment of premenstrual dysphoric disorder with a new drospirenone-containing oral contraceptive formulation. Contraception 2005; 72:414–21.

76. Apter D, Borsos A, Baumgartner W et al. Effect of an oral contraceptive containing drospirenone and ethinylestradiol on general

well-being and fluid-related symptoms. Eur J Contracept Reprod Health Care 2003; 8:37–51.

77. Borenstein J, Yu HT, Wade S et al. Effect of an oral contraceptive containing ethinyl estradiol and drospirenone on premenstrual symptomatology and health-related quality of life. J Reprod Med 2003; 48:79–85.

78. Freeman EW, Rickels K, Sondheimer SJ. Fluvoxamine for premenstrual dysphoric disorder: a pilot study. J Clin Psychiatry 1996; 57:56–60.

79. Blake F, Salkovskis P, Gath D et al. Cognitive therapy for premenstrual syndrome: a controlled trial. J Psychosom Res 1998; 45:307–18.

80. Harrison WM, Endicott J, Nee J. Treatment of premenstrual dysphoria with alprazolam. A controlled study. Arch Gen Psychiatry 1990; 47:270–5.

81. Borenstein J, Chiou CF, Dean B et al. Estimating direct and indirect costs of premenstrual syndrome. J Occup Environ Med 2005; 47:26–33.

6

Comorbidity of premenstrual syndrome and premenstrual dysphoric disorder with other psychiatric conditions

Kimberly A Yonkers and Kara Lynn McCunn

INTRODUCTION

Premenstrual syndrome (PMS) is a relatively common condition that is experienced by approximately 30% of reproductive-aged women.[1,2] Those with clinically significant PMS regularly experience mood and/or physical symptoms during the few days to 2 weeks prior to the onset of menses. By definition, symptoms remit within a few days after initiation of the menstrual flow, leaving women asymptomatic for the remainder of the follicular phase. Common symptoms include low mood, anxiety, and irritability but physical symptoms such as breast pain and bloating are also widespread.[3] Behaviorally, women may experience changes in sleep, appetite, energy, concentration, or physical dexterity.

Premenstrual dysphoric disorder (PMDD) occurs in approximately 3–8% of women,[4,5] differs from PMS in severity, and may diverge in the symptoms experienced. As with PMS, the diagnosis of PMDD also stipulates that symptoms are experienced only during the luteal phase but women must endorse difficulties with at least one emotional symptom (e.g. low mood, irritability, etc.)[6] and symptoms must be severe enough to interfere with some aspect of psychosocial functioning. The provisional diagnosis of PMDD has been placed in the mood disorders section of the Diagnostic and Statistical Manual of Mental Disorders, fourth edition (DSM-IV) because of the prominent role of mood symptoms in the condition.[6] Criteria for clinically significant PMS[7] and PMDD[6] stipulate that the temporal pattern of symptom onset and offset be confirmed through several months of longitudinal, daily ratings. For both diagnoses, but especially PMDD, symptoms should not be 'merely an exacerbation' of another general medical or psychiatric condition.

Several aspects of the above definitions make it difficult to determine the common comorbidity of PMS and PMDD. First, it is challenging to conduct epidemiological studies that are representative of general populations when daily ratings are required in order to make a diagnosis. Completing these reports entails enrolling subjects who are willing to take on the task of charting symptoms daily and are compliant with such record-keeping. Women may not be able to comply for a number of reasons. For example, it may be that women who are very symptomatic from either a premenstrual or a comorbid condition have greater difficulty adhering to such a task, which would result in biased estimates of the premenstrual condition. On the other hand, there is substantial recall bias in reporting premenstrual symptoms,[8,9] so, if retrospective reports are used, they may mischaracterize chronic symptoms as symptoms that are limited to the premenstrual phase of the cycle. Secondly, operationalizing what is 'merely an exacerbation' of another condition, as stipulated in the DSM-IV definition, is complex. A woman suffering from a severe premenstrual condition can experience some symptoms throughout the menstrual cycle and continue to feel those symptoms along with additional ones during the premenstrual phase of the cycle. Whereas some clinicians would say that an underlying disorder is worsened or exacerbated during the premenstrual phase of the cycle, others might say that there are two processes ongoing: a chronic condition and a premenstrual condition.[10] These issues are further complicated by the fact that mood and anxiety disorders are prevalent in women and peak during the woman's reproductive years.[11–13] Therefore, there is a high likelihood of comorbidity simply because of the frequency of mood and anxiety disorders on the one hand and premenstrual syndromes on the other hand. Finally, there are no unique blood tests or other markers for PMS, PMDD, or indeed any mood or anxiety disorders. Emotional symptoms of low mood, disinterest, irritability, and anxiety occur as part of many mood and anxiety disorders, as well as PMS and PMDD, and are not unique to any of the various conditions. The feature that most highly differentiates a premenstrual condition from other mood or anxiety disorders is the temporal linkage of symptom expression to the premenstrual phase of the menstrual cycle, rather than patient characteristics or signs and symptoms. Given these limitations, we organize this chapter by comorbid condition and provide prevalence estimates for premenstrual worsening of other psychiatric illnesses as well as lifetime comorbidity. Further, we indicate whether data on comorbidity rely on retrospective assessments of a premenstrual condition or were made after completion of daily ratings.

PMDD AND UNIPOLAR DEPRESSIVE DISORDERS

Women are at approximately twice the risk of developing major depressive disorder (MDD) compared with men. The National Epidemiologic Survey on Alcoholism and Related Conditions, a survey of more then 43 000 adults, found that the 12-month prevalence of MDD in women is 6.87% and the lifetime prevalence 17.10%.[14]

The high rate of MDD in women increases the likelihood that women with MDD will also have PMDD or PMS. It is the case that high rates of comorbidity between either PMS or PMDD and past episodes of MDD have been documented by a number of groups (see Yonkers,[15] Kim et al,[16] and Breaux et al[17] for reviews). Among women who have prospectively confirmed PMS or PMDD and are not in a current episode of MDD, approximately 30–70% of them will have had a prior episode of MDD.[18–25] Especially if rates are on the higher end of this range, estimates such as these suggest shared vulnerability between MDD and PMDD. However, these estimates are drawn from clinical samples of women with PMDD rather than non-treatment-seeking individuals and, because patients with a larger number of psychiatric conditions are more likely to seek treatment, rates of comorbidity between the two conditions may be inflated.

Conversely, estimates of *concurrent* non-seasonal depressive disorders with PMDD are lower and fall between 12% and 25%.[16] Part of the reason may be that the symptoms required for the two conditions overlap and, when an individual is symptomatic and suffering from MDD, it may be difficult to detect premenstrual worsening because of a 'ceiling effect'. Some researchers

who compared rates of concurrent mood disorders in women who did vs did not prospectively confirm a diagnosis of PMS or PMDD, find higher rates of MDD in the latter group although not all studies concur.[17,26–28] It is more difficult to detect cyclic symptom changes in women who have moderate to severe symptoms than in those who do not. Furthermore, women who retrospectively endorse PMS or PMDD, but do not confirm daily ratings of symptoms, seem particularly likely to have MDD or a minor depressive syndrome that accounts for their complaint. Rather than having comorbid conditions, they may instead misattribute symptoms to the premenstrual phase of the cycle, when they are, in fact, chronic. The onset of menses can be a marker that women may use as a reference point, increasing the likelihood of recall bias. Alternatively, women may have premenstrual exacerbation of a chronic mood disorder that might be difficult to fully appreciate as separate from the underlying condition. Estimates show that up to 70% of women in clinical cohorts, who have a depressive disorder, also identify problems with premenstrual symptom exacerbation.[29–33] In a recent report, premenstrual worsening of depressive symptoms were retrospectively reported by 64% of a large cohort (n = 433) of premenopausal women participating in an antidepressant treatment trial,[33] suggesting a substantial clinical problem.

The comorbidity between seasonal affective disorder (SAD) and PMDD can be probed by assessing daily ratings in SAD women during the summer. This sidesteps potential problems with the ceiling effect, since individuals with SAD are typically not symptomatic during summer. In one such study,[34] 46% of women with SAD but only 2% of healthy controls confirmed symptoms consistent with PMDD after daily ratings, suggesting a strong association between the SAD and a premenstrual disorder.

Symptom deterioration among women with depressive disorders is also found among women who are not necessarily treatment-seeking. In a comprehensive and well-designed study, researchers explored premenstrual exacerbation of depressive symptoms in a community cohort by examining daily ratings over one to two menstrual cycles.[35] The point prevalence for full or subclinical depressive illness in the cohort of women was 6.5%. Of that group, slightly over one-half (58%) felt worse premenstrually. The majority of women experienced deterioration in only one depressive symptom, which was most commonly sleep (21%) and least commonly thoughts of death or suicide (2%). Importantly, women taking antidepressant medication were as likely as those who were not taking antidepressants to experience premenstrual exacerbation. Given that the medication most often used to treat depression was a serotonin reuptake inhibitor, medications routinely used to treat PMDD without comorbid depression, it is clear that other clinical strategies are needed to help women with depression and premenstrual symptom-worsening.

Difficulties with premenstrual symptoms or a premenstrual disorder also predict future episodes of affective illness.[36–38] Over time, women with premenstrual complaints at baseline are more likely to develop new illness onsets[37,38] or recurrences[36] of MDD.

It may also be that the types of premenstrual symptoms expressed are influenced by a woman's vulnerability to past depressive disorders. Women with prior depression tend to experience time-limited depressive episodes premenstrually[39] rather than other symptom constellations (e.g. anxiety, etc.).[40]

Investigations of biological processes that are common to both depressive disorders and PMDD are few. In an older study that evaluated consecutive cortisol levels over 24 hours in subjects with MDD, PMDD, and controls,[41] subjects with MDD had the highest cortisol levels, controls had the lowest, and women with PMDD were in between the two. This suggests some degree of shared diathesis among women with PMDD and MDD.

In a study that compared plasma γ-aminobutyric acid levels (pGABA) in PMDD subjects with and without a history of MDD, subjects with PMDD and a history of MDD had low pGABA levels throughout the menstrual cycle whereas women with PMDD and no history of MDD had low pGABA only during the premenstrual phase of the cycle.[42] This study suggests a biological deficit in common between women with MDD and PMDD, but the deficit only occurs premenstrually if a woman has no comorbid history of MDD.

PREMENSTRUAL SYMPTOMS AND BIPOLAR DISORDER

Whereas there appears to be a strong relationship between unipolar mood disorders and PMDD, the relationship between PMDD and bipolar disorder is less clear. Early work that used retrospective reports to determine premenstrual exacerbation of bipolar disorder suggested higher rates of premenstrual problems among women with bipolar disorder than controls[30,43] or women with other illnesses.[44] However, this has not been confirmed in a study that used prospective ratings to explore linkages between the premenstrual phase of the cycle and clinical deterioration.[45] In the latter study, 25 women with rapid cycling bipolar disorder were assessed over 3–50 months and, although mood fluctuated over time, it was not more problematic premenstrually.

PREMENSTRUAL SYMPTOMS AND ANXIETY DISORDERS

Anxiety disorders are quite prevalent, with 28.8% of Americans experiencing at least one episode of an anxiety disorder in their lifetime.[46] The anxiety disorders include panic disorder, agoraphobia, social phobia, obsessive compulsive disorder (OCD), post-traumatic stress disorder, acute stress disorder, generalized anxiety disorder, and specific phobia. Women are also more susceptible to these disorders, with an odds ratio of 1.6.[46]

Obsessive compulsive disorder

Among women attending a PMS clinic, rates for concurrent OCD are three- (9% vs 3%)[47] to fourfold higher (16.1% vs 3.9%)[48] than rates of OCD diagnosed in community women. Diagnoses of OCD in these studies were generated by structured lay interview but reports of PMS were based upon retrospective report. However, these rates are similar (13%) to that found by Fava and colleagues in a study of women from a gynecological clinic who kept daily ratings and also underwent a structured interview.[49]

Several groups evaluated possible premenstrual worsening or a comorbid premenstrual condition in women with OCD. These studies typically assessed premenstrual symptoms in clinical cohorts of women with established OCD.[50–52] Premenstrual symptom deterioration was not uncommon, in that 20–50% of women describe such difficulties. Differences in these estimates are attributable to instability of figures arising from small cohorts, differences in questions used to assess premenstrual symptom worsening, and the retrospective nature of the reports. In studies that queried women about a spectrum of symptoms, estimates of premenstrual symptom exacerbation were higher.[52] It is interesting that most symptoms of exacerbation were depression and dysphoria,[50,51] although in some instances the underlying illness of OCD worsened.[52] In the recent report by Vulink and colleagues, a subset of their subjects was assessed longitudinally across the menstrual cycle and the symptom scores on the Yale Brown Obsessive Compulsive Scale showed worsening. They found that about 13% of subjects with OCD were comorbid with PMDD.[52] This is a slightly lower estimate of comorbidity with PMDD than found by Williams and Koran (21%).[50]

Panic disorder

Studies assessing possible concurrent panic disorder in women with PMS or PMDD show a wide range of estimates. Again, using retrospective reports for PMS or PMDD and structured interviews for panic disorder, between <1% and 9% of women in gynecological settings or PMS clinics also meet criteria for panic disorder.[23,47,48] Interestingly, among women who prospectively confirm premenstrual difficulties, a concurrent diagnosis of panic has been found in 16%[21] and 25% of women.[49]

Premenstrual worsening of panic has received considerable study. Several small studies showed that panic disordered-women commonly reported premenstrual worsening of panic symptoms but do not confirm such deterioration with prospective ratings.[53-55] These reports were limited by small sample sizes. A fourth, somewhat larger, but still modest study found premenstrual worsening of panic among 20 women with panic disorder.[56] Interestingly, women with panic disorder experienced not only worsening of panic attack frequency but also mood symptoms during the premenstrual phase. The increased dysphoria experienced by women with PMS or PMDD study is similar to that noted in studies of women with obsessive compulsive disorder.[52] Mood symptoms commonly occur with anxiety disorders but are not criterion items of anxiety disorders. Thus, it is possible that women with panic or OCD and premenstrual mood symptoms have at least two conditions contributing to their morbidity: a chronic anxiety disorder and their premenstrual condition.

The relationship between panic disorder and PMDD has been investigated from a biological perspective (see Vickers and McNally for a review[57]). Reproducibly, women with PMDD have very high rates of panic attacks after being exposed to a challenge agent. Although PMDD women do not panic at as high a rate as those who suffer from panic disorder, rates of panic are higher than for other psychiatric disorders, including other mood disorders. To date, research has shown that women with PMDD are more likely to panic than controls when exposed to lactate,[58-60] carbon dioxide,[61] cholecystokinin-tetrapeptide,[62] and flumazenil.[63] Given that approximately 50–60% of women with PMDD will experience a panic attack with these provocative agents, it has been suggested that there may be shared biological mechanisms in PMDD and panic.[62,63] An alternative explanation is that psychological mediators, including catastrophic misinterpretations of bodily sensations and heightened anxiety sensitivity, in the two disorders.[57]

Generalized anxiety disorder

In women who retrospectively reported premenstrual difficulties, over a quarter also met criteria for generalized anxiety disorder (GAD).[47] Studies that included prospective ratings to confirm premenstrual symptoms and structured diagnostic interviews find rates of nearly 10%[23] and 38%.[49] Premenstrual worsening of GAD has also been reported,[64] although how commonly it occurs is not known.

SCHIZOPHRENIA

Although very rare, periodic psychosis during the premenstruum has been described in numerous case reports and case series. These reports describe symptoms in adult women and adolescents that are limited to the premenstrual or menstrual phase of the cycle.[65] Some argue that the low reported incidence is due to under-recognition of the problem.[66] Although the literature does not support adding psychotic symptoms to the diagnostic criteria of PMDD, they should be considered a possible associated feature.[65] Routine screening for these symptoms may provide additional evidence for the existence of premenstrual psychosis.

There have been two prospective studies examining premenstrual symptom exacerbation in patients with schizophrenia using the Daily Rating Form (DRF) and the Brief Psychiatric Rating Scale (BPRS). One study utilized retrospective and prospective reports of 39 women hospitalized with schizophrenia. The prospective results showed an increase in affective symptoms during the menstrual but not premenstrual phase. The retrospective data was collected using the Premenstrual Affective Form and showed an increase in affective symptoms in the premenstruum.[67] The second study observed 30 patients with schizophrenia over one menstrual cycle. The data were analyzed for the 24 subjects who completed the DRF correctly. This study showed an increase in premenstrual symptoms that were affective and behavioral in nature.[68] Neither investigation found a significant change in psychotic symptoms during the menstrual or premenstrual phase.[67,68] As with a number of the other comorbid conditions reviewed above, these reports suggest that women with schizophrenia may experience comorbid PMS symptoms and 'merely' premenstrual exacerbation of schizophrenia.

There are observational data that support the theory of premenstrual exacerbation of schizophrenia. A study of 285 premenopausal women with schizophrenia showed that there was an increase in psychiatric admissions during the 3 days before and after the beginning of menses.[69] A smaller study with 33 patients showed similar results.[70] However, these studies did not analyze which symptoms led to admission, and it is possible that affective symptoms rendered the baseline psychotic symptoms even more difficult to tolerate than usual. Future work may be able to confirm onset of additional symptoms as well as worsening of core schizophrenia symptoms and resolve this question.

SUMMARY

The most common psychiatric comorbidity among women with either PMS or PMDD is with other unipolar mood disorders. While this may be because both types of conditions occur frequently in women, work suggests shared biological vulnerability. Anxiety disorders are also common, but the relationship between these conditions and either PMS and PMDD is less well studied. Interestingly, women with PMDD are at high risk of panic given the same provocations that lead to panic in women with panic disorder. Schizophrenia may worsen premenstrually in some women and isolated psychotic symptoms in the premenstruum are rare but have been reported.

Identifying comorbidity is important because it may influence morbidity and treatment. Community studies show that morbidity is increased when women with psychiatric illness also have either PMS or PMDD.[35] Changes to an agent that is effective for both MDD and PMDD may be warranted for women who have MDD and PMDD. Similarly, worsening of mood symptoms in a woman with schizophrenia while she is premenstrual may require addition of an agent to treat the premenstrual condition. The existence of concurrent PMDD should be explored in women who have other psychiatric illnesses that do not respond to usual treatments, since this can be a source of non-response.

REFERENCES

1. Borenstein J, Dean B, Endicott J et al. Health and economic impact of the premenstrual syndrome. J Reprod Med 2003; 48:515–24.
2. Deuster P, Adera T, South-Paul J. Biological, social, and behavioral factors associated with premenstrual syndrome. Arch Fam Med 1999; 8:122–8.
3. Wood C, Larsen L, Williams R. Menstrual characteristics of 2343 women attending the Shepard Foundation. Aust N Z J Obstet Gynaecol 1979; 19:107–10.
4. Rivera-Tovar AD, Frank E. Late luteal phase dysphoric disorder in young women. Am J Psychiatry 1990; 147:1634–6.
5. Soares C, Cohen L, Otto M, Harlow B. Characteristics of women with premenstrual dysphoric disorder (PMDD) who did or did not report history of depression: a preliminary report from the Harvard Study of Moods and Cycles. J Womens Health Gend Based Med 2001; 10:873–8.
6. American Psychiatric Association. Diagnostic and Statistical Manual of Mental Disorders, 4th edn – DSM-IV. Washington DC: American Psychiatric Association; 1994.
7. ACOG. ACOG issues guidelines on diagnosis and treatment of PMS. 2003.
8. Rubinow DR, Roy-Byrne P, Hoban MC, Gold PW, Post RM. Prospective assessment of menstrually related mood disorders. Am J Psychiatry 1984; 141(5):684–6.
9. Rubinow DR, Roy-Byrne PP. Premenstrual syndromes: overviews from a methodologic perspective. Am J Psychiatry 1984; 141: 163–72.
10. Yonkers KA, White K. Premenstrual exacerbation of depression: one process of two? J Clin Psychiatry 1992; 53:289–92.
11. Kessler R. Epidemiology of women and depression. J Affect Disord 2003; 74(1):5–13.
12. Kessler RC, McGonagle KA, Swartz M et al. Sex and depression in the National Comorbidity Survey. I: Lifetime prevalence, chronicity and recurrence. J Affect Disord 1993; 29:85–96.
13. Kessler R, Mcgonagle K, Zhao S et al. Lifetime and 12-month prevalence of DSM-III-R psychiatric disorders in the United States. Results from the National Comorbidity Survey. Arch Gen Psychiatry 1994; 51:8–19.
14. Hasin DS, Goodwin RD, Stinson FS, Grant BF. Epidemiology of major depressive disorder: results from the National Epidemiologic Survey on Alcoholism and Related Conditions. Arch Gen Psychiatry 2005; 62(10):1097–106.
15. Yonkers K. The association between premenstrual dysphoric disorder and other mood disorders. J Clin Psychiatry 1997; 58(Suppl 0).
16. Kim D, Gyulai L, Freeman E et al. Premenstrual dysphoric disorder and psychiatric comorbidity. Arch Womens Ment Health 2004; 7:37–47.
17. Breaux C, Hartlage S, Gehlert S. Relationships of premenstrual dysphoric disorder to major depression and anxiety disorders: a re-examination. J Psychosom Obstet Gynecol 2000; 21:17–24.
18. Critchlow D, Bond AJ, Wingrove J. Mood disorder history and personality assessment in premenstrual dysphoric disorder. J Clin Psychiatry 2001; 62:688–93.
19. Freeman EW, Rickels K, Sondheimer SJ et al. Nefazodone in the treatment of premenstrual syndrome: a preliminary study. J Clin Psychopharmacol 1994; 14(3):180–6.
20. Freeman EW, Rickels K, Sondheimer SJ, Polansky M. A double-blind trial of oral progesterone, alprazolam, and placebo in treatment of severe premenstrual syndrome. JAMA 1995; 274:51–7.
21. Harrison WM, Endicott J, Nee J, Glick H, Rabkin JG. Characteristics of women seeking treatment for premenstrual syndrome. Psychosomatics 1989; 30:405–11.
22. Harrison WM, Endicott J, Nee J. Treatment of premenstrual dysphoria with alprazolam. A controlled study. Arch Gen Psychiatry 1990; 47:270–5.
23. Pearlstein TB, Frank E, Rivera-Tovar A et al. Prevalence of axis I and axis II disorders in women with late luteal phase dysphoric disorder. J Affect Disord 1990; 20:129–34.
24. Pearlstein TB, Stone AB. Long-term fluoxetine treatment of late luteal phase dysphoric disorder. J Clin Psychiatry 1994; 55:332–5.
25. Yonkers KA, Halbreich U, Freeman E et al. Symptomatic improvement of premenstrual dysphoric disorder with sertraline treatment. JAMA 1997; 278:983–8.
26. Dejong R, Rubinow DR, Roy-Byrne P et al. Premenstrual mood disorder and psychiatric illness. Am J Psychiatry 1985; 142(11): 1359–61.
27. West C. The characteristics of 100 women presenting to a gynecological clinic with premenstrual complaints. Acta Obstet Gynecol Scand 1989; 68:743–7.
28. De Ronchi D, Muro A, Marziani A, Rucci P. Personality disorders and depressive symptoms in late luteal phase dysphoric disorder. Pyschother Psychosom 2000; 69:27–34.
29. Coppen A. The prevalence of menstrual disorders in psychiatric patients. Br J Psychiatry 1965; III:155–67.
30. Diamond SB, Rubinstein AA, Dunner DL, Fieve RR. Menstrual problems in women with primary affective illness. Compr Psychiatry 1976; 17:541–8.

31. Halbreich U, Endicott J. Relationship of dysphoric premenstrual changes to depressive disorder. Acta Psychiatr Scand 1985; 71: 331–8.

32. Kashiwagi T, Mcclure JN, Wetzel RD. Premenstrual affective syndrome and psychiatric disorder. Dis Nerv Syst 1976; 37:116–19.

33. Kornstein S, Harvey A, Rush A et al. Self-reported premenstrual exacerbation of depressive symptoms in patients seeking treatment for major depression. Psychol Med 2005; 35:683–92.

34. Praschak-Rieder N, Willeit M, Neumeister A et al. Prevalence of premenstrual dysphoric disorder in female patients with seasonal affective disorder. J Affect Disord 2001; 63:239–42.

35. Hartlage S, Brandenburg D, Kravitz H. Premenstrual exacerbation of depressive disorders in a community-based sample in the United States. Psychosom Med 2004; 66:698–706.

36. Graze KK, Nee J, Endicott J. Premenstrual depression predicts future major depressive disorder. Acta Psychiatr Scand 1990; 81:201–5.

37. Schuckit M, Daly V, Herrman G, Hineman S. Premenstrual symptoms and depression in a university population. Dis Nerv Syst 1975; 37:516–17.

38. Wetzel RD, Reich T, Mcclure JN, Wald JA. Premenstrual affective syndrome and affective disorder. Br J Psychiatry 1975; 127:219–21.

39. Bancroft J, Rennie D, Warner P. Vulnerability to perimenstrual mood change: the relevance of a past history of depressive disorder. Psychosom Med 1994; 56:225–31.

40. Halbreich U. Premenstrual dysphoric disorders: a diversified cluster of vulnerability traits to depression. Acta Psychiatr Scand 1997; 95:169–76.

41. Mortola JF, Liu JH, Gillin JC et al. Pulsatile rhythms of adrenocorticotropin (ACTH) and cortisol in women with endogenous depression: evidence for increased ACTH pulse frequency. J Clin Endocrinol Metab 1987; 65:962–8.

42. Halbreich U, Petty F, Yonkers K et al. Low plasma γ-aminobutyric acid levels during the late luteal phase of women with premenstrual dysphoric disorder. Am J Psychiatry 1996; 153:718–20.

43. Price WA, Dimarzio LR. Premenstrual tension syndrome in rapid-cycling bipolar affective disorder. J Clin Psychiatry 1986; 47(8): 415–17.

44. Roy-Byrne PP, Rubinow DR, Hoban MC et al. Premenstrual changes: a comparison of five populations. Psychiatry Res 1986; 17:77–85.

45. Leibenluft E, Ashman SB, Feldman-Naim S, Yonkers KA. Lack of relationship between menstrual cycle phase and mood in a sample of women with rapid cycling bipolar disorder. Biol Psychiatry 1999; 46(4):577–80.

46. Kessler RC, Berglund P, Demler O et al. Lifetime prevalence and age-of-onset distributions of DSM-IV disorders in the National Comorbidity Survey Replication [see comment] [erratum appears in Arch Gen Psychiatry 2005; 62(7):768 Note: Merikangas, Kathleen R [added]]. Arch Gen Psychiatry 2005; 62(6):593–602.

47. Chandraiah S, Levenson J, Collins J. Sexual dysfunction, social maladjustment, and psychiatric disorders in women seeking treatment in a premenstrual syndrome clinic. Int J Psychiatry Med 1991; 21(2):189–204.

48. Stout AL, Steege JF, Blazer DG, George LK. Comparison of lifetime psychiatric diagnoses in Premenstrual Syndrome Clinic and community samples. J Nerv Ment Dis 1986; 174:517–22.

49. Fava M, Pedrazzi F, Guaraldi GP et al. Comorbid anxiety and depression among patients with late luteal phase dysphoric disorder. J Anx Disord 1992; 6:325–35.

50. Williams KE, Koran LM. Obsessive-compulsive disorder in pregnancy, the puerperium and the premenstruum. J Clin Psychiatry 1997; 58(7):330–4.

51. Labad J, Menchon JM, Alonso P et al. Female reproductive cycle and obsessive-compulsive disorder. J Clin Psychiatry 2005; 66(4):428–35.

52. Vulink NC, Denys D, Bus L, Westenberg HG. Female hormones affect symptom severity in obsessive-compulsive disorder. Int Clin Psychopharmacol 2006; 21(3):171–5.

53. Cameron OG, Kuttesch D, McPhee K, Curtis GC. Menstrual fluctuation in the symptoms of panic anxiety. J Affect Disord 1988; 15:169–74.

54. Cook BL, Noyes R, Garvey MJ et al. Anxiety and the menstrual cycle in panic disorder. J Affect Disord 1990; 19:221–6.

55. Stein MB, Schmidt PJ, Rubinow DR, Uhde TW. Panic disorder and the menstrual cycle: panic disorder patients, healthy control subjects, and patients with premenstrual syndrome. Am J Psychiatry 1989; 146(10):1299–303.

56. Kaspi S, Otto M, Pollack M et al. Premenstrual exacerbation of symptoms in women with panic disorder. J Anx Disord 1994; 8(2):131–8.

57. Vickers K, McNally RJ. Is premenstrual dysphoria a variant of panic disorder? A review. Clin Psychol Rev 2004; 24:933–56.

58. Facchinetti F, Romano G, Fava M, Genassani AR. Lactate infusion induces panic attacks in patients with premenstrual syndrome. Psychosom Med 1992; 54:288–96.

59. Sandberg D, Endicott J, Harrison W et al. Sodium lactate infusion in late luteal phase dysphoric disorder. Psychiatry Res 1993; 46: 79–88.

60. Schwartz GE, Goetz RR, Klein DF et al. Tidal volume of respiration and 'sighing' as indicators of breathing irregularities in panic disorder patients. Anxiety 1996; 2(3):145–8.

61. Harrison W, Sandberg D, Gorman J et al. Provocation of panic with carbon dioxide inhalation in patients with premenstrual dysphoria. Psychiatry Res 1989; 27:183–92.

62. Le Melledo JM, Bradwejn J, Koszycki D, Bichet D. Premenstrual dysphoric disorder and response to cholecystokinin-tetrapeptide. Arch Gen Psychiatry 1995; 52:605–6.

63. Le Melledo J, Van Driel M, Coupland N et al. Response to flumazenil in women with premenstrual dysphoric disorder. Am J Psychiatry 2000; 157(6):821–3.

64. McLeod DR, Hoehn-Saric R, Foster GV, Hipsley PA. The influence of premenstrual syndrome on ratings of anxiety in women with generalized anxiety disorder. Acta Psychiatr Scand 1993; 88:248–51.

65. Severino SK, Yonkers KA. A literature review of psychotic symptoms associated with the premenstruum. Psychosomatics 1993; 34(4):299–306.

66. Kranidiotis LS, Rajendran JP. Goserelin for menstrual psychosis. J Obstet Gynaecol 2006; 26(2):183.

67. Harris AH. Menstrually related symptom changes in women with schizophrenia. Schizophrenia Res 1997; 27:93–9.

68. Choi SH, Kang SB, Joe SH. Changes in premenstrual symptoms in women with schizophrenia: a prospective study. Psychosom Med 2001; 63:822–9.

69. Bergemann N, Parzer P, Nagl I et al. Acute psychiatric admission and menstrual cycle phase in women with schizophrenia. Arch Womens Ment Health 2002; 5(3):119–26.

70. Lande RG, Karamchandani V. Chronic mental illness and the menstrual cycle. J Am Osteopath Assoc 2002; 102(12):655–9.

7

The clinical presentation and course of premenstrual symptoms

Ellen W Freeman

INTRODUCTION

The premenstrual syndromes (PMS) are characterized by symptoms that are limited to the luteal phase of the menstrual cycle, occur for several days to 2 weeks before menses, and remit during the menstrual flow. Over 300 symptom complaints have been linked to the condition.[1] Although a diagnosis of PMS is clearly hampered by the absence of a biological marker, the more immediate problem is the absence of accepted, evidence-based diagnostic criteria to evaluate the numerous undifferentiated menstrual cycle complaints that may be presented to the clinician. This chapter addresses the clinical presentation and course of premenstrual symptoms, the current diagnostic criteria, and considerations in evaluating premenstrual symptoms of women who seek medical treatment for PMS.

NOMENCLATURE OF PMS

The term PMS as used by both clinicians and the general public is generic, imprecise, and commonly applied to numerous symptoms that range from the mild and normal physiological changes of the menstrual cycle to clinically significant symptoms that limit or impair normal functioning. When the severity of the symptoms is not identified, up to 90% of menstruating women report PMS symptoms.[2,3] Only a small minority of women report severe premenstrual symptoms that impair functioning. Three to eight percent of women meet the stringent criteria for premenstrual dysphoric disorder (PMDD), a severe dysphoric form of PMS.[4–6] In addition to the number of women who meet criteria for PMDD, another 19–21% of women may be only one symptom short of meeting the PMDD criteria as identified in both a population-based study and a clinical study of women seeking treatment for premenstrual symptoms.[4,5] These results are consistent with epidemiological studies that have identified approximately 20% of women with moderate to severe PMS.[5,7,8] In this chapter, the term PMS is used to indicate a clinically significant disorder that affects approximately 20% of menstruating women in addition to those diagnosed with PMDD.

PMS SYMPTOMS

Numerous symptoms have traditionally been attributed to PMS. The symptoms are diverse and range over mood, behavioral, cognitive, autonomic, allergy, gastrointestinal, fluid retention, and pain domains. Many healthy women describe premenstrual symptoms but view them as normal and not troublesome.[9] The plethora of over 300 premenstrual complaints is due in part to the absence of a clear diagnosis that distinguishes PMS from either normal or other comorbid conditions. Numerous physical and psychiatric disorders are exacerbated premenstrually or occur as a comorbid disorder with PMS.[10]

When a careful diagnosis is made to distinguish PMS from other conditions, a much smaller group of symptoms appear to be typical of the disorder. Among women who have been screened for PMS, mood and anxiety symptoms are the primary complaint (irritability, anxiety, tension, mood swings, feeling out of control, depression) and account for much of the functional impairment.[11] Other symptoms usually accompany the mood symptoms, most commonly behavioral symptoms such as decreased interest, fatigue, poor concentration, and poor sleep and physical symptoms such as breast tenderness and abdominal swelling.

There is no consensus on the key symptoms of PMS or whether there are core symptoms that define the clinical syndrome. There is some evidence that irritability and tension are the cardinal symptoms of PMS.[8,12,13] Depressive symptoms such as low mood, fatigue, appetite changes, sleep difficulties, and poor concentration are also frequent complaints of women with PMS. While these are symptoms of anxiety and depressive disorders, studies in recent years have provided strong evidence that severe PMS is a distinct disorder and not a simple variant of either depression or anxiety.[14,15] Such evidence includes:

1. The rapid response to selective serotonin reuptake inhibitors (SSRIs) within hours or a day or two, as demonstrated by the efficacy of luteal phase dosing, rather than the 1–4 weeks that may be required for depression.[12,16,17]
2. The maximal response of PMS patients to SSRIs at low doses, with little or no additional improvement at the high end of the dose ranges, which may due to factors other than the inhibition of 5-hydroxytryptamine (5-HT) reuptake that is believed to improve major depressive disorder.[18,19]
3. The predominance of irritability symptoms together with physical symptoms such as breast soreness and swelling, symptoms that are not characteristic of depression but respond to SSRI treatment for PMS.[16]
4. The lack of association between the response to SSRIs and a history of depression or depressive symptoms in PMS patients.[20,21]
5. The positive response of PMS patients to gonadotropin-releasing hormone (GnRH) agonist treatment, which is not effective for depressive disorders,[22,23] and the poor response of PMS patients to the antidepressant bupropion or to most tricyclic antidepressants, which have less selective serotonergic activity but are very effective for depressive disorders.[20,24–26]
6. The chronic course of PMS, which is unlikely to remit without treatment and appears to have swift return of symptoms after discontinuation of medication.[4,27–30]
7. The positive response of PMS/PMDD patients to panic provocation in laboratory studies, but neither a history of panic disorder nor a biological abnormality shared with panic disorder patients has been identified.[15]

Prevalence

Surveys indicate that premenstrual syndrome is among the most common health problems reported by women of reproductive age.[31] Current estimates of the prevalence of severe PMS range from 12.6% to 31% of menstruating women.[5] The severe, dysphoric form, termed premenstrual dysphoric disorder, is limited to 5–8% of menstruating women.[4] In another community-based study, 8% of menstruating women had severe premenstrual symptoms and 14% had moderate premenstrual symptoms that were significantly associated with functional impairment.[8] Using PMDD criteria to define cases in population-based data indicated that, in addition to the 5–8% who met criteria for PMDD, another 18% were only one symptom short of the five symptoms required for the diagnosis.[4] These estimates consistently suggest that approximately 20% of women experience premenstrual symptoms that are severely distressing or impair functioning and are consistent with the numbers of women who believe they need treatment for PMS as reported in other survey studies.[3,32–34]

COURSE OF PMS

PMS is a chronic disorder that occurs in ovulating women. The symptoms appear to gradually worsen with age until ovarian activity declines and ultimately ends at menopause. In a population-based study, severe PMS was highly stable over time, and full remissions of untreated cases were quite rare.[4] A recent follow-up study of PMS patients likewise found that the symptoms of women with untreated, clinically significant PMS were stable across menstrual cycles.[11]

The peak symptom levels of PMS in our clinical samples occur between the late twenties and late thirties. The mean age in these samples is in the early thirties and seldom includes adolescents.[35] The mean age at onset of PMS is around 26 years old, as reported by the women in clinical treatment samples, but the well-known biases of recall must be considered in these retrospective reports.[36]

In contrast, population-based data from adolescent women (aged 14–24 years old) indicate that 5.8% of these young women met criteria for PMDD and an additional 18.6% were 'near threshold cases'.[4] These estimates strongly suggest that severe PMS starts in the teen years and early twenties. It is noteworthy that this proportion appears to be similar across the reproductive years, as indicated in another population-based sample of women aged 36–44 years old, where 6.4% had a confirmed diagnosis of PMDD, only slightly more than the 5.8% with PMDD among women aged 14–24 years old.[6]

PMS is understood to occur in ovulatory menstrual cycles, and therefore ends with the cessation of ovulation at menopause. Clinical data show that the overall severity of PMS decreases in the fifth decade, possibly because ovulation is less frequent as women enter the menopausal transition.[35] These findings were supported in a population-based cohort study of women who reported that their PMS symptoms significantly decreased after age 40 years old.[37] New symptoms that occur in the transition to menopause may be difficult to distinguish from those of PMS/PMDD. Another study found that a higher-than-expected percentage of perimenopausal women with an onset of depression also had premenstrual dysphoria.[38] Several studies have shown that women with a history of PMS were more likely to experience symptoms in the transition to menopause that were not limited to the luteal phase of the menstrual cycle, particularly hot flashes, depressed mood, poor sleep, and decreased libido.[37–39]

PMS AND DIAGNOSTIC CRITERIA

The diagnosis of PMS continues to lack widely accepted criteria and remains controversial, in spite of the many women who seek medical treatment for the disorder.[31,32] At this time, three proffered diagnoses differ considerably in their criteria and utility for assessment in clinical practice.

The WHO International Classification of Diseases, 10th edition (ICD-10) lists premenstrual tension syndrome (PMTS) as a gynecological disorder.[40] This diagnosis requires no specific symptoms or number of symptoms, and provides no requirement for level of severity, differential diagnosis, or exclusion criteria, resulting in no systematic criteria for PMS. The non-specificity of this diagnosis is consistent with the view that there are over 300 premenstrual complaints associated with PMS but fails to differentiate severe PMS either from normal premenstrual changes or from other psychiatric or physical disorders with similar presenting complaints.

In contrast to the non-specificity of the ICD-10 diagnosis of PMTS, criteria for a severe, dysphoric form of PMS, termed premenstrual dysphoric disorder, were included for further research in the Diagnostic and Statistical Manual of Mental Disorders, 4th edition (DSM-IV).[41] The PMDD criteria require five of 11 specified symptoms at a severe level in the premenstrual phase of the cycle, symptom remission in the follicular phase of the cycle, marked functional impairment, absence of other diagnoses that would account for the symptoms, and prospective confirmation of the symptoms for at least two consecutive menstrual cycles.

The symptoms included in the PMDD diagnosis are depressed mood, anxiety/tension, mood swings, anger/irritability, decreased interest, difficulty concentrating, fatigue, appetite changes, sleep difficulties, feeling out of control, and physical symptoms. Of the five symptoms

required to meet the PMDD criteria, at least one must be among the first four emotional symptoms listed above, and all physical symptoms, regardless of the number, are considered a single symptom for meeting the diagnostic criteria.

The PMDD criteria have been used by many researchers in recent years. These criteria mark a major step in providing specific parameters for a diagnosis of premenstrual symptoms, and the use of PMDD criteria has contributed to identifying effective treatments and increasing scientific information about the disorder. However, the clinical application of the PMDD criteria is limited by its psychiatric focus and complexity and only a small minority of women who seek treatment for premenstrual symptoms meet the PMDD criteria. Moreover, there is no data-based evidence for the assumptions of the diagnosis, and responses to treatment do not differ between women diagnosed with PMDD and women who do not meet the PMDD criteria but have severe PMS.[20,21]

In contrast to the psychiatric emphasis of PMDD, a third diagnostic approach was recently offered by the American College of Obstetricians and Gynecologists (ACOG).[42] The ACOG criteria for PMS require only one of 10 specified symptoms during the 5 days before menses, remission during the menstrual flow without recurrence of the symptoms until at least cycle day 13, identifiable impairment or distress, absence of other diagnoses that would account for the symptom(s), and prospective confirmation of the symptom(s) for three menstrual cycles.

The symptoms included in the ACOG criteria are depression, angry outbursts, irritability, anxiety, confusion, social withdrawal, breast tenderness, abdominal bloating, headache, and swelling of extremities.

The ACOG criteria avoid the symptom count required for the PMDD diagnosis and instead emphasize overall severity as demonstrated by distress or impaired functioning. As with the PMDD and ICD-10 criteria, the extent to which these criteria appropriately diagnose women who seek treatment for PMS has not been demonstrated.

Each of these three diagnoses attempts to provide parameters for a diagnosis of PMS. Importantly, all lack a standard approach to operationalizing their proposed criteria. The severity of the symptoms, the degree of distress or interference with functioning, and the predominant symptoms of the patient's complaint can vary widely depending on the methods applied to operationalize the diagnostic criteria. This was demonstrated in a recent study, which showed that the method selected to determine severity thresholds for PMDD resulted in widely divergent samples.[43] The study also showed that the interference criterion contributes little to the diagnosis of PMDD, in part due to the high correlation between symptom severity and self-reported impairment.

PMS symptoms and assessment tools

PMS is diagnosed on the basis of the *timing* and *severity* of the symptoms and the degree of distress or functional impairment. PMS symptoms must be limited to the luteal phase of the menstrual cycle and subside during the menstrual flow. These factors, together with an assessment of whether other physical or psychiatric disorders may account for the symptoms, are more important for the diagnosis than the particular symptoms, which are typically non-specific and must be assessed for their relationship to the menstrual cycle.

Most women who seek medical treatment describe multiple symptoms, with the primary symptoms and most distressing problems usually focused on the mood and behavioral symptoms. Physical symptoms are widely experienced by women around menstruation, but many women do not perceive problems with these symptoms. Physical symptoms alone in the luteal phase, without other mood or behavioral symptoms, are seldom sufficient for a clinical diagnosis of PMS. Physical symptoms, particularly pain around menses, often point to primary dysmenorrhea or endometriosis, which are distinct and a separate diagnosis from PMS.

Referral patterns can influence the diagnosis. Gynecologists may focus on the physical symptoms that are associated with the menstrual cycle, while psychiatrists may focus on the mood problems. Patients who have severe psychological problems may go to gynecologists rather than psychiatrists in order to avoid the label of a psychiatric illness.

The pattern of luteal phase symptoms that remit during menses is clearly demonstrated with daily symptom reports from PMS patients charted over the menstrual cycle.[44,45] The effect size of the overall symptom scores compared between PMS patients and normal controls for each day of the menstrual cycle exceeds 1.6 from approximately cycle day 17 through cycle day 1.[45] It is important to note the magnitude of this difference between PMS patients and non-patients in the most symptomatic time period. Women, overall, report increasing symptoms in the week before menses and decreasing symptoms in the week following day 1 of menses,[45,46] but the severity of the symptoms in women with PMS significantly exceeds the symptom levels of women without PMS.

The key diagnostic tool for evaluating premenstrual symptoms is the daily symptom report. The criteria for PMDD and the ACOG PMS diagnosis require that the reported symptoms are confirmed and linked to the menstrual cycle in the requisite pattern by the prospective daily symptom reports maintained for at least two menstrual cycles. Numerous daily symptom reports that are appropriate for the diagnosis of PMS are identified in the literature[47] (see Chapter 4). No one of these forms is considered the 'gold standard.' Rather, it is important to select a symptom rating form that includes the symptoms required for the target diagnosis (e.g. PMDD) and will encourage compliance of the patients. It is also important that the rating scale is sufficient to indicate the severity of each symptom and not simply an indication of their presence or absence.

Steiner et al developed a simple questionnaire to use at the office visit, named the Premenstrual Symptoms Screening Tool (PSST) for clinicians.[48] Use of this form successfully identifies PMDD patients and suggests the utility of a brief retrospective report of PMS symptoms, although its validation against prospective daily reports is needed. The daily rating form that has been used most frequently in studies of PMDD is the Daily Record of Severity of Problems (DRSP).[49] Other forms that were designed to assess PMS/PMDD and have been used in multiple research studies include the Daily Symptom Report (DSR), the Calendar of Premenstrual Experiences (COPE), and visual analog scales where the selected symptoms are each rated on a line that represents a linear scale.[45,50,51]

The primary reason for obtaining prospective information about the symptoms is that many women who state they have PMS fail to confirm the required pattern when they report their symptoms daily. Consequently, daily symptom reports have become a requirement in research studies, although clinicians frequently avoid their use, in part because they are cumbersome and time-consuming for both the patient and the clinician. Rating symptoms for several menstrual cycles also delays the initiation of therapy, which some patients are unwilling to accept. Nonetheless, daily symptom reports provide diagnostic information and are particularly helpful in pointing to other problems when the reports show that symptoms occur randomly or throughout the menstrual cycle. When there is evidence that symptoms are not limited to the luteal phase of the cycle, it is likely that other medical or psychiatric problems are present, and treatment of PMS alone will be inappropriate and/or ineffective.

The daily symptom reports are also an important educational tool for patients. By systematically recording their symptoms, many women learn to recognize their symptom patterns over the menstrual cycle, confirm for themselves whether they do or do not have PMS, and gain an increased sense of control in managing their symptoms. During this diagnostic interval before initiating drug treatment, patients can also be encouraged to try self-help strategies that are widely recommended for PMS to determine whether a non-medical approach is helpful.[52]

Diagnostic procedures

There are no laboratory tests or physical findings that indicate a diagnosis of PMS. Laboratory tests should not be routinely performed for this diagnosis, although laboratory tests that indicate or confirm other possible disorders are useful if suggested by the individual woman's symptom presentation or medical findings. A gynecological examination is not mandatory, but may be important for ruling out other disorders. Patients may consider a pelvic examination unnecessarily intrusive, particularly in the absence of physical symptoms. Menstrual cycles that are irregular or outside the normal range are an indication for further gynecological evaluation. Specific information on functional impairment is helpful for determining the impact of the symptoms. A medical history with emphasis on reproductive events, other physical disorders that might account for the symptoms, mood disorders, and family history of PMS and mood disorders should be obtained.

Premenstrual exacerbations and comorbidities

Other disorders need to be identified if present. Primary dysmenorrhea is often confused or included with PMS but is a distinct diagnosis. Dysmenorrhea is characterized by pelvic pain or backache that may occur for several days but typically peaks on the first day of the menstrual flow. Primary dysmenorrhea is linked to prostaglandins originating in secretory endometrium and is relieved by prostaglandin inhibitors in the great majority of dysmenorrheic women. Pelvic pain, backache, or complaints of dyspareunia may also signal endometriosis, particularly in women who previously had pain-free menses for an extended period of time. Symptoms of endometriosis can be present throughout the month and are not limited to the luteal phase, although women can also have extensive endometriosis with little or no pain. Migraine is associated with ovulatory cycles, as indicated by its onset at menarche (10.7%), attacks in the time around menses (60% of cases), and disappearance during pregnancy (67% of cases), and may be a modulator of PMS.[53,54] Menstrually related migraine attacks appear longer and less responsive to the treatments than non-menstrual attacks and consequently may require different treatment considerations.[55]

Many women who seek treatment for PMS have a depression or anxiety disorder that is exacerbated premenstrually.[56,57] The extent of premenstrual exacerbation is suggested in the large STAR-D study of major depressive disorder, where 64% of the premenopausal women not taking oral contraceptives reported premenstrual worsening of their depression.[58] The mood symptoms that are predominant in PMS include depression, anxiety, tension, and irritability, but these symptoms are ongoing in mood and anxiety disorders and are not limited to the luteal phase of the menstrual cycle. One approach to differentiating PMS and mood disorders is to evaluate the patient at least once in the *postmenstrual* phase of the cycle when premenstrual symptoms have remitted. Clinically significant mood or anxiety symptoms in the postmenstrual phase strongly suggest a psychiatric or other medical diagnosis.

There are numerous other conditions whose symptoms may be confused with PMS or may be exacerbated premenstrually. Physical conditions such as uterine fibroids, endometriosis, adenomyosis, chronic pelvic pain, ovarian cysts, pelvic inflammatory disease, seizure disorders, thyroid disorders, asthma, allergies, diabetes, hepatic dysfunction, lupus, anemia, chronic fatique syndrome, fibromyalgia, and infections may worsen premenstrually. Other psychiatric conditions that may be comorbid or exacerbated premenstrually include substance abuse, eating disorders, and schizophrenia. It can be difficult to determine whether the symptoms are an exacerbation of a comorbid condition or PMS symptoms (that occur only in the luteal phase) superimposed on another condition. In either case, the usual recommendation is to treat the underlying condition first, then assess the response to treatment and possibly increase the dose premenstrually and/or add medication for the symptoms that arise in the premenstrual phase.

SUMMARY

Guidelines and criteria for diagnosis of PMS have advanced in the past decade. Appropriate diagnosis has become increasingly important as effective treatments have been identified for PMS, and the majority of patients can obtain relief from their symptoms. However, it is still difficult for primary care clinicians to evaluate a disorder that is linked with hundreds of possible symptoms, lacks widely accepted criteria, and depends upon the patient's maintaining daily reports of the symptoms for several months. A greater consensus on the diagnostic criteria for PMS is needed, together with an empirical demonstration that the criteria appropriately diagnose women who seek treatment for PMS. Further studies of the utility of well-designed retrospective reports of the symptom complaints that can be administered at the office visit are also needed. Continued advances in the diagnosis of

PMS will contribute to reducing the healthcare costs that are incurred by the large numbers of women who seek medical care for this distressing disorder.

REFERENCES

1. Halbreich U, Borenstein J, Pearlstein T et al. The prevalence, impairment, impact, and burden of premenstrual dysphoric disorder (PMS/PMDD). Psychoneuroendocrinology 2003; 28:1–23.

2. Andersch B, Wenderstam C, Hahn L et al. Prevalence of premenstrual symptoms in a Swedish urban population. J Psychosom Obstet Gynaecol 1986; 5:39–49.

3. Johnson SR, McChesney C, Bean JA. Epidemiology of premenstrual symptoms in a nonclinical sample. I. Prevalence, natural history and help-seeking behavior. J Reprod Med 1988; 33:340–6.

4. Wittchen HU, Becker E, Lieb R et al. Prevalence, incidence and stability of premenstrual dysphoric disorder in the community. Psychol Med 2002; 32:119–32.

5. Steiner M, Macdougall M, Brown E. The premenstrual symptoms screening tool (PSST) for clinicians. Arch Womens Ment Health 2003; 6:203–9.

6. Cohen LS, Soares CN, Otto MW et al. Prevalence and predictors of premenstrual dysphoric disorder (PMDD) in older premenopausal women. The Harvard Study of Moods and Cycles. J Affect Disord 2002; 70:125–32.

7. Sveindottir H, Backstrom T. Prevalence of menstrual cycle symptom cyclicity and premenstrual dysphoric disorder in a random sample of women using and not using oral contraceptives. Acta Obstet Gynecol Scand 2000; 79:405–13.

8. Angst J, Sellaro R, Merikangas KR et al. The epidemiology of perimenstrual psychological symptoms. Acta Psychiatr Scand 2001; 104:110–16.

9. Sveinsdottir H, Lundman B, Norberg A. Women's perceptions of phenomena they label premenstrual tension: normal experiences reflecting ordinary behaviour. J Adv Nurs 1999; 30:916–25.

10. Steiner M, Pearlstein T, Cohen LS et al. Expert guidelines for the treatment of severe PMS, PMDD, and comorbidities: the role of SSRIs. J Womens Health (Larchmt) 2006; 15:57–69.

11. Bloch M, Schmidt PJ, Rubinow DR. Premenstrual syndrome: evidence for symptom stability across cycles. Am J Psychiatry 1997; 154:1741–6.

12. Eriksson E. Serotonin reuptake inhibitors for the treatment of premenstrual dysphoria. Int Clin Psychopharmacol 1999; 14:S27–33.

13. Eriksson E, Andersch B, Ho H-P et al. Premenstrual dysphoria: an illustrative example of how serotonin modulates sex-steroid-related behavior. CNS Spectr 2001; 6:141–9.

14. Landen M, Eriksson E. How does premenstrual dysphoric disorder relate to depression and anxiety disorders? Depress Anxiety 2003; 17:122–9.

15. Vickers K, McNally RJ. Is premenstrual dysphoria a variant of panic disorder? A review. Clin Psychol Rev 2004; 24:933–56.

16. Dimmock PW, Wyatt KM, Jones PW et al. Efficacy of selective serotonin-reuptake inhibitors in premenstrual syndrome: a systematic review. Lancet 2000; 356:1131–6.

17. Wyatt KM, Dimmock PW, O'Brien PM. Selective serotonin reuptake inhibitors for premenstrual syndrome. Cochrane Database Syst Rev 2002; 4:CD001396.

18. Endicott J, Amsterdam J, Eriksson E et al. Is premenstrual dysphoric disorder a distinct clinical entity? J Womens Health Gend Based Med 1999; 8:663–79.

19. Pinna G, Costa E, Guidotti A. Fluoxetine and norfluoxetine stereospecifically and selectively increase brain neurosteroid content at doses that are inactive on 5-HT reuptake. Psychopharmacology 2006; 186:362–72.

20. Freeman EW, Rickels K, Sondheimer SJ et al. Continuous or intermittent dosing with sertraline for patients with severe premenstrual syndrome or premenstrual dysphoric disorder. Am J Psychiatry 2004; 161:343–51.

21. Freeman EW, Rickels K, Sondheimer SJ et al. Differential response to antidepressants in women with premenstrual syndrome/premenstrual dysphoric disorder: a randomized controlled trial. Arch Gen Psychiatry 1999; 56:932–9.

22. Brown CS, Ling FW, Andersen RN et al. Efficacy of depot leuprolide in premenstrual syndrome: effect of symptom severity and type in a controlled trial. Obstet Gynecol 1994; 84:779–86.

23. Freeman EW, Sondheimer SJ, Rickels K. Gonadotropin-releasing hormone agonist in treatment of premenstrual symptoms with and without ongoing dysphoria: a controlled study. Psychopharmacol Bull 1997; 33:303–9.

24. Pearlstein TB, Stone AB, Lund SA. Comparison of fluoxetine, bupropion, and placebo in the treatment of premenstrual dysphoric disorder. J Clin Psychopharmacol 1997; 17:261–6.

25. Eriksson E, Hedberg A, Andersch B, Sundblad C. The serotonin reuptake inhibitor paroxetine is superior to the noradrenaline reuptake inhibitor maprotiline in the treatment of premenstrual syndrome. Neuropsychopharmacology 1995; 12:167–76.

26. Taghavi E, Menkes DB, Howard RC et al. Premenstrual syndrome: a double-blind controlled trial of desipramine and metylscopolamine. Int Clin Psychopharmacol 1995; 10:119–22.

27. Yonkers KA, Barnett LK, Carmody T et al. Serial discontinuation of SSRI treatment for PMDD. Biol Psychiatry 1998; 43:1S–133S.

28. Pearlstein TB, Stone AB. Long-term fluoxetine treatment of late luteal phase dysphoric disorder. J Clin Psychiatry 1994; 55:332–5.

29. Elks ML. Open trial of fluoxetine therapy for premenstrual syndrome. South Med J 1993; 86:503–7.

30. Freeman EW, Sondheimer SJ, Rickels K et al. A pilot naturalistic follow-up of extended sertraline treatment for severe premenstrual syndrome. J Clin Psychopharmacol 2004; 24:351–3.

31. Brown WJ, Doran FM. Women's health: consumer views for planning local health promotion and health care priorities. Aust N Z J Public Health 1996; 20:149–54.

32. Singh BB, Berman BM, Simpson RL et al. Incidence of premenstrual syndrome and remedy usage: a national probability sample study. Altern Ther Health Med 1998; 4:75–9.

33. Corney RH, Stanton R. A survey of 658 women who report symptoms of premenstrual syndrome. J Psychosom Res 1991; 35:471–82.

34. Campbell EM, Peterkin D, O'Grady K et al. Premenstrual symptoms in general practice patients: prevalence and treatment. J Reprod Med 1997; 42:637–46.

35. Freeman EW, Rickels K, Schweizer E et al. Relationships between age and symptom severity among women seeking medical treatment for premenstrual symptoms. Psychol Med 1995; 25:309–15.

36. Hurt SW, Schnurr PP, Severino SK et al. Late luteal phase dysphoric disorder in 670 women evaluated for premenstrual complaints. Am J Psychiatry 1992; 149:525–30.

37. Freeman EW, Sammel MD, Rinaudo PJ et al. Premenstrual syndrome as a predictor of menopausal symptoms. Obstet Gynecol 2004; 103:960–6.

38. Richards M, Rubinow DR, Daly RC et al. Premenstrual symptoms and perimenopausal depression. Am J Psychiatry 2006; 163:133–7.

39. Schmidt PJ, Haq N, Rubinow DR. A longitudinal evaluation of the relationship between reproductive status and mood in perimenopausal women. Am J Psychiatry 2004; 161:2238–44.

40. WHO. International Classification of Diseases, 10th edn. Geneva: World Health Organization; 1996.

41. American Psychiatric Association. Diagnostic and Statistical Manual of Mental Disorders, 4th edition. Washington, DC. American Psychiatric Association; 1994.

42. American College of Obstetricians and Gynecologists (ACOG). Premenstrual Syndrome. Washington, DC: ACOG; 2000.

43. Smith MJ, Schmidt PJ, Rubinow DR. Operationalizing DSM-IV criteria for PMDD: selecting symptomatic and asymptomatic cycles for research. J Psychiatr Res 2003; 37:75–83.

44. Pearlstein T, Yonkers KA, Fayyad R et al. Pretreatment pattern of symptom expression in premenstrual dysphoric disorder. J Affect Disord 2005; 85:275–82.

45. Freeman EW, DeRubeis RJ, Rickels K. Reliability and validity of a daily diary for premenstrual syndrome. Psychiatry Res 1996; 65:97–106.

46. Meaden PM, Hartlage SA, Cook-Karr J. Timing and severity of symptoms associated with the menstrual cycle in a community-based sample in the Midwestern United States. Psychiatry Res 2005; 134:27–36.

47. Haywood A, Slade P, King H. Assessing the assessment measures for menstrual cycle symptoms: a guide for researchers and clinicians. J Psychosom Res 2002; 52:223–37.

48. Steiner M, Macdougall M, Brown E. The premenstrual symptoms screening tool (PSST) for clinicians. Arch Womens Ment Health 2003; 6:203–9.

49. Endicott J, Nee J, Harrison W. Daily Record of Severity of Problems (DRSP): reliability and validity. Arch Womens Ment Health 2006; 9:41–9.

50. Feuerstein M, Shaw WS. Measurement properties of the calendar of premenstrual experience in patients with premenstrual syndrome. J Reprod Med 2002; 47:279–89.

51. Steiner M, Streiner DL. Validation of a revised visual analog scale for premenstrual mood symptoms: results from prospective and retrospective trials. Can J Psychiatry 2005; 50:327–32.

52. Dell DL. Premenstrual syndrome, premenstrual dysphoric disorder, and premenstrual exacerbation of another disorder. Clin Obstet Gynecol 2004; 47:568–75.

53. Granella F, Sances G, Zanferrari C et al. Migraine without aura and reproductive life events: a clinical epidemiological study in 1300 women. Headache 1993; 33:385–9.

54. Martin VT, Wernke S, Mandell K et al. Symptoms of premenstrual syndrome and their association with migraine headache. Headache 2006; 46:125–37.

55. Granella F, Sances G, Allais G et al. Characteristics of menstrual and nonmenstrual attacks in women with menstrually related migraine referred to headache centres. Cephalalgia 2004; 24:707–16.

56. Kim DR, Gyulai L, Freeman EW et al. Premenstrual dysphoric disorder and psychiatric co-morbidity. Arch Womens Ment Health 2004; 7:37–47.

57. Hsiao MC, Hsiao CC, Liu CY. Premenstrual symptoms and premenstrual exacerbation in patients with psychiatric disorders. Psychiatry Clin Neurosci 2004; 58:186–90.

58. Kornstein SG, Harvey AT, Rush AJ et al. Self-reported premenstrual exacerbation of depressive symptoms in patients seeking treatment for major depression. Psychol Med 2005; 35:683–92.

Derby Hospitals NHS Foundation
Trust
Library and Knowledge Service

8

Physiology of the menstrual cycle

Robert L Reid and Dean A Van Vugt

INTRODUCTION

Ovulatory menstrual bleeding can be considered the final curtain call on a precisely choreographed play that, each month, sees hypothalamic, pituitary, and gonadal hormones interact in an effort to optimize circumstances for reproduction. In non-contracepting women, when not interrupted by pregnancy or lactation, this play can be expected to run for some 40 years.

Estimates suggest that a century ago women would experience fewer than 100 menstrual cycles in a lifetime because of repeated interruptions for pregnancy followed by lengthy intervals of breast-feeding. In contrast, today's woman can expect to experience many more menstrual cycles in her lifetime in part due to earlier menarche, later menopause, and widespread use of effective contraception resulting in fewer pregnancies.

The fetal ovary is reported to contain some seven million germ cells in the fifth month of gestation. Most of these are lost before birth, with the newborn female having only 1–2 million oocytes remaining. By puberty the number of oocytes has dropped to 500 000 and it is from this pool that one egg matures and an additional 1000 oocytes are lost each month until the oocyte pool is ultimately depleted and menopause begins.[1,2] In the final 5 years before menopause the remaining oocytes show increasing resistance to gonadotropic stimulation, resulting in menstrual cycles which are irregular, unpredictable, and punctuated by transient signs and symptoms of menopause. Although the phase from menarche to menopause is often referred to as 'the reproductive years' it is now clear that the competence of oocytes declines steadily with age and that pregnancy is an uncommon event after age 40 years old. In the absence of contraception or other endocrine disruption to menstrual cyclicity (e.g. excessive weight loss or gain, thyroid dysfunction, hyperprolactinemia, etc.), the modern woman can expect to have 400–450 menstrual cycles in her lifetime.[3]

PUBERTAL ONSET OF HYPOTHALAMIC ACTIVITY

The hypothalamic decapeptide gonadotropin-releasing hormone (GnRH) regulates the synthesis and secretion of the pituitary gonadotropins – luteinizing hormone (LH) and follicle-stimulating hormone (FSH) – that are ultimately responsible for ovarian activation. A hypothalamic 'pulse generator' regulates the pulsatile release of GnRH. Throughout childhood, central mechanisms block the release of GnRH. Typically around the age of 11 or 12 years old, this central restraint declines – initially resulting in nocturnal pulses of GnRH and ultimately in 24-hour GnRH pulsatile secretion. These GnRH pulses, in turn, lead to pituitary release of LH and FSH and subsequent activation of ovarian steroidogenesis.[4]

Kisspeptins (named for the famous Hershey 'kiss' chocolate produced in the place of their discovery – Hershey, Pennsylvania) represent the most exciting new research development in our understanding of puberty. The kisspeptins are a family of proteins derived from the metastasis repressor gene which are ligands for GPR54, a G-protein receptor.[5] Mutation in this receptor has been found in humans with delayed puberty and hypogonadotropic hypogonadism.[6,7] Administration of kisspeptin-10, the most potent ligand of GPR54, advanced pubertal onset in female rats and stimulated GnRH secretion in peripubertal non-human primates.[7,8] Metastasis repressor gene and GPR54 gene expression is increased in the hypothalamus of female peripubertal monkeys.[9] Together, these findings are strong evidence that GPR54 signaling is critical to the initiation of puberty.

OVARIAN STEROIDOGENESIS

A 'two cell – two gonadotropin' hypothesis has allowed a better understanding of the changing steroidogenesis that results during the menstrual cycle (Figure 8.1).

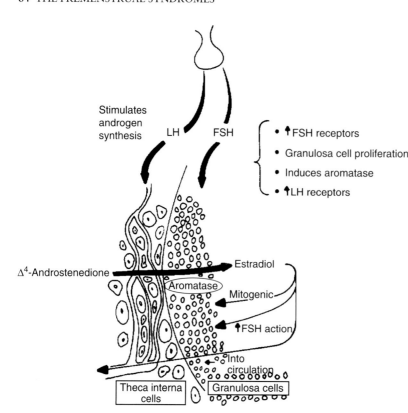

Figure 8.1 The 'Two cell – two gonadotropin' hypothesis of ovarian steroidogenesis. (Reproduced with permission from Reid RL and Van Vugt DA.[4])

Under the influence of LH, the well-vascularized theca cells synthesize androstenedione and testosterone. These androgens diffuse through the basement membrane of the follicle to reach the avascular granulosa cell layer where they form the substrate for estrogen production.[10]

FSH exerts its effects primarily on the granulosa cells that line the inside of the antral follicle, causing (1) mitosis and a rapid increase in granulosa cell numbers, (2) an increase in cell surface FSH and LH receptors, and (3) the acquisition of aromatase activity by granulosa cells.[11] As aromatase within this follicle converts androgens to estrogen, estrogen is released into the circulation and exerts negative feedback at the hypothalamus and pituitary to inhibit FSH secretion. As the menstrual cycle progresses, there is gradual reduction in FSH release. Each of these effects is critical to the process of achieving monofollicular ovulation in primates.

Follicular growth starts out as an FSH-independent process. Primordial follicle development is slow and highly variable, at times taking 120 days to develop into 2 mm preantral follicles. This process is almost certainly regulated by intraovarian peptides in a paracrine fashion.[10] The final 15 days of follicular growth depends on a cyclical rise in FSH.

Follicular development in this final stage (representing the 'follicular phase' of the menstrual cycle) has been divided into three stages: 'recruitment', 'selection', and 'dominance'. The phase of 'recruitment' starts a day or two before menstruation and concludes by day 4 of the follicular phase. The onset of this phase is initiated by the demise of the corpus luteum from the preceding cycle. The hypothalamus and pituitary are released from the restraining effects of progesterone and inhibins produced within the corpus luteum, resulting in a rapid rise in FSH and the 'recruitment' of a new cohort of antral follicles to enter the maturation process. By day 5, one follicle from this cohort starts to gain a competitive advantage over the other recruited follicles. Which follicle will be selected is probably more a matter of chance than of destiny. Analogous to pups around a food bowl – one pup, by chance, gets slightly larger than the others. This results in a competitive advantage that allows that pup to continue to gain over its litter mates. As one follicle gets a slight 'head start' in its growth it becomes slightly more sensitive than neighboring follicles to FSH. Its competitive advantage comes from the fact that it releases into circulation increasing amounts of estrogen, that in turn suppresses the pituitary release of FSH needed to allow continued growth of smaller follicles in the cohort. Since the slightly larger follicle has acquired more granulosa cells, more FSH and LH receptors, and more aromatase activity, it is better able to survive the falling FSH levels. Recent evidence indicates that FSH and LH receptors share a common intracellular cyclic AMP pathway; hence, the 'selected' follicle can develop in response to either FSH or LH, unlike smaller follicles in the cohort, which have few LH receptors. For the remainder of the cohort, the drop in FSH at such an early stage in development results in their gradual demise by day 8 of the cycle. At the same time, the selected follicle appears to release certain proteins that have paracrine effects. Vascular endothelial growth factor (VEGF) results in an increased density of capillaries around the dominant follicle and thereby enhances delivery of FSH, LH, and steroidogenic substrates necessary for final development of the dominant follicle.[10] Ultimately, this 'dominant' follicle undergoes exponential growth over the final 5–6 days of the follicular phase, culminating in ovulation around day 14.

INTERPLAY BETWEEN OVARIAN AND PITUITARY HORMONES

Both the frequency and amplitude of GnRH pulses change throughout the menstrual cycle in response to feedback effects of the gonadal steroids estrogen and progesterone on hypothalamic neuroregulators such as dopamine and endogenous opioid peptides.

The hypothalamic GnRH pulse generator produces one pulse per hour in the absence of ovarian restraint.[12] During the luteal–follicular transition when estradiol, progesterone, and inhibin levels fall, pulses of GnRH occur every 90–120 minutes. In the mid to late follicular phase, GnRH frequency increases to one pulse per hour, favoring LH secretion, while FSH is inhibited by rising levels of estradiol and inhibin B from the dominant follicle. Differential regulation of FSH and LH secretion late in the follicular phase is accomplished by at least two different mechanisms.[13] First, estradiol and inhibin A feedback to the pituitary gonadotrope to augment LH and inhibit FSH secretion.[14] Secondly, a changing (more rapid) pattern of GnRH pulses favors LH release.[15] The LH surge onsets most often between midnight and 8 am and is unlikely to occur before the follicle diameter has achieved 15 mm and or serum estradiol reaches 600 pmol/L.[16]

The LH surge induces resumption of meiosis, luteinization of the granulosa cells that line the interior of the dominant follicle, and a series of inflammatory events that precipitate follicular rupture.[17] The LH surge lasts for approximately 48 hours and ovulation occurs about 36 hours after the onset and 12 hours from the peak serum LH concentration. Granulosa cells are decidualized by high concentrations of LH and acquire the ability to produce progesterone. After ovulation, this production of progesterone by the corpus luteum influences opioidergic, noradrenergic, and γ-aminobutyric acid (GABA) systems within the hypothalamus, slowing GnRH pulse frequency to one pulse every 3–5 hours.[18] Corpus luteal production of estradiol and inhibin A reduces FSH release into the circulation, resulting in accumulating pituitary stores of FSH. When the corpus luteum eventually undergoes demise, the subsequent FSH release starts recruitment of a new cohort of follicles.[19] LH pulses (as a marker for GnRH pulse frequency) have been examined through frequent sampling of blood at different phases of the menstrual cycle in women with premenstrual syndrome (PMS) and controls, with no significant differences being detected.[20]

OVARIAN STEROID FLUCTUATIONS DURING THE MENSTRUAL CYCLE

The menstrual cycle is typically described in two phases: the *follicular phase*, a 10–14 day period leading up to ovulation; the *luteal phase*, the 12–14 day phase from ovulation until the onset of menstrual bleeding (Figure 8.2[21]). Low levels of estradiol are present from immediately prior to menstrual bleeding until the dominant follicle begins to grow.

Late in the second week of the menstrual cycle, estradiol concentrations reach approximately 1000 pmol/L. Coincident with follicular rupture, there is a transient but abrupt fall in estradiol levels for a 24–48-hour period. This abrupt midcycle drop in estradiol has been associated with endometrial destabilization and bleeding in some women[22] and transient PMS-like mood symptoms in others.[23] Ovulatory pain has been termed 'mittelschmerz' while the periovulatory mood disturbance is recorded as 'mittelwahn' in the older literature on PMS. Thereafter, the corpus luteum increases production of both estradiol and progesterone for the next 10–12 days of the luteal phase.

Rapid vascularization of the corpus luteum appears to be guided by angiogenic factors from the follicular fluid.[18] Continued pulsatile release of LH is critical to the maintenance of corpus luteal function throughout its natural lifetime.[24] Wide fluctuations in circulating progesterone result as the corpus luteum secretes pulses of the steroid into the blood stream.[25] In the absence of human chorionic gonadotropin (hCG) stimulation of the corpus luteum, steroidogenesis in the corpus luteum declines after 10–12 days. Circulating progesterone concentrations swing markedly during the luteal phase, with elevations following every LH pulse.[15]

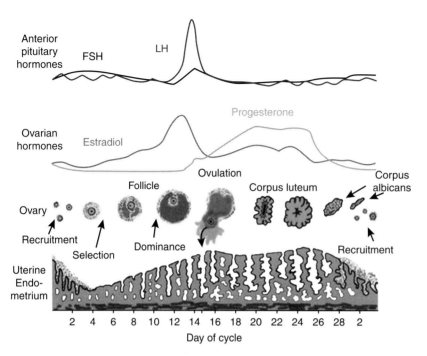

Figure 8.2 The changing levels of pituitary and ovarian hormones throughout the human menstrual cycle. FSH, follicle-stimulating hormone; LH, luteinizing hormone. (Reproduced with permission from Parrish.[21])

In its phase of peak steroidogenic activity, the corpus luteum appears as a swollen vascular area on the surface of the ovary. When surgically incised, the center appears yellowish orange due to the high concentration of cholesterol, which forms the substrate for steroidogenesis.

In conception cycles, the embryo migrates at the morula stage into the endometrial cavity about 4 days after ovulation. The following day, the embryo sheds its zona pellucida and develops a loose adherence to the endometrium. Implantation in the human can only occur during a 6–10 day 'window of implantation' and if this happens the hCG from the early pregnancy with its biological similarity to LH can maintain the activity of the corpus luteum until approximately 7–8 weeks from the last menstrual period when placental steroidogenesis takes over.[26,27] (Figure 8.3[25]).

When pregnancy does not ensue, a new cohort of follicles is recruited and the former corpus luteum involutes slowly over several months. Grossly, the old corpus luteum has the appearance of an inactive whitish area of scar tissue known as the corpus albicans.

TESTOSTERONE LEVELS

The physiological roles of androgens in women remain poorly understood. About 50% of testosterone and androstenedione come from the ovary, with the remainder originating in the adrenal gland.

Data on total and free testosterone levels throughout the normal menstrual cycle are limited due to challenges with conducting assays at the low levels normally found in women.[28] In a recent study using very sensitive detection methods, androgen levels were monitored on a daily basis throughout a complete menstrual cycle in 34 healthy women between the ages of 25 and 40 years old (Figure 8.4). Serum testosterone levels increased gradually, from 1.04 ± 0.76 nmol/L in the menstrual phase to 1.52 ± 1.03 nmol/L at 3 days before the LH surge. Total testosterone levels fell slightly to 1.1 nmol/L in the midluteal phase. Free testosterone levels mirrored those of total testosterone in the follicular phase, but were maintained without the modest midluteal decline seen with total testosterone. Mean testosterone levels during the follicular and luteal phases were not significantly different (1.21 ± 1.21 vs 1.18 ± 1.21).[29]

Serial measurements of testosterone and free testosterone across the menstrual cycle between women with prospectively defined PMS and controls revealed no significant differences.[30]

ENDOMETRIAL CHANGES DURING THE MENSTRUAL CYCLE

Under the influence of rising levels of estradiol, the endometrium shows extensive glandular mitotic activity as stromal and glandular tissues proliferate in the

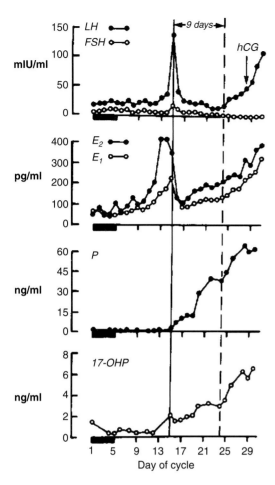

Figure 8.3 Hormonal changes during a conception cycle and the first week of pregnancy. LH, luteinizing hormone; FSH, follicle-stimulating hormone; E_2, estradiol; E_1, estrone; P, progesterone; 17-OHP, 17-hydroxyprogesterone. (Reproduced with permission from Yen.[26])

follicular phase. In the luteal phase, the predominance of progesterone results in decidualization of the endometrium – the increase in vascularity and secretory vacuoles that would be integral to implantation and early embryonic development. Cytosolic vacuoles containing prostaglandins rupture and release their contents when progesterone levels fall late in the luteal phase. These prostaglandins, in turn, cause blood vessels within the endometrium to constrict, resulting in ischemic necrosis and sloughing of the superficial endometrium. The basal layer of endometrium is preserved and the deeper glands constitute the source for new endometrial cells that resurface the denuded endometrial cavity. Bleeding typically subsides as small vessels that supply the endometrium constrict and develop a platelet and fibrin plug. Aberrations of coagulation (either congenital, like von Willebrand's disease, or acquired, such as idiopathic thrombocytopenic purpura) or fibrinolysis can result in exaggerated flow in some women. More commonly, women with pathological abnormalities of the endometrium (endometrial polyps) or myometrium (leiomyomata) will report unusually heavy menstrual flow. In the normal situation the endometrium is rapidly resurfaced in the 5–6 days after menstruation abates.

Synchronous time-limited shedding of the endometrium results when progesterone levels decline in ovulatory women and asynchronous (incomplete) sloughing of endometrium may result from temporary declines in estrogen that occur in ovulatory cycles coincident with ovulation[22] but more commonly at unpredictable times in anovulatory women. Accordingly, the pattern of menstruation will usually confirm whether or not a woman is ovulatory. Regular predictable cycles with an intermenstrual interval of 24–35 days are the hallmark of ovulatory menstrual cycles, whereas unpredictable bleeding at intervals of weeks to months that lasts for different durations (sometimes several weeks) is highly predictive of anovulatory or oligo-anovulatory cycles.

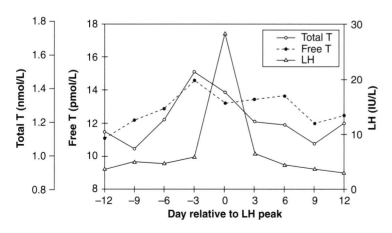

Figure 8.4 Graph showing mean serum concentrations of testosterone (Total T) and free testosterone (Free T) related to luteinizing hormone (LH) levels during the menstrual cycle in 34 healthy women. (Reproduced with permission from Sinha-Hikim et al.[29])

REFERENCES

1. Macklon NS, Fauser BC. Follicle-stimulating hormone and advanced follicle development in the human. Arch Med Res 2001; 32:595–600.

2. Richardson SJ, Senikas V, Nelson JF. Follicular depletion during the menopausal transition: evidence for accelerated loss and ultimate exhaustion at menopause. J Clin Endocrinol Metab 1987; 65:1231–7.

3. Eaton SB, Pike MC, Short RV et al. Women's reproductive cancers in evolutionary context. Q Rev Biol 1994; 69(3):353–67.

4. Reid RL, Van Vugt DA. Neuroendocrine events that regulate the menstrual cycle. Contemp Ob/Gyn 1987; 30(3):147–55.

5. Lee DK, Nguyen T, O'Neill GP et al. Discovery of a receptor related to the galanin receptors. FEBS Lett 1999; 446:103–7.

6. de Roux N, Genin E, Carel JC et al. Hypogonadotropic hypogonadism due to loss of function of the KiSS1-derived peptide receptor GPR54. Proc Natl Acad Sci USA 2003; 100:10972–6.

7. Seminara SB, Messager S, Chatzidaki EE et al The GPR54 gene as a regulator of puberty. N Engl J Med 2003; 349:1614–27.

8. Navarro VM, Fernandez-Fernandez R, Castellano JM et al. Advanced vaginal opening and precocious activation of the reproductive axis by KiSS-1 peptide, the endogenous ligand of GPR54. J Physiol (Lond) 2004; 561:379–86.

9. Shahab M, Mastronardi C, Seminara SB et al. Increased hypothalamic GPR54 signaling: a potential mechanism for initiation of puberty in primates. Proc Natl Acad Sci USA 2005; 102:2129–34.

10. Chabbert-Buffet N, Bouchard P. The normal human menstrual cycle. Rev Endocr Metab Disord 2002; 3:173–83.

11. Zeleznik AJ. Follicle selection in primates: 'Many are called but few are chosen'. Biol Reprod 2001; 65:655–9.

12. Marshall JC, Dalkin AC, Haisenleder DJ et al. Gonadotropin releasing hormone pulses: regulators of gonadotropin synthesis and ovulatory cycles. Rec Prog Hormone Res 1991; 47:155–87.

13. McCartney CR, Gingrich MB, Hu Y et al. Hypothalamic regulation of cyclic ovulation: evidence that the increase in gonadotropin-releasing hormone pulse frequency during the follicular phase reflects the gradual loss of the restraining effects of progesterone. J Clin Endocrinol Metab 2002; 87:2194–200.

14. Nippoldt TB, Reame NE, Kelch RP, Marshall JC. The roles of estradiol and progesterone in decreasing luteinizing hormone pulse frequency in the luteal phase of the menstrual cycle. J Clin Endocrinol Metab 1989; 69(1):67–76.

15. Marshall JC, Griffin ML. The role of changing pulse frequency in the regulation of ovulation. Hum Reprod 1993; 8 (Suppl 2):57–61.

16. Cahill DJ, Wardle PG, Harlow CR et al. Onset of the preovulatory luteinizing hormone surge: diurnal timing and critical follicular prerequisites. Fertil Steril 1998; 70(1):56–9.

17. Tsafriri A, Chun SY, Reich R. Follicular rupture and ovulation. In: Adashi EY, Leung PCK, eds. The Ovary. New York: Raven Press; 1993: 227–44.

18. Buffet NC, Bouchard P. The neuroendocrine regulation of the human ovarian cycle. Chronobiol Int 2001; 18(6): 893–919.

19. Marshall JC, Eagleson CA, McCartney CR. Hypothalamic dysfunction. Mol Cell Endocrinol 2001; 18:29–32.

20. Reame NE, Marshall JC, Kelch RP. Pulsatile LH secretion in women with premenstrual syndrome (PMS): evidence for normal neuroregulation of the menstrual cycle. Psychoneuroendocrinology 1992; 17(2/3):205–13.

21. Parrish J. With permission from the author. Internet reference: http://www.wisc.edu/anscirepro/ May 30, 2006.

22. Bromberg YM, Bercovici B. Occult intermenstrual bleeding about the time of ovulation. Fertil Steril 1956; 7:71–9.

23. Reid RL. Endogenous opioid activity and the premenstrual syndrome. Lancet 1983; 2(8353):786.

24. Stouffer RL. Progesterone as a mediator of gonadotrophin action in the corpus luteum: beyond steroidogenesis. Hum Reprod Update 2003; 9(2):99–117.

25. Filicori M, Butler JP, Crowley WF Jr. Neuroendocrine regulation of the corpus luteum in the human. Evidence for pulsatile progesterone secretion. J Clin Invest 1984; 73:1638–47.

26. Yen SSC. The endocrinology of pregnancy. In: Creasy RK, Resnick R, eds. Maternal and Fetal Medicine: Principle and Practice. Philadelphia: WB Saunders, 1984:341.

27. Kodaman PH, Taylor HS. Hormonal regulation of implantation. Obstet Gynecol Clin N Am 2004; 31:745–66.

28. Rivera-Woll LM, Papalia M, Davis SR et al. Androgen insufficiency in women: diagnostic and therapeutic implications. Hum Reprod Update 2004; 10(5):421–34.

29. Sinha-Hikim I, Arver S, Beall G et al. The use of a sensitive equilibrium dialysis method for the measurement of free testosterone levels in healthy cycling women and in human immunodeficiency virus-infected women. J Clin Endocrinol Metab 1998; 83:1312–18.

30. Bloch M, Schmidt PJ, Su TP et al. Pituitary adrenal hormones and testosterone across the menstrual cycle in women with premenstrual syndrome and controls. Biol Psychiatry 1998; 43:897–903.

9

Neurotransmitter physiology: the basics for understanding premenstrual syndrome

Andrea J Rapkin and John Kuo

INTRODUCTION

The concept that severe premenstrual affective, behavioral, and physical symptoms could be triggered by ovulation and the rise and fall of ovarian sex steroids in the luteal phase of the menstrual cycle was an advance over previous notions that the symptoms resulted from 'agitated menstrual blood seeking escape from the womb'. Still, the explicit psychoneuroendocrine etiology of premenstrual syndrome (PMS) remains unknown, and more than two decades of research have demonstrated that a simple alteration of hormones, neuropeptides, or neurotransmitters cannot completely explain the occurrence of the symptoms. The purpose of this chapter is to provide an overview of the three leading hypotheses that currently attempt to explain the biological basis of PMS. To this end, we will discuss the monoamine neurotransmitter serotonin (5-hydroxytryptamine, 5-HT); the GABAergic neurotransmitter system, in particular, the $GABA_A$ receptor complex; and the pro-opiomelanocortin (POMC) pathway, in particular, the endogenous opiate peptide, β-endorphin.

GABA NEUROTRANSMITTER SYSTEM

Clinical background

The symptoms of PMS are more severe in the 5–7 days before menses, as progesterone levels decline in the late luteal phase of the menstrual cycle. The first neuroendocrine hypothesis therefore logically stated that progesterone deficiency or withdrawal could elicit the symptoms of PMS. However, the mood deterioration generally begins in parallel with the rise in the production of progesterone by the corpus luteum, suggesting hormone withdrawal cannot explain the symptoms.[1]

Progesterone deficiency was also excluded by studies demonstrating that progesterone concentrations are not lower in women with PMS compared with controls.[2–4] Furthermore, PMS symptoms were found to be more severe in cycles with higher concentrations of both estradiol and progesterone.[5] Finally, a series of double-blind placebo-controlled treatment trials failed to demonstrate progesterone supplementation to be more efficacious than placebo.[6–8]

Since ovulation and probably progesterone production trigger the symptoms of PMS, investigations proceeded into the neuroactive metabolites of progesterone and their role in the genesis of PMS symptoms. Progesterone is metabolized in the ovary and the brain to form the potent neuroactive steroids, 3α-hydroxy-5α-pregnan-20-one (allopregnanolone) and 3α-hydroxy-5β-pregnan-20-one (pregnanolone), positive allosteric modulators of the γ-aminobutyric acid (GABA) neurotransmitter system in the brain. The contribution of this receptor system to the genesis of the premenstrual symptoms is also discussed in further detail in Chapter 13.

GABA physiology

GABA, the main inhibitory neurotransmitter in the mammalian brain, is the most widely distributed amino acid neurotransmitter in the central nervous system (CNS), crucial for the regulation of anxiety, vigilance, alertness, stress, and seizures.[9] Most neurons are sensitive to GABA. GABA is derived from glucose metabolism: α-ketoglutarate formed by the Krebs (tricarboxylic acid) cycle is transaminated by GABA-oxoglutarate transaminase (GABA-T) to the amino acid, glutamate.[10] Found exclusively in GABAergic neurons, glutamic acid decarboxylase (GAD) catalyzes the rate-limiting decarboxylation of glutamate to GABA.[11] GABA is then stored in vesicles concentrated in the presynaptic terminal until it is released by a nerve impulse.

GABA postsynaptic receptors are classified into three subtypes: $GABA_A$, $GABA_B$, and $GABA_C$ receptors.[12] The type A ($GABA_A$) receptor is a basic control mechanism fundamental to the functioning of the CNS, and is the site of action for endogenous neuroactive hormonal steroids as well as exogenous agents such as benzodiazepines, barbiturates, alcohol, and anticonvulsants that regulate mood and behavior.[9,13] The $GABA_A$ receptors are plasma membrane-bound protein complexes that form an ion-permeable channel. Specifically, $GABA_A$ receptor activation by GABA results in rapid and transient responses entailing the opening of a chloride anion channel leading to neuronal chloride influx, decreasing the likelihood of depolarization by excitatory neurotransmitters. This hyperpolarization is inhibitory since it represents a move away from the action potential threshold.

The $GABA_A$ receptor is distributed ubiquitously throughout the brain. Benzodiazepines, barbiturates, steroid hormones, and ethanol are all positive allosteric modulators or agonists of this receptor. Binding of such a modulator shifts the GABA response curve to the left, enhances the effect of synaptically released GABA, and potentiates the GABA response. Inhibitory compounds such as the β-carbolines shift the GABA concentration response curve to the right and are termed negative modulators or inverse agonists.[9,14,15] Antagonists such as bicuculline bind to the GABA binding site but do not open the chloride channel. The 3α-hydroxy-5α-pregnan-20-one (allopreganolone), corticosterone, and testosterone metabolites, barbiturates, benzodiazepines, and probably ethanol all have separate extracellularly directed binding sites on the $GABA_A$ receptor, which can increase neuronal inhibition. Some steroids, such as pregnenolone sulfate and dehydroepiandrosterone (DHEA) can act as negative modulators; penicillin, picrotoxin, calcium, and bicuculline also decrease the GABA response and inhibit $GABA_A$ receptor chloride channel flux[9] (Figure 9.1).

Classically, activation of steroid hormone receptors results in transcription and translation of specific genes. However, in contrast to the slower (hours to days) genomic effects of most cytosolic steroid hormone receptors, GABA release through neurosteroid modulation of the $GABA_A$ membrane receptor is direct and rapid (within minutes). Synaptic GABA transmitter inactivation is primarily through reuptake. In addition, both glia and neurons possess these proteins and reuptake GABA. Once GABA is taken up, it can be enzymatically inactivated.[16]

$GABA_A$, but not $GABA_C$ and $GABA_B$, receptors have been associated with alterations in mood, cognition, and affect. Ovarian and adrenal steroids are potent

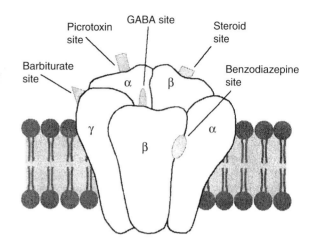

Figure 9.1 Theoretical model of the $GABA_A$ receptor complex and its various ligand binding sites. (Reprinted from N-Wihlbäck et al,[37] with kind permission from Springer Science and Business Media.)

modulators of the GABAergic system in the brain. Increasing plasma concentrations of progesterone and corticosterone give rise to higher brain concentrations of neurosteroids, which suggests that plasma progesterone and corticosterone are significant sources of substrate for neurosteroid formation.[17] Neurosteroidogenesis begins with the conversion of cholesterol to pregnenolone by the cytochrome P450 side chain cleavage enzyme located in the inner mitochondrial membrane of glial cells[18] (Figure 9.2). In the brain, pregnenolone can be converted by the 3β-hydroxysteroid dehydrogenase isomerase (3β-HSD) into progesterone, which is also a neuroactive steroid because in nanomolar concentrations it can bind to intracellular (nuclear) progesterone receptors and control the transcription of specific genes in neurons or glial cells.[18] The main pathway of progesterone metabolism in the brain and the ovary is its conversion into 5α-dihydroprogesterone catalyzed by type I 5α-reductase and the conversion of 5α-dihydroprogesterone into 3α,5α-TH PROG (allopregnanolone) catalyzed by the 3α-hydroxysteroid oxide reductase (3α-HSD). Endogenously produced 3α,5α-TH PROG plays an important physiological modulatory role in tuning the sensitivity of $GABA_A$ receptors to GABA or to other agents (e.g. benzodiazepines) that act by binding to $GABA_A$ receptors.[17,19,20]

The $GABA_A$ receptor is most commonly composed of α, β, δ and/or γ-subunits, the specific composition of which confers flexibility and partially explains the specificity for neurosteroid activity[20,21] (see Figure 9.1). The α2 subunit of the $GABA_A$ receptor is mainly

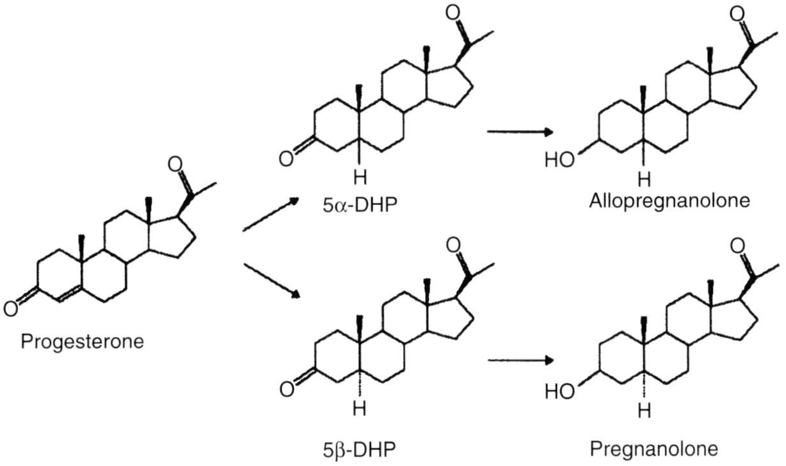

Figure 9.2 Synthesis of progesterone metabolites. (Reprinted from N-Wihlbäck et al,[37] with kind permission from Springer Science and Business Media.)

expressed in brain regions associated with emotional stimulus, such as the hippocampus and amygdala.[22] Receptors containing the δ subunit in combination with the α_4 subunit, are highly sensitive to the ovarian-, adrenal-, and brain-derived neurosteroid allopregnanolone and to the adrenal- and brain-derived neurosteroid 3α,5α-tetrahydrodeoxycorticosterone (3α,5α-THDOC).[20]

Acute stress, pregnancy, or progesterone exposure in a rodent model simulating the luteal phase of the menstrual cycle all result in increased neurosteroid production, which confers short-term changes in GABA$_A$ receptor composition, e.g. up-regulation of α_4, δ, and γ subunit expression. This GABA$_A$ plasticity results in temporarily decreased sensitivity to GABA and GABA agonists. For example, after withdrawal of allopregnanolone, there is a marked decrease in GABA$_A$-gated chloride influx in hippocampal neurons and increased neuronal excitability.[23–28] Progesterone therefore indirectly, through its metabolite allopregnanolone, increases the expression of the α_4, γ_2, and δ subunits of the GABA$_A$ receptor.

The α_4 subunit of the GABA$_A$ receptor has been linked to anxiety.[29] Increased α_4 subunit is observed in the rat model in the postpartum state and after withdrawal from progesterone, and has been associated with anxiety-like reaction in the maze plus and prod burial tests.[23,29–31] Expression of the γ_2 subunit is also altered by pregnancy and postpartum states, estrous and menstrual cycle fluctuations in progesterone, and even administration of oral contraceptives.[31–33] During the rodent ovarian cycle, elevated expression of the δ subunit of the GABA$_A$ receptor results in decreased seizure susceptibility and lowered anxiety levels.[28] Thus, exposure to the progesterone metabolite allopregnanolone alters the subunit composition of the GABA$_A$

receptor, rendering the receptor temporarily insensitive to modulation by neurosteroids.[24,26,34–36]

GABA$_A$ receptor, neurosteroids, and mood symptoms

These alterations of GABA$_A$ receptor isoforms, which result in reduced neurosteroid sensitivity, are very likely to be important in the etiology of PMS, postpartum mood disorders, and even the adverse psychological effects of progesterone and progestins.[37] CNS concentration of these neuroactive metabolites, duration of exposure, as well as genetic predisposition are important determinants of GABA$_A$ receptor agonist effect. Acute treatment with allopregnanolone has been shown to have anxiolytic, antidepressive, and anticonvulsant effects[38,39] and decreased neuroactive steroids have been associated with anxious and depressive behavior.[40,41] That allopregnanolone may play a role in affecting mood is apparent from the fact that improvement of unipolar depression by fluoxetine treatment lasting 8–10 weeks was correlated with a normalization of endogenous CSF allopregnanolone content, which was significantly decreased prior to fluoxetine treatment.[41] Decreased GABA synthesis and activity in the brain have also been associated with depression and mood disorders.[42] Helpless, chronically stressed and anxious rodents have significantly decreased GABA$_A$ receptor expression, GABA$_A$ receptor-medicated chloride ion flux, and decreased sensitivity to GABA$_A$ receptor modulators.[43–46]

Similarly, human patients with mood disorders and PMS have been shown to be insensitive to modulatory effects of benzodiazepines and have altered GABA$_A$ receptor expression and function.[37,47,48] Studies of plasma neuroactive steroids in PMS have been contradictory with some[49,50] but not others,[51–53] suggesting a deficiency of allopregnanolone. However, analogous to the rodent model of progesterone exposure, decreased sensitivity to $GABA_A$ agonists, including neuroactive steroids, has been demonstrated in the luteal phase in women with PMS.[54,55] Women with PMS demonstrate decreased pregnanolone responsiveness possibly due to altered sensitivity of $GABA_A$ receptors[54] and there is some evidence to suggest that patients with mood disorders are also insensitive to modulatory effects of benzodiazepines.[47,48]

The length of allopregnanolone exposure thus plays a critical role in the regulation and function of the $GABA_A$ receptor. Whereas acute, short-term allopregnanolone exposure decreases anxiety, chronic exposure to elevated allopregnanolone can produce decreased expression and binding to the $GABA_A$ receptor as well as uncoupling of the receptor from several anxiolytic modulators, leading to increased anxiety.[56,57] Progesterone metabolite effects on mood and behavior also appear to be biphasic in nature.[37] In high concentrations, pregnanolone and allopregnanolone produce anxiolytic, sedative, antiepileptic, and anesthetic effects.[58–60] At lower physiological levels, though, allopregnanolone can cause anxiety, aggression, impulsive behavior, and negative mood in predisposed individuals.[29,61,62] In sum, $GABA_A$ receptor function and modulation probably varies throughout the menstrual cycle and probably contributes to the negative mood symptoms experienced by many women during the luteal phase.

SEROTONIN NEUROTRANSMITTER SYSTEM

Clinical background

Depression is one of the most serious symptoms of PMS. The monoamine theory of depression posits deficiency of norepinephrine and also the indole amine, serotonin (5-HT). Serotonergic dysfunction has been implicated in the etiology of PMS, and currently, one of the treatments of first choice for severe PMS/PMDD (premenstrual dysphoric disorder) is a serotonergic antidepressant. However, the absence of biological markers for depression in women with PMS (e.g. failure of dexamethasone to suppress cortisol),[63,64] reduced platelet monoamine oxidase (MAO) B,[65] and the rapid response to serotonergic antidepressants suggest that PMS is not a subset of depressive or anxiety disorders and that the neurophysiology is likely to differ. The serotonin hypothesis is also hampered by incomplete understanding of the neurophysiology of the serotonergic system, as well as the lack of a complete response to serotonergic medications by all women with PMS.

Serotonin physiology

Serotonin (5-HT, 5-hydroxytryptamine) is synthesized within serotonergic neurons and in several types of peripheral cells.[66] The brain accounts for about 1% of the total body stores of 5-HT. The amino acid tryptophan is transported to the CNS via an active transport pump.[67] Two enzymes sequentially alter tryptophan: tryptophan hydroxylase is the rate-limiting step in the formation of 5-HT, producing 5-hydroxytryptophan (5-HTP); then the L-aromatic amino acid decarboxylase decarboxylates the hydroxylated tryptophan, resulting in serotonin (5-HT).[68,69]

5-HT cannot cross the blood–brain barrier; thus, CNS neurons must synthesize the amine. Tryptophan is present in high levels in plasma, and changes in dietary tryptophan can substantially alter brain levels of 5-HT.[70] The availability of dietary tryptophan is important in regulating 5-HT synthesis.[71] Since other large neutral aromatic amino acids compete for transport into the CNS, brain levels of tryptophan are also dependent upon plasma concentrations of other competing neutral amino acids.[67] 5-HT is then stored in vesicles concentrated in the presynaptic terminal until it is released by a nerve impulse (Figure 9.3).

Impulse-modulating and release-modulating receptors, designated $5\text{-}HT_{1A}$ somatodendritic autoreceptor and $5\text{-}HT_{1D}$ terminal autoreceptor, are located on the cell body and the nerve terminal, respectively, and detect the presence of 5-HT and then regulate the release and firing rate of 5-HT neurons.[66,72] Drugs that block the $5HT_{1D}$ autoreceptor increase 5-HT release and are under development. The serotonergic neuron also has a terminal autoreceptor, the α_2 heteroreceptor, that, when occupied by norepinephrine, turns off serotonin release (Figure 9.4), as well as an α_1 heteroreceptor on the cell body that can enhance serotonin release.[73] 5-HT that is released into the synapse is inactivated primarily by reuptake through the high-affinity presynaptic membrane serotonin transporter (SERT) or 'reuptake pumps'. SERT is an important clinical target for therapeutic drugs, such as selective serotonin reuptake inhibitors (SSRIs).[74] The enzymatic degradation of 5-HT is catalyzed by the MAO enzyme located within the serotonergic neuron, producing 5-hydroxyindoleacetic acid (5-HIAA). Low cerebrospinal fluid (CSF) 5-HIAA has been found in patients with antisocial, borderline, self-destructive personality disorders and poor impulse control and those who are prone to aggressive outbursts and violent suicide.[73,75,76]

However, as noted above, the MAO inhibitors and tricyclic antidepressants, both of which increase all three monoamine neurotransmitters, but particularly norepinephrine, and which were effective for the

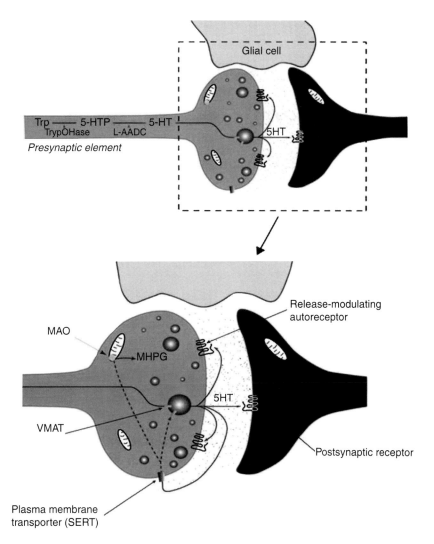

Figure 9.3 Basic neurophysiology of a serotonergic neuron. (Reprinted from Deutch and Roth,[16] Section II, Chapter 7, page 177. © 2002, with permission from Elsevier.)

treatment of depression, were not useful for the treatment of PMS. These agents are not selective for serotonin. Also, SSRIs increase serotonin acutely, particularly in the region of the $5\text{-}HT_{1A}$ autoreceptor, but there is a 3–8 week delay for the antidepressant effect of the serotonin-augmenting drugs when used for the treatment of depression, but not however for PMS and PMDD.[77,78] The delayed treatment response in affective disorder has been explained by the neurotransmitter receptor theory, suggesting that monoamine depletion results in 5HT receptor up-regulation and symptoms of depression. Prolonged drug exposure would then be necessary to desensitize the $5\text{-}HT_{1A}$ autoreceptors and to down-regulate postsynaptic

receptors. A neurophysiological explanation for the rapid response to SSRIs in PMDD remains unknown.

5-HT postsynaptic receptors are classified into four subtypes, $5\text{-}HT_1$ to $5\text{-}HT_4$, with further subdivision of the 5-HT1 subtypes:[79] the most important for mood regulation include the $5\text{-}HT_{1A}$, $5\text{-}HT_{2A}$, and $5\text{-}HT_{2C}$.[80–82] The $5\text{-}HT_3$ receptor is especially important as a chemoreceptor that controls emesis, and $5\text{-}HT_3$ and $5\text{-}HT_4$ receptors help to regulate gastrointestinal motility and appetite.[83,84] Side effects of serotonergic drugs such as SSRIs are generally related to the stimulation of the 5-HT 2A, 2C, 3, and 4 receptor subtypes. Acute stimulation of 2A and 2C receptors in various brain and peripheral regions can lead to agitation, restlessness,

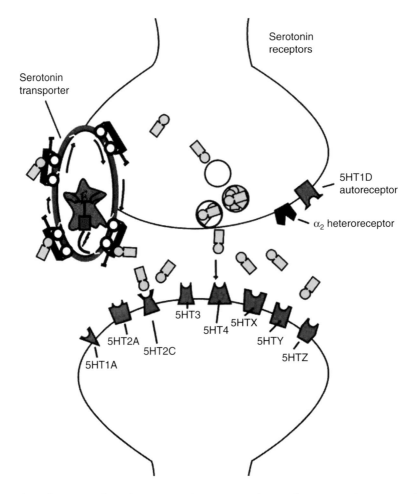

Figure 9.4 Illustration of presynaptic and postsynaptic receptor subtypes for seronergic neurons. (Reprinted from Stahl SM,[73] Chapter 5, page 172. © 2000. Reprinted with the permission of Cambridge University Press.)

myoclonus, nocturnal awakenings, and sexual dysfunction.[73] 5-HT$_3$ and 5-HT$_4$ receptors may be responsible for the gastrointestinal side effects of nausea, cramps, and diarrhea.[83]

Cell bodies containing serotonin are found primarily in the raphe nucleus of the brainstem and in nerve endings diffusely distributed throughout the brain.[66] 5-HT has been implicated in modulation of circadian rhythms, eating, mood, sleep, and arousal.[85] Projections from the raphe nucleus to the frontal cortex are important in mood regulation.[86] Projections to the basal ganglia help control movements and obsessions and compulsions.[87] Those to the limbic area are implicated in anxiety and panic reactions, whereas those to the hypothalamus regulate appetite and eating disorders.[88,89] Serotonergic neurons in the brainstem regulate sleep.[90] Projections down the spinal cord are involved in spinal

reflexes for sexual responses of orgasm and ejaculation.[91] 5-HT also has hormone-like effects when released into the bloodstream, regulating smooth muscle contraction and affecting platelet aggregation and immune systems. A deficiency of the serotonergic system could cause depression, anxiety, panic, obsessions, compulsions, and cravings for food.[86–89]

Serotonergic activity in the brain is also affected by estrogen and progesterone. Sex steroids can modify serotonin availability at the neuronal synapse.[92] Estrogen augments serotonin by increasing degradation of MAO and catechol O-methyltransferase (COMT), regulating the availability of free tryptophan in the brain, enhancing serotonin transport, and increasing the density of 5-HT-binding sites in brain regions affecting mood and cognition.[93] This is important, since MAO and COMT degrade 5-HT and determine its synaptic availability.

Estrogen has also been shown to improve the clinical effect of SSRIs.[94]

By contrast, progesterone increases MAO and COMT enzyme activity, acts as an antiestrogen, and down-regulates estrogen receptors.[93] Exogenously administered synthetic and natural progestins can induce negative mood, but this effect is dependent upon relative estrogen and progesterone dosages.[93,95,96] In summary, progesterone increases MAO, which decreases 5-HT availability and depressed mood, whereas estrogen decreases MAO activity, thus increasing 5-HT availability with resulting antidepressant effect.[97] It may be that these inter-relationships of sex steroids and serotonergic function are an oversimplification of the true picture and there may be some contradictions that will become evident as more research becomes available.

Serotonin, affective symptoms and PMS

Clinical substantiation for the role of serotonin in premenstrual disorders is supported by various lines of evidence, including:

1. Similarity between symptoms of PMS and those triggered by serotonin depletion paradigms,[4,98,99] such as depression and impulsive/aggressive behavior, irritability, anxiety, food cravings, and weight gain.
2. Decreased luteal phase platelet uptake of serotonin,[100] decreased luteal phase whole blood 5-HT at baseline,[101] and after either oral[102] or intravenous L-tryptophan challenge.[103]
3. Lack of significant improvement of PMS symptoms with antidepressants that augment only norepinepherine but not serotonin.
4. Numerous double-blind placebo-controlled trials demonstrating the efficacy of serotonergic agents administered continuously or solely in the luteal phase for the treatment of the severe form of PMS, premenstrual dysphoric disorder (PMDD).[104,105]

It must be remembered that extrapolation of therapeutic response to causality must always be viewed with caution.

SEROTONIN, GABA, AND PMS

There is evidence to support a link between the GABAergic and serotonergic neurotransmitter systems, and this link may be relevant to depressive disorders and PMS. SSRI treatment for major depression increases GABA concentration, especially in the occipital cortex.[106,107] GABA has been shown to regulate the activity of 5-HT neurons in the dorsal raphe nucleus through allopregnanolone-potentiated GABA$_A$-mediated inhibition.[108] Additionally, serotonergic neurons often terminate at inhibitory GABAergic interneurons in the hippocampus, suggesting a direct interaction.[109] 5-HT1a and 5-HT3 receptors have been localized to GABA interneurons in the cortex and hippocampus.[110,111] In the piriform cortex, 5-HT1a has been shown to increase the firing rate of GABAergic neurons.[112] Futhermore, in-vivo administration of a 5-HT1A receptor agonist enhances GABA$_A$-stimulated chloride ion influx.[113] In 5-HT1A receptor knock-out mice, there is an alteration of GABA$_A$ receptor subunits, receptor binding is reduced, and the mice develop benzodiazepine-resistant anxiety.[114] There clearly is a complex interaction between GABA and 5-HT neurons that may partially explain their influence on premenstrual mood and behavior.

ENDOGENOUS OPIOID PEPTIDES

Clinical background

The endorphin hypothesis of PMS was based on the recognition that some of the symptoms of PMS resembled those of opiate addiction and withdrawal, i.e. fatigue, depression, tension, anxiety, irritability, headaches, and pain sensitivity. It was hypothesized that women could become addicted to their own endogenous opiate peptides (EOPs).[115] One study demonstrated prevention of PMS symptoms with full-cycle treatment with naltrexone, an opioid antagonist used for opiate addiction.[116]

Endogenous opioid peptide physiology

Endogenous opioids include endorphins, enkephalins, dynorphins, and other peptides. Pro-opiomelanocortin (POMC) is the 31-kDa glycopeptide precursor that is cleaved to a number of smaller peptides, including endorphins, enkephalin, adrenocorticotropic hormone (ACTH), and melanocyte-stimulating hormone (MSH).[117] Proteolytic processing of POMC to certain small fractions appears to be tissue-specific, depending on the region of the brain.[118] POMC has been demonstrated in the anterior and intermediate lobes of the pituitary gland, hypothalamus, brain, sympathetic nervous system, lungs, adrenal medulla, gastrointestinal tract, reproductive tract, and placenta.[119–121] Proenkephalin A is a precursor for enkephalins, whereas proenkephalin B is the precursor for dynorphins. Proenkephalin A has been found in the adrenal medulla, posterior pituitary gland, brain, spinal cord, and gastrointestinal tract.[121] Proenkaphalin B is found in the brain and gastrointestinal tract.[121]

These endogenous opioid peptides bind to a multiplicity of opioid receptors, with different opiates possessing different selectivity for particular receptors.[121] Five opioid receptor types have been proposed, consisting of the μ, δ, κ, ε, and σ receptors.[122,123] Morphine binds preferentially to the μ-receptor, enkephalins to the δ-receptor, β-endorphin to the ε receptor, and dynorphin to the κ receptor.[124] The distribution of morphine and enkephalin receptors in the brain has been investigated with equal numbers in the cerebral cortex and striatum, twice as many morphine receptors as enkephalin receptors in the limbic system, hippocampus, and brainstem, and four times greater morphine receptors in the thalamus and hypothalamus.[125]

Specifically, β-endorphin is a polypeptide containing 31 amino acids with 5–10 times the potency of morphine. Endorphins regulate gonadotropin secretion and mediate pain response. Although widely distributed in the body, endorphins have the highest concentration within the arcuate nucleus and median eminence of the hypothalamus and the intermediate lobe of the pituitary gland.[126,127] The medial basal hypothalamus, which incorporates the arcuate nucleus, is an area also highly concentrated in gonodotropin-releasing hormone (GnRH)- and dopamine-containing cells.[128] High concentrations of β-endorphin have been found in the hypophyseal portal blood, suggesting that endogenous opioids of hypothalamic origin are secreted into the portal blood and may directly regulate pituitary peptide hormone secretion.[129] However, most studies support the notion that endogenous opioids probably decrease pituitary gonadotropin secretion by exerting effects on hypothalamic GnRH secretion, where endorphins are located in close proximity to GnRH-secreting cells, rather than direct pituitary stimulation.[130–132]

The concentration of β-endorphin in the hypophyseal portal blood varies in relation to the menstrual cycle. Studies in female monkeys have shown that β-endorphin is present in high concentrations during the mid-to-late follicular phase and the luteal phase, but undetectable at the time of menses and after ovariectomy.[133] Chronic administration of estrogen or estrogen with progesterone in ovariectomized monkeys restored detectable levels of β-endorphin in the hypophyseal portal blood.[134] These results suggest that ovarian steroids effect the release of hypothalamic β-endorphin into the hypophyseal portal blood, and cyclic changes in sex steroids during the menstrual cycle may affect anterior pituitary gonadotropin secretion through a mechanism involving β-endorphins.

In normal human subjects, opiate administration results in a significant decrease in luteinizing hormone (LH) secretion and an increase in prolactin secretion.[135] Naloxone, a competitive opioid antagonist, blocks the different subtypes of opioid receptors with different affinities, and has the greatest affinity for the μ and ε receptors. Naloxone administered in the late follicular and mid-luteal phases of the menstrual cycle in women increases the frequency and amplitude of LH pulses and circulating LH concentration, which suggests that endogenous opiates are involved in the regulation of LH secretion during the high estrogen and estrogen–progesterone phases of the menstrual cycle.[136,137] However, naloxone has no discernible effect on LH release during the early follicular phase when ovarian steroid secretion is minimal, further suggesting that gonadal steroids modify endogenous opiate activity.[136,138] The mid-cycle rise of estrogen and progesterone probably induces central opioid activity. Endogenous opioid activity is low in oophorectomized women, but estrogen treatment increases opioid activity and the addition of a progestin further increases the opioid activity. For example, in oophorectomized women treated with chronic conjugated estrogens or conjugated estrogens with medroxyprogesterone acetate, serum LH increases during naloxone infusion to levels found in ovulatory women.[139] In summary, evidence suggests that β-endorphin is an important determinant in modulating gonadotropin secretion during the menstrual cycle.

Endogenous opioid peptides, affective symptoms, and PMS

Differences in β-endorphin levels during the menstrual cycle have been established comparing women with PMS to controls. The β-endorphin levels are significantly lower during the luteal phase in women experiencing PMS.[140,141] Additionally, in control women, central opioid tone is enhanced during the mid luteal phase and becomes minimal in the late luteal phase, but women with PMS have low central opioid activity during the mid and late luteal phase as indicated by the loss of naloxone-induced LH release.[142–144] Low opioid tone has been associated with dysphoria, retarded motor activity, emotional liability, and lethargy, symptoms that are similar to those of PMS.[145,146] Therefore, attenuated central opioid tone may play a role in the pathophysiology of PMS.

There has also been evidence to suggest that endogenous opioid peptides may inhibit LH secretion through influence on the hypothalamic serotonergic system. Specifically, endogenous opiates seem to induce the release of serotonin and increase its turnover.[147–151] A dysfunction in this opioid–serotonin relationship could also contribute to the development of PMS symptoms, with decreased central opioid activity leading to lowered serotonin levels and mood deterioration.

In conclusion, it appears that the genesis of the symptoms of PMS may entail alterations of the serotogenic, GABA, and the endorphin systems. There is a growing body of evidence for the interaction of these networks in production of severe premenstrual symptoms. SSRIs, the current treatment of choice for PMDD, increase the activity of the enzymes required for the formation of allopregnanolone and, as a result, brain and CSF allopregnanolone concentrations.[41,152,153] Another serotonergic compound, L-tryptophan was also shown to increase peripheral allopregnanolone in women with PMS.[154] Reduced luteal phase GABAergic sensitivity in women with PMS was normalized after the administration of an SSRI.[54]

The connection between the GABA$_A$ receptor system, serotonin, and EOPs was recently highlighted by an investigation of LH response to an estrogen challenge, suggesting increased GnRH activity in women with PMS.[155] After estrogen exposure, GnRH is restrained tonically by GABA and by endogenous opioid peptides[41] and serotonin modulates the GABA$_A$ receptor complex.[155,156] Clearly, the fluctuation of sex steroids across the menstrual cycle profoundly affects all three candidate systems and it is likely that genetically programmed and environmentally driven differences are responsible for the defining features of each individual's affective, behavioral, and physical premenstrual state.

REFERENCES

1. Backström T. Neuroendocrinology of premenstrual syndrome. In: Pitkin RM, Scott JR, eds. Clinical Obstetrics and Gynecology. Philadelphia: JB Lippincott, 1992; 35:612–28.
2. O'Brien PM, Selby C, Symonds EM. Progesterone, fluid and electrolytes in premenstrual syndrome. Br Med J 1980; 280(6224):1161–3.
3. Backström T, Sanders D, Leask RM et al. Mood, sexuality, hormones and the menstrual cycle. II. Hormone levels and their relationship to premenstrual syndrome. Psychosom Med 1983; 45(6):503–7.
4. Rubinow DR, Hoban MC, Grover GN et al. Changes in plasma hormones across the menstrual cycle in patients with menstrually related mood disorder and in control subjects. Am J Obstet Gynecol 1988; 158(1):5–11.
5. Hammarback S, Damber J-E, Backström T. Relationship between symptom severity and hormone changes in patients with premenstrual syndrome. J Clin Endocrinol Metab 1989; 68(1):125–30.
6. Sampson GA. Premenstrual syndrome. A double-blind controlled trial of progesterone and placebo. Br J Psychiatry 1979; 135:209–15.
7. Rapkin AJ, Chang LC, Reading AE. Premenstrual syndrome: A double-blind placebo controlled study of treatment with progesterone vaginal suppository. J Obstet Gynaecol 1987; 7:217–20.
8. Freeman E, Rickels K, Sondheimer SJ et al. Ineffectiveness of progesterone suppository treatment for premenstrual syndrome. JAMA 1990; 264(3):349–53.
9. Rabow LE, Russek SJ, Farb DH. From ion currents to genomic analysis: recent advances in GABA$_A$ receptor research. Synapse 1995; 21(3):189–274.
10. Peng L, Hertz L, Huang R et al. Utilization of glutamine and of TCA cycle constituents as precursors for transmitter glutamate and GABA. Dev Neurosci 1993; 15:367–77.
11. Sherif FM. GABA-transaminase in brain and blood platelets: basic and clinical aspects. Prog Neuropsychopharmacol Biol Psychiatry 1994; 18:1219–33.
12. Watanabe M, Maemura K, Kanbara K, Tamayama T, Mayasaki H. GABA and GABA receptors in the central nervous system and other organs. Int Rev Cytol 2002; 213:1–47.
13. Olsen RW, Tobin AJ. Molecular biology of the GABA$_A$ receptors. FASEB J 1990; 4(5):1469–80.
14. Majewska MD, Harrison NL, Schwartz RD et al. Steroid hormone metabolites are barbiturate-like modulators of the GABA receptor. Science 1986; 232:1004–7.
15. Belelli D, Lambert JJ. Neurosteroids: endogenous regulators of the GABA(A) receptor. Nat Rev Neurosci 2005; 6:565–75.
16. Deutch AY, Roth RH. Neurotransmitters. In: Squire LR, Bloom FE, McConnell SK et al, eds. Fundamental Neuroscience, 2nd edn. New York: Academic Press; 2003:163–96.
17. Rupprecht R. Neuroactive steroids: mechanisms of action and neuropsychopharmacological properties. Psychoneuroendocrinology 2003; 28(2):139–68.
18. Guidotti A, Dong E, Matsumoto K et al. The socially-isolated mouse: a model to study the putative role of allopregnanolone and 5α-dihydroprogesterone in psychiatric disorders. Brain Res Brain Res Rev 2001; 37:110–15.
19. Majewska MD. Neurosteroids: endogenous bimodal modulators of the GABA-A receptor. Mechanism of action and physiological significance. Prog Neurobiol 1992; 38(4):379–95.
20. Belelli D, Herd MB, Mitchell EA et al. Neuroactive steroids and inhibitory neurotransmission: mechanisms of action and physiological relevance. Neuroscience 2006; 138(3):821–9.
21. Luddens H, Wisden W. Function and pharmacology of multiple GABA$_A$ receptor subunits. Trends Pharmacol Sci 1991; 12:49–51.
22. Wisden W, Laurie DJ, Monyer H et al. The distribution of 13 GABA$_A$ receptor subunit mRNAs in the rat brain. I. Telencephalon, diencephalon, mesencephalon. J Neurosci 1992; 12:1040–62.
23. Smith SS, Gong QH, Li X et al. Withdrawal from 3alpha-OH-5alpha-pregnan-20-one using a pseudopregnancy model alters the kinetics of hippocampal GABA$_A$-gated current and increases the GABA$_A$ receptor alpha4 subunit in association with increased anxiety. J Neurosci 1998; 18:5275–84.
24. Smith S, Gong Q, Hsu F et al. GABA(A) receptor alpha4 subunit suppression prevents withdrawal properties of an endogenous steroid. Nature 1998; 392(6679):926–30.
25. Gulinello M, Smith SS. Anxiogenic effects of neurosteroid exposure: sex differences and altered GABA$_A$ receptor pharmacology in adult rats. J Pharmacol Exp Ther 2003; 305(2):541–8.
26. Concas A, Mostallino M, Porcu P et al. Role of brain allopregnanolone in the plasticity of gamma-aminobutyric acid type A receptor in rat brain during pregnancy and after delivery. Proc Natl Acad Sci USA 1998; 95(22):13284–9.
27. Moran MH, Goldberg M, Smith SS. Progesterone withdrawal. II: insensitivity to the sedative effects of a benzodiazepine. Brain Res 1998; 807:91–100.
28. Maguire JL, Stell BM, Rafizadeh M et al. Ovarian cycle-linked changes in GABA(A) receptors mediating tonic inhibition alter seizure susceptibility and anxiety. Nat Neurosci 2005; 8(6):797–804.
29. Gulinello M, Gong QH, Li X et al. Short-term exposure to a neuroactive steroid increases alpha4 GABA(A) receptor subunit

levels in association with increased anxiety in the female rat. Brain Res 2001; 910:55–66.

30. Biggio G, Follesa P, Sanna E et al. GABA$_A$-receptor plasticity during long-term exposure to and withdrawal from progesterone. Int Rev Neurobiol 2001; 46:207–41.

31. Concas A, Follesa P, Barbaccia ML et al. Physiological modulation of GABA(A) receptor plasticity by progesterone metabolites. Eur J Pharmacol 1999; 375:225–35.

32. Follesa P, Floris S, Tuligi G et al. Molecular and functional adaptation of the GABA(A) receptor complex during pregnancy and after delivery in the rat brain. Eur J Neurosci 1998; 10:2905–12.

33. Follesa P, Porcu P, Sogliano C et al. Changes in GABA$_A$ receptor gamma 2 subunit gene expression induced by long-term administration of oral contraceptives in rats. Neuropharmacology 2002; 42:325–36.

34. Smith SS. Withdrawal properties of a neuroactive steroid: implications for GABA$_A$ receptor gene regulation in the brain and anxiety behavior. Steroids 2002; 67(6):519–28.

35. Concas A, Serra M, Atsoggiu T et al. Foot-shock stress and anxiogenic beta-carbolines increase t-[35S]butylbicyclo-phosphorothionate binding in the rat cerebral cortex, an effect opposite to anxiolytics and gamma-aminobutyric acid mimetics. J Neurochem 1988; 51:1868–76.

36. Sundström Poromaa I, Smith S, Gulinello M. GABA receptors, progesterone and premenstrual dysphoric disorder. Arch Womens Ment Health 2003; 6(1):23–41.

37. N-Wihlbäck AC, Sundström-Poromaa I, Bäckström T. Action by and sensitivity to neuroactive steroids in menstrual cycle related CNS disorders. Psychopharmacology (Berl) 2006; 186(3):388–401.

38. Bitran D, Klibansky DA, Martin GA. The neurosteroid pregnanolone prevents the anxiogenic-like effect of inescapable shock in the rat. Psychopharmacology (Berl) 2000; 151(1):31–7.

39. Molina-Hernandez M, Tellez-Alcantara NP. Antidepressant-like actions of pregnancy, and progesterone in Wistar rats forced to swim. Psychoneuroendocrinology 2001; 26:479–91.

40. Steimer T, Driscoll P, Schulz PE. Brain metabolism of progesterone, coping behaviour and emotional reactivity in male rats from two psychogenetically selected lines. J Neuroendocrinol 1997; 9:169–75.

41. Uzunova V, Sheline Y, Davis JM et al. Increase in the cerebrospinal fluid content of neurosteroids in patients with unipolar major depression who are receiving fluoxetine or fluvoxamine. Proc Natl Acad Sci USA 1998; 95(6):3239–44.

42. Brambilla P, Perez J, Barale F et al. GABAergic dysfunction in mood disorders. Mol Psychiatry 2003; 8:721–37.

43. Drugan RC, Morrow AL, Weizman R et al. Stress-induced behavioral depression in the rat is associated with a decrease in GABA receptor-mediated chloride ion flux and brain benzodiazepine receptor occupancy. Brain Res 1989; 487:45–51.

44. Gruen RJ, Wenberg K, Elahi R et al. Alterations in GABA$_A$ receptor binding in the prefrontal cortex following exposure to chronic stress. Brain Res 1995; 684:112–14.

45. Serra M, Pisu MG, Littera M et al. Social isolation-induced decreases in both the abundance of neuroactive steroids and GABA(A) receptor function in rat brain. J Neurochem 2000; 75:732–40.

46. Majewska MD, Harrison R, Schwartz R. Steroid hormone metabolites are barbiturate-like modulators of the GABA receptor. Science 1986; 232:1004.

47. Sanacora G, Mason GF, Krystal JH. Impairment of GABAergic transmission in depression: new insights from neuroimaging studies. Crit Rev Neurobiol 2000; 14:23–45.

48. Malizia AL, Cunningham VJ, Bell CJ et al. Decreased brain GABA(A)-benzodiazepine receptor binding in panic

disorder: preliminary results from a quantitative PET study. Arch Gen Psychiatry 1998; 55:715–20.

49. Rapkin A, Morgan M, Goldman L et al. Progesterone metabolite allopregnanolone in women with premenstrual syndrome. Obstet Gynecol 1997; 90(5):709–14.

50. Monteleone P, Luisi S, Tonetti A et al. Allopregnanolone concentrations and premenstrual syndrome. Eur J Endocrinol 2000; 142:269–73.

51. Schmidt PJ, Purdy RH, Moore PH Jr et al. Circulating levels of anxiolytic steroids in the luteal phase in women with premenstrual syndrome and in control subjects. J Clin Endocrinol Metab 1994; 79(5):1256–60.

52. Wang M, Seippel L, Purdy RH et al. Relationship between symptom severity and steroid variation in women with premenstrual syndrome: study on serum pregnenolone, pregnenolone sulfate, 5 alpha-pregnane-3,20-dione and 3 alpha-hydroxy-5 alpha-pregnan-20-one. J Clin Endocrinol Metab 1996; 81(3):1076–82.

53. Girdler SS, Straneva PA, Light KC et al. Allopregnanolone levels and reactivity to mental stress in premenstrual dysphoric disorder. Biol Psychiatry 2001; 49(9):788–97.

54. Sundström I, Andersson A, Nyberg S et al. Patients with premenstrual syndrome have a different sensitivity to a neuroactive steroid during the menstrual cycle compared to control subjects. Neuroendocrinology 1998; 67(2):126–38.

55. Sundström I, Nyberg S, Bäckström T. Patients with premenstrual syndrome have reduced sensitivity to midazolam compared to control subjects. Neuropsychopharmacology 1997; 17(6):370–81.

56. Friedman L, Gibbs TT, Farb DH. Gamma-aminobutyric acid A receptor regulation: chronic treatment with pregnanolone uncouples allosteric interactions between steroid and benzodiazepine recognition sites. Mol Pharmacol 1993; 44:191–7.

57. Yu R, Follesa P, Ticku MK. Down-regulation of the GABA receptor subunits mRNA levels in mammalian cultured cortical neurons following chronic neurosteroid treatment. Brain Res Mol Brain Res 1996; 41:163–8.

58. Carl P, Hogskilde S, Nielsen JW et al. Pregnanolone emulsion. A preliminary pharmacokinetic and pharmacodynamic study of a new intravenous anaesthetic agent. Anaesthesia 1990; 45:189–97.

59. Bitran D, Hilvers RJ, Kellogg CK. Anxiolytic effects of 3 alpha-hydroxy-5 alpha[beta]-pregnan-20-one: endogenous metabolites of progesterone that are active at the GABAA receptor. Brain Res 1991; 561:157–61.

60. Landgren S, Aasly J, Backstrom T et al. The effect of progesterone and its metabolites on the interictal epileptiform discharge in the cat's cerebral cortex. Acta Physiol Scand 1987; 131:33–42.

61. Andreen L, Sundstrom-Poromaa I, Bixo M et al. Relationship between allopregnanolone and negative mood in postmenopausal women taking sequential hormone replacement therapy with vaginal progesterone. Psychoneuroendocrinology 2005; 30:212–24.

62. Miczek KA, Fish EW, DeBold JF. Neurosteroids, GABA$_A$ receptors, and escalated aggressive behavior. Horm Behav 2003; 44(3):242–57.

63. Roy-Byrne PP, Rubinow DR, Gwirtsman H et al. Cortisol response to dexamethasone in women with premenstrual syndrome. Neuropsychobiology 1986; 16(2–3):61–3.

64. Roca CA, Schmidt PJ, Altemus M et al. Differential menstrual cycle regulation of hypothalamic–pituitary–adrenal axis in women with premenstrual syndrome and controls. J Clin Endocrinol Metab 2003; 88(7):3057–63.

65. Rapkin AJ, Buckman TD, Sutphin MS et al. Platelet monoamine oxidase B activity in women with premenstrual syndrome. Am J Obstet Gynecol 1988; 159:1536–40.

66. Jacobs BL, Azmitia EC. Structure and function of the brain serotonin system. Physiol Rev 1992; 72:165–229.

67. Leathwood PD. Tryptophan availability and serotonin synthesis. Proc Nutr Soc 1987; 46:143–56.

68. Hamon M, Bourgoin S, Artaud F et al. The respective roles of tryptophan uptake and tryptophan hydroxylase in the regulation of serotonin synthesis in the central nervous system. J Physiol (Paris) 1981; 77:269–79.

69. Boadle-Biber MC. Regulation of serotonin synthesis. Prog Biophys Mol Biol 1993; 60:1–15.

70. Fernstrom JD, Wurtman RJ. Brain serotonin content: physiological dependence on plasma tryptophan levels. Science 1971; 173:149–52.

71. Fernstrom JD. Role of precursor availability in control of monoamine biosynthesis in brain. Physiol Rev 1983; 63:484–546.

72. Aghajanian GK, Sprouse JS, Rasmussen K. Electrophysiology of central serotonin receptor subtypes. In: Saunders-Bush E, ed. The Serotonin Receptors. Clifton, NJ: The Humana Press; 1988:225–52.

73. Stahl SM. Depression and bipolar disorders. In: Grady MM, ed. Essential Psychopharmacology: Neuroscientific Basis and Practical Applications, 2nd edn. New York: Cambridge University Press; 2000:135–97.

74. White KJ, Walline CC, Barker EL. Serotonin transporters: implications for antidepressant drug development. AAPS J 2005; 7:E421–33.

75. Deakin JF. Depression and antisocial personality disorder: two contrasting disorders of 5-HT function. J Neural Transm Suppl 2003; 64:79–93.

76. Roggenbach J, Muller-Oerlinghausen B, Franke L. Suicidality, impulsivity and aggression – is there a link to 5HIAA concentration in the cerebrospinal fluid? Psychiatry Res 2002; 113:193–206.

77. Wikander I, Sundblad C, Andersch B et al. Citalopram in premenstrual dysphoria: is intermittent treatment during luteal phases more effective than continuous medication throughout the menstrual cycle? J Clin Psychopharmacol 1998; 18:390–8.

78. Artigas F, Romero L, de Montigny C et al. Acceleration of the effect of selected antidepressant drugs in major depression by 5-HT1A antagonists. Trends Neurosci 1996; 19:378–83.

79. Hoyer D, Clarke DE, Fozard JR et al. International Union of Pharmacology classification of receptors for 5-hydroxytryptamine (serotonin). Pharmacol Rev 1994; 46:157–203.

80. Caliendo G, Santagada V, Perissutti E et al. Derivatives as 5HT1A receptor ligands – past and present. Curr Med Chem 2005; 12:1721–53.

81. Anguelova M, Benkelfat C, Turecki G. A systematic review of association studies investigating genes coding for serotonin receptors and the serotonin transporter: I. Affective disorders. Mol Psychiatry 2003; 8:574–91.

82. Millan MJ. Serotonin 5-HT2C receptors as a target for the treatment of depressive and anxious states: focus on novel therapeutic strategies. Therapie 2005; 60:441–60.

83. Gershon MD. Review article: serotonin receptors and transporters – roles in normal and abnormal gastrointestinal motility. Aliment Pharmacol Ther 2004; 20:S3–14.

84. Gandara DR, Roila F, Warr D et al. Consensus proposal for 5-HT3 antagonists in the prevention of acute emesis related to highly emetogenic chemotherapy. Dose, schedule, and route of administration. Support Care Cancer 1998; 6:237–43.

85. Pucadyil TJ, Kalipatnapu S, Chattopadhyay A. The serotonin1A receptor: a representative member of the serotonin receptor family. Cell Mol Neurobiol 2005; 25:553–80.

86. Graeff FG, Guimaraes FS, De Andrade TG et al. Role of 5-HT in stress, anxiety, and depression. Pharmacol Biochem Behav 1996; 54(1):129–41.

87. Jenike MA, Rauch SL, Cummings JL et al. Recent developments in neurobiology of obsessive-compulsive disorder. J Clin Psychiatry 1996; 57:492–503.

88. Charney DS. Neuroanatomical circuits modulating fear and anxiety behaviors. Acta Psychiatr Scand Suppl 2003; 417:38–50.

89. Meguid MM, Fetissov SO, Varma M et al. Hypothalamic dopamine and serotonin in the regulation of food intake. Nutrition 2000; 16:843–57.

90. Dugovic C. Role of serotonin in sleep mechanisms. Rev Neurol (Paris) 2001; 157:S16–19.

91. Giuliano F, Clement P. Physiology of ejaculation: emphasis on serotonergic control. Eur Urol 2005; 48:408–17.

92. Hirschfeld RM. History and evolution of the monoamine hypothesis of depression. J Clin Psychiatry 2000; 61 (Suppl 6):4–6.

93. Schechter D. Estrogen, progesterone, and mood. J Gend Specif Med 1999; 2:29–36.

94. Schneider LS, Small GW, Hamilton SH et al. Estrogen replacement and response to fluoxetine in a multicenter geriatric depression trial. Fluoxetine Collaborative Study Group. Am J Geriatr Psychiatry 1997; 5:97–106.

95. Klaiber EL, Broverman DM, Vogel W et al. Individual differences in changes in mood and platelet monoamine oxidase (MAO) activity during hormonal replacement therapy in menopausal women. Psychoneuroendocrinology 1996; 21:575–92.

96. Magos AL, Brewster E, Singh R et al. The effects of norethisterone in postmenopausal women on oestrogen replacement therapy: a model for the premenstrual syndrome. Br J Obstet Gynaecol 1986; 93:1290–6.

97. Spinelli MG. Depression and hormone therapy. Clin Obstet Gynecol 2004; 47:428–36.

98. Roca CA, Schmidt PJ, Smith MJ et al. Effects of metergoline on symptoms in women with premenstrual dysphoric disorder. Am J Psychiatry 2002; 159(11):1876–81.

99. Menkes DB, Coates DC, Fawcett JP. Acute tryptophan depletion aggravates premenstrual syndrome. J Affect Disord 1994; 32(1):37–44.

100. Taylor DL, Mathew RJ, Ho BT et al. Serotonin levels and platelet uptake during premenstrual tension. Neuropsychobiology 1984; 12:16–8.

101. Rapkin AJ, Edelmuth E, Chang LC et al. Whole-blood serotonin in premenstrual syndrome. Obstet Gynecol 1987; 70:533–7.

102. Rapkin A, Chang LC, Reading A. Tryptophan loading test in premenstrual syndrome. J Obstet Gynecol 1989; 10:140–4.

103. Rasgon N, McGuire M, Tanavoli S et al. Neuroendocrine response to an intravenous L-tryptophan challenge in women with premenstrual syndrome. Fert Steril 2000; 73(1):144–9.

104. Dimmock PW, Wyatt KM, Jones PW et al. Efficacy of selective serotonin-reuptake inhibitors in premenstrual syndrome: a systematic review. Lancet 2000; 356:1131–6.

105. Wyatt KM, Dimmock PW, O'Brien PM. Selective serotonin reuptake inhibitors for premenstrual syndrome. Cochrane Database Syst Rev 2002; 4:CD001396.

106. Sanacora G, Mason GF, Rothman DL et al. Increased occipital cortex GABA concentrations in depressed patients after therapy with selective serotonin reuptake inhibitors. Am J Psychiatry 2002; 159:663–5.

107. Bhagwagar Z, Wylezinska M, Taylor M et al. Increased brain GABA concentrations following acute administration of a selective serotonin reuptake inhibitor. Am J Psychiatry 2004; 161:368–70.

108. Kaura V, Ingram CD, Gartside SE, Young AH, Judge SJ. The progesterone metabolite allopregnanolone potentiates GABA(A) receptor-mediated inhibition of 5-HT neuronal activity. Eur Neuropsychopharmacol 2007; 17(2):108–15.

109. Gulyas AI, Acsady L, Freund TF. Structural basis of the cholinergic and serotonergic modulation of GABAergic neurons in the hippocampus. Neurochem Int 1999; 34:359–72.

110. Morales M, Battenberg E, de Lecea L et al. The type 3 serotonin receptor is expressed in a subpopulation of GABAergic neurons in the rat neocortex and hippocampus. Brain Res 1996; 731:199–202.

111. Willins DL, Deutch AY, Roth BL. Serotonin 5-HT2A receptors are expressed on pyramidal cells and interneurons in the rat cortex. Synapse 1997; 27:79–82.

112. Gellman RL, Aghajanian GK. Pyramidal cells in piriform cortex receive a convergence of inputs from monoamine activated GABAergic interneurons. Brain Res 1993; 600:63–73.

113. Soderpalm B, Andersson G, Enerback C et al. In vivo administration of the 5-HT1A receptor agonist 8-OH-DPAT interferes with brain GABA(A)/benzodiazepine receptor complexes. Neuropharmacology 1997; 36:1071–7.

114. Sibille E, Pavlides C, Benke D et al. Genetic inactivation of the serotonin(1A) receptor in mice results in downregulation of major GABA(A) receptor alpha subunits, reduction of GABA(A) receptor binding, and benzodiazepine-resistant anxiety. J Neurosci 2000; 20:2758–65.

115. Vargyas J, Lobo R, Mishell DB. Brain opioid activity in the premenstrual syndrome. Fertil Steril 1984; 42:324.

116. Chuong CJ, Coulam CB, Bergstralh EJ et al. Clinical trial of naltrexone in premenstrual syndrome. Obstet Gynecol 1988; 72(3 Pt 1):332–6.

117. Krieger DT, Liotta AS, Brownstein MJ et al. ACTH, beta-lipotropin, and related peptides in brain, pituitary, and blood. Recent Prog Horm Res 1980; 36:277–344.

118. Facchinetti F, Petraglia F, Genazzani AR. Localization and expression of the three opioid systems. Semin Reprod Endocrinol 1987; 5:103.

119. Eipper BA, Mains RE. Structure and biosynthesis of pro-adrenocorticotropin/endorphin and related peptides. Endocr Rev 1980; 1:1–27.

120. Evans CJ, Erdelyi E, Weber E et al. Identification of pro-opiomelanocortin-derived peptides in the human adrenal medulla. Science 1983; 221:957–60.

121. Yen SS, Quigley ME, Reid RL et al. Neuroendocrinology of opioid peptides and their role in the control of gonadotropin and prolactin secretion. Am J Obstet Gynecol 1985; 152:485–93.

122. Miller RJ. Multiple opiate receptors for multiple opioid peptides. Med Biol 1982; 60:1–6.

123. Grossman A. Brain opiates and neuroendocrine function. Clin Endocrinol Metab 1983; 12:725–46.

124. Seifer DB, Collins RL. Current concepts of beta-endorphin physiology in female reproductive dysfunction. Fertil Steril 1990; 54:757–71.

125. Chang KJ, Cooper BR, Hazum E et al. Multiple opiate receptors: different regional distribution in the brain and differential binding of opiates and opioid peptides. Mol Pharmacol 1979; 16:91–104.

126. Wilkes MM, Watkins WB, Stewart RD et al. Localization and quantitation of beta-endorphin in human brain and pituitary. Neuroendocrinology 1980; 30:113–21.

127. Watkins WB, Yen SS, Moore RY. Presence of beta-endorphin-like immunoreactivity in the anterior pituitary gland of rat and man and evidence for the differential localization with ACTH. Cell Tissue Res 1981; 215:577–89.

128. Silverman AJ, Antunes JL, Abrams GM et al. The luteinizing hormone-releasing hormone pathways in rhesus (Macaca mulatta) and pigtailed (Macaca nemestrina) monkeys: new observations on thick, unembedded sections. J Comp Neurol 1982; 221:309–17.

129. Wardlaw SL, Wehrenberg WB, Ferin M et al. High levels of beta-endorphin in hypophyseal portal blood. Endocrinology 1980; 106:1323–6.

130. Ferin M, Wehrenberg WB, Lam NY et al. Effects and site of action of morphine on gonadotropin secretion in the female rhesus monkey. Endocrinology 1982; 111:1652–6.

131. Rasmussen DD, Liu JH, Wolf PL et al. Endogenous opioid regulation of gonadotropin-releasing hormone release from the human fetal hypothalamus in vitro. J Clin Endocrinol Metab 1983; 57:881–4.

132. Blank MS, Roberts DL. Antagonist of gonadotropin-releasing hormone blocks naloxone-induced elevations in serum luteinizing hormone. Neuroendocrinology 1982; 35:309–12.

133. Wehrenberg WB, Wardlaw SL, Frantz AG et al. Beta-Endorphin in hypophyseal portal blood: variations throughout the menstrual cycle. Endocrinology 1982; 111:879–81.

134. Wardlaw SL, Wehrenberg WB, Ferin M et al. Effect of sex steroids on beta-endorphin in hypophyseal portal blood. J Clin Endocrinol Metab 1982; 55:877–81.

135. Reid RL, Hoff JD, Yen SS et al. Effects of exogenous beta h-endorphin on pituitary hormone secretion and its disappearance rate in normal human subjects. J Clin Endocrinol Metab 1981; 52:1179–84.

136. Quigley ME, Yen SS. The role of endogenous opiates in LH secretion during the menstrual cycle. J Clin Endocrinol Metab 1980; 51:179–81.

137. Ropert JF, Quigley ME, Yen SS. Endogenous opiates modulate pulsatile luteinizing hormone release in humans. J Clin Endocrinol Metab 1981; 52:583–5.

138. Blankstein J, Reyes FI, Winter JS et al. Endorphins and the regulations of the human menstrual cycle. Clin Endocrinol (Oxf) 1981; 14:287–94.

139. Shoupe D, Montz FJ, Lobo RA. The effects of estrogen and progestin on endogenous opioid activity in oophorectomized women. J Clin Endocrinol Metab 1985; 60:178–83.

140. Reid RL, Yen SS. Premenstrual syndrome. Am J Obstet Gynecol 1981; 139:85–104.

141. Chuong CJ, Coulam CB, Kao PC et al. Neuropeptide levels in premenstrual syndrome. Fertil Steril 1985; 44:760–5.

142. Chuong CJ, Hsi BP. Effect of naloxone on luteinizing hormone secretion in premenstrual syndrome. Fertil Steril 1994; 61(6):1039–44.

143. Rapkin AJ, Shoupe D, Reading A et al. Decreased central opioid activity in premenstrual syndrome: luteinizing hormone response to naloxone. J Soc Gynecol Investig 1996; 3:93–8.

144. Facchinetti F, Martignoni E, Petraglia F et al. Premenstrual fall of plasma beta-endorphin in patients with premenstrual syndrome. Fertil Steril 1987; 47:570–3.

145. Mendelson JH, Ellingboe J, Keuhnle JC et al. Effects of naltrexone on mood and neuroendocrine function in normal adult males. Psychoneuroendocrinology 1978; 3:231–6.

146. Cohen MR, Cohen RM, Pickar D et al. Behavioural effects after high dose naloxone administration to normal volunteers. Lancet 1981; 2:1110.

147. Van Loon GR, De Souza EB. Effects of beta-endorphin on brain serotonin metabolism. Life Sci 1978; 23:971–8.

148. Brase DA. Roles of serotonin and gamma-aminobutyric acid in opioid effects. Adv Biochem Psychopharmacol 1979; 20:409–28.

149. Foresta C, Scanelli G, Tramarin A et al. Serotonin but not dopamine is involved in the naloxone-induced luteinizing hormone release in man. Fertil Steril 1985; 43:447–50.

150. Vugt DA, Meites J. Influence of endogenous opiates on anterior pituitary function. Fed Proc 1980; 39:2533–8.

151. Haubrich DR, Blake DE. Modification of serotonin metabolism in rat brain after acute or chronic administration of morphine. Biochem Pharmacol 1973; 22:2753–9.

152. Mellon SH, Griffin LD. Neurosteroids: biochemistry and clinical significance. Trends Endocrinol Met 2002; 13(1):35–43.

153. Guidotti A, Uzunov DP, Costa E. Fluoxetine treatment selectively causes brain accumulation of allopregnanolone (ALLO). Biol Psychiatry 1996; 39(7):592–3.

154. Rasgon N, Serra M, Biggio G et al. Neurosteroid-serotonergic interaction: responses to an intravenous L-tryptophan challenge in women with premenstrual dysphoric disorder. Eur J Endocrinol 2001; 145:25–33.

155. Eriksson O, Bäckström T, Stridsberg M et al. Differential response to estrogen challenge test in women with and without premenstrual dysphoria. Psychoneuroendocrinology 2006; 31:415–27.

156. Tunnicliff G, Schindler NL, Crites GJ et al. The GABA(A) receptor complex as a target for fluoxetine action. Neurochem Res 1999; 24(10):1271–6.

10

Pathophysiology I: role of ovarian steroids

David R Rubinow and Peter J Schmidt

INTRODUCTION

A comprehensive review of the early endocrine studies of premenstrual syndrome (PMS) was performed by Reid and Yen[1] and, as described elsewhere,[2] most of these studies suffered from methodologic flaws, including the use of inadequate diagnostic criteria. PMS is a time-oriented not a symptom-oriented diagnosis and requires prospective demonstration that symptom appearance is confined primarily to the luteal phase of the woman's menstrual cycle. Since 1983, the use of two sets of diagnostic guidelines – Diagnostic and Statistical Manual of Mental Disorders, fourth edition (DSM-IV),[3] and National Institute of Mental Health (NIMH) Premenstrual Syndrome Workshop Guidelines, unpublished work[4] – has permitted greater homogeneity of samples across studies, a requirement for comparison, and generalization of results obtained. Data subsequently generated provide little if any evidence for a role of hormone excess or deficiency in the etiology of PMS.

Hormonal studies in women with PMS have employed several different strategies:

- examination of symptoms after the administration of hormones hypothesized to be deficient in women with PMS
- measurement of basal hormone levels at selected points in the menstrual cycle
- evaluation of dynamic endocrine function employing frequent serial monitoring of hormone secretion or endocrine challenge paradigms
- manipulation of menstrual cycle physiology in order to examine the plasticity of the linkage between the menstrual cycle and PMS symptoms.

The most frequently employed strategy has been the comparison of luteal phase basal hormone levels with those from the follicular phase in women with PMS or with comparable values from a non-PMS control group.

In this chapter we focus on the roles of ovarian steroids in the pathophysiology of PMS. Additionally, we include studies investigating hypothalamic–pituitary–adrenal (HPA) axis function in PMS, since this axis is regulated by ovarian steroids, and abnormalities of HPA axis function are reported in PMS. First, we provide background information reviewing the physiology of ovarian steroids and their cellular mechanisms of action. Secondly, we describe examples of the neuromodulatory actions of gonadal steroids in both preclinical and human studies. Thirdly, we focus on the regulatory effects of gonadal steroids on systems relevant to the pathophysiology of PMS and affective adaptation, including a section on the regulatory effects of ovarian steroids on HPA axis function. Finally, we present studies on the role of ovarian hormones in PMS categorized on the basis of the research strategies employed.

GONADAL STEROID HORMONES

Synthesis and metabolism

Gonadal steroids, like all steroid hormones, are derivatives of cholesterol. Steroidogenic acute regulatory protein (STAR) is the critical regulator of cholesterol's availability within the mitochondria, where it is converted by the enzyme cholesterol desmolase to pregnenolone.[5,6] Pregnenolone then serves as the precursor for the whole family of steroid hormones, individual members of which are generated through the actions of a relatively small number of enzymes with multiple sites of action (Figure 10.1). The resulting end products of this cascade are determined by the tissue in which the metabolism is occurring and the enzymes present in that tissue. For example, testosterone may be the end product and act directly at the androgen receptor, or it may be reduced to a form with greater affinity for the androgen receptor (dihydrotestosterone), converted to

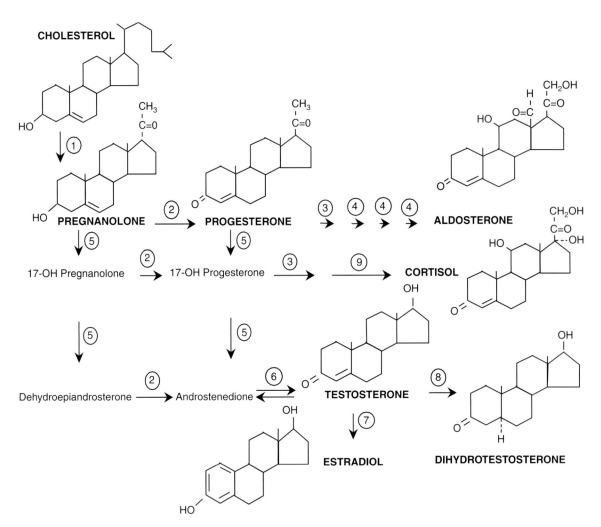

Figure 10.1 Synthetic pathways for steroid hormones. Circled numbers identify synthetic enzymes: **1**, cytochrome P450 (CYP) 11A (cholesterol desmolase); **2**, 3β-hydroxysteroid dehydrogenase; **3**, CYP21 (21-hydroxylase); **4**, CYP11B2 (11β-hydroxylase, 18-hydroxylase, 18-oxidase); **5**, CYP17 (17α-hydroxylase, 17,20-lyase); **6**, 17β-hydroxysteroid dehydrogenase (or oxidoreductase); **7**, aromatase; **8**, 5α-reductase; **9**, CYP11B1 (11β-hydroxylase).

a form with less affinity for the androgen receptor (androsterone), or aromatized to estradiol and act through the estrogen receptor.

As steroid hormones are highly homologous and serve as precursors for one another, the manner in which steroids are metabolized can markedly change the amplitude or nature of the steroid signal. Steroid metabolic enzymes, then, can contribute to the variance in a steroid signal in several ways. First, enzymes regulate the activation and potency of steroid hormones: seen, for example, with the enzyme (5α-reductase), which converts testosterone into dihydrotestosterone (DHT), an androgen with

fourfold greater affinity for the androgen receptor and fivefold greater stability.[7] Secondly, enzymes determine the receptor system that is activated: seen, for example, in the conversion by aromatase of testosterone (acting at the androgen receptor) to estradiol (acting at estrogen receptors α and/or β). Thirdly, the metabolism of steroids can facilitate or inhibit the accumulation of metabolites that may be neurotoxic: seen, for example, with the ability of 5α-reductase to shunt testosterone away from the pathway, leading to accumulation of estradiol, which can function as a neurotoxin.[8,9] Fourthly, enzymes may produce steroid metabolites that have a completely different neuromodulatory profile from that of the parent hormones: seen, for example, with the conversion of progesterone to the neurosteroid allopregnanolone or DHT to the neurosteroid androsterone (by 5α-reductase and 3α-hydroxysteroid oxidoreductase [3α-HSOR]), both potent modulators of the γ-aminobutyric acid (GABA) receptor chloride ionophore.[10,11] Since many of the enzymes have multiple steroid substrates, a single enzyme's activity may regulate the relative amounts of different behaviorally active metabolites: for example, 3α-HSOR both inactivates the androgen DHT (at the androgen receptor) and produces the neurosteroids allopregnanolone and androsterone.[12] Not only will different metabolic profiles activate or inhibit different receptor systems but also the consequence of the activation of a given steroid receptor will differ depending upon which hormones are present. Estradiol and cortisol, for example, exert opposing effects on AP1-modulated genes through interactions with the cointegrator CBP/P300.[13] A steroid hormone, then, may produce markedly different effects, depending upon its metabolism and the hormonal context in which it is acting. Finally, abnormalities of these metabolic enzymes occur secondary to genotypic variation and, therefore, one metabolic product could be selectively favored over others. Several genetically based abnormalities of steroid metabolism exist, and investigators speculate that similar variants in the enzymes required for neurosteroid synthesis may underlie behavioral disorders, including PMS.

Mechanisms of actions

The classic action of steroid hormones occurs after the steroid binds (activates) its intracellular receptor, which, after undergoing phosphorylation and release from heat shock proteins, binds (usually as a dimer) to a hormone response element on a gene and directs or modifies transcription of that gene. Once the ligand–receptor complex binds to the hormone response element (which is located on or near the promoter of the gene), the result can be either the initiation or repression of transcription of messages coding for an array of proteins, including synthetic and metabolic enzymes for neurotransmitters, neuropeptides, receptor proteins (both membranous and intracellular), transporters, and second messengers.

Several factors may influence the genomic actions of gonadal steroids and account for their widespread and variable effects. First, isoforms of both the androgen and progesterone receptors exist, and each isoform has different transcriptional effects. Two separate estrogen receptors, α and β, exist and are coded for by genes on the 6th and 14th chromosomes, respectively. These estrogen receptors have different distributions in the brain,

different transcriptional actions, and even possess additional isoforms (e.g. insertional and deletional variants of ER α and β). Secondly, the activated steroid receptor regulates transcription by binding protein intermediaries called coregulators (both stimulatory and inhibitory). Coregulators are expressed in a tissue-specific fashion, and their differential localization may contribute to functional variability in the effects of the same hormone in different tissues despite the presence of similar concentrations of both ligand and receptor. Thirdly, activated hormone receptors can influence the transcription of genes that do not possess hormone response elements through interactions with other cellular proteins called cointegrators, which enable hormones to regulate genes at transcription factor binding elements (e.g. AP-1, SP-1 sites). Fourthly, steroid hormone receptors can be activated by a variety of neurotransmitters (e.g. dopamine through D_1 receptor) and growth factors, even in the absence of steroid hormones. In this fashion environmental events (e.g. stressors) can impact the response to a steroid hormone signal. Finally, hormones may influence each other's activity by competing for cofactors or by producing opposing regulatory effects on genes through integrator proteins.

The relatively slow, 'genomic' effects of gonadal steroids have been expanded in two dimensions: time, with a variety of rapid (seconds to minutes) effects observed; and targets, which now include ion channels and a variety of second messenger systems. For example, estradiol (E_2), in just minutes, increases firing of neurons in the cerebral cortex and hippocampus (CA1)[14] and decreases firing in medial preoptic neurons.[15] The activity of membrane receptors like the glutamate and GABA receptors is acutely modulated by gonadal steroids (estradiol and the 5α-reduced metabolite of progesterone, allopregnanolone, respectively).[10,16] Estradiol binds to and modulates the Maxi-K potassium channel,[17] increases cyclic adenosine monophosphate (cAMP) levels,[18] regulates membrane G proteins ($G_{\alpha i}$, $G_{\alpha q}$; $G_{\alpha s}$)[19] (Manji et al, unpublished work), inhibits L-type calcium channels (via non-classical receptor),[20] and immediately activates the mitogen-activated protein kinase (MAPK) pathway (albeit in a receptor-mediated fashion).[21] The effects observed are tissue- and even cell-specific (e.g. estradiol increases MAPK in neurons but decreases it in astrocytes).[22,23] Finally, both estradiol and progesterone[24,25] phosphorylate dopamine- and cAMP-regulated phosphoprotein-32 (DARPP-32), which is an important regulator of the phosphorylation state of many cellular proteins and, therefore, an important regulator of neural function.[26] The increase in the number of described mechanisms by which gonadal steroids can impact on cell function has paralleled the rapid growth in their observed effects. Consequently, with each of these newly identified actions (which are usually, but sometimes inaccurately, called 'non-genomic'), one needs to examine multiple factors prior to inferring the mechanism of action:

- the duration required to see the effect
- the impact on the effect of inhibitors of transcription and protein synthesis
- the presence (or absence) of intracellular steroid hormone receptors
- the stereospecificity of ligand binding (to see if effects are mediated through a classical receptor)
- the effect of hormone receptor blockers
- the ability of the ligand to initiate the action from the cell membrane (i.e. when entry into the cell is blocked).

This last requirement acknowledges the presence on the membrane of binding sites for gonadal steroids that increasingly seem to be physiologically relevant.[27]

NEUROMODULATORY EFFECTS OF OVARIAN STEROIDS

The best support for the importance of the neuromodulatory actions of gonadal steroids is found in their dramatic and widely ranging effects on the brain. In fact, gonadal steroids have been shown to play a role in all stages of neural development, including neurogenesis, synaptogenesis, neural migration, growth, differentiation, survival, and death.[28] These effects occur largely as a consequence of the ability of gonadal steroids to modulate genomic transcription. As transcriptional regulators, the receptors for gonadal steroids direct or modulate the synthesis of the synthetic and metabolic enzymes as well as receptor proteins for many neurotransmitters and neuropeptides.[29] The advances of the past 15 years, however, have demonstrated that the cellular effects of gonadal steroids are far more complex and wide-reaching than suggested by their originally described genomic actions.

Gonadal steroids regulate cell survival. Neuroprotective effects of E_2 have been described in neurons grown in serum-free media or those exposed to glutamate, amyloid, hydrogen peroxide, or glucose deprivation.[14] Some of these effects appear to lack stereospecificity (i.e. are not classical receptor-mediated effects) and may be attributed to the antioxidant properties of E_2,[30,31] although data from one report are consistent with a receptor-mediated effect.[32] Gonadal steroids may also modulate cell survival through effects on cell survival proteins (e.g. Bcl-2, BAX), MAPK, Akt or even amyloid precursor protein metabolism.[22,23,33,34]

Some actions of gonadal steroids on brain appear to be context- and developmental stage-dependent. Toran-Allerand[35] has shown that estrogen displays reciprocal interactions with growth factors and their receptors (e.g. p51 and neurotrophins, trkA) in such a way as to regulate, throughout development, the response to estrogen stimulation: estrogen stimulates its own receptor early in development, inhibits it during adulthood, and stimulates it again in the context of brain injury. Additionally, we have demonstrated that the ability to modulate serotonin receptor subtype and GABA receptor subunit transcription in rat brain with exogenous administration of gonadal steroids or gonadal steroid receptor blockade is largely dependent on the developmental stage (e.g. last prenatal week vs fourth postnatal week) during which the intervention occurs[36] (Zhang et al, unpublished data).

Finally, the effects of gonadal steroids do not occur in isolation but, rather, in exquisite interaction with the environment. Juraska,[37] for example, demonstrated that the rearing environment (enriched vs impoverished) dramatically influences sex differences in dendritic branching in the rat cortex and hippocampus. Further, the size of the spinal nucleus of the bulbocavernosus and the degree of adult male sexual behavior in rats is in part regulated by the amount of anogenital licking they receive as pups from their mothers, an activity that is elicited from the dames by the androgen the pups secrete in their urine.[38]

The vicissitudes of gonadal steroids and their receptors, therefore, both direct neural architecture and provide the means by which the response of the central nervous system (CNS) to incoming stimuli may be altered. The extent to which these effects underlie or contribute to differential pharmacological efficacy or behavioral differences observed across individuals is unclear but is of considerable potential relevance for PMS and other reproductive endocrine-related mood disorders.

ROLE OF OVARIAN STEROIDS IN MODULATING THE SYSTEMS INVOLVED IN AFFECTIVE ADAPTATION AND PREMENSTRUAL SYNDROME

Neuroregulation

Results from animal studies demonstrate that ovarian steroids influence several of the neuroregulatory systems thought to be involved in both the pathophysiology of affective disorders and PMS.[39–41] Preclinical studies have documented the myriad of effects of ovarian steroids on neurotransmitter system activities, including regulation of synthetic and metabolic enzyme production as well as receptor and transporter protein activity. The modulatory effects of ovarian steroids on the serotonin (5-hydroxytryptamine; 5-HT) system have been extensively studied, reflecting in part interest in the higher prevalence of depression in women and the efficacy of selective serotonin reuptake inhibitors in PMS. In some, but not all (reviewed in Rubinow et al[42]), experimental paradigms, estradiol has been observed to inhibit serotonin reuptake transporter (SERT) mRNA,[43] decrease activity of the $5HT_{1A}$ receptor (down-regulation and uncoupling from its G protein),[44,45] increase $5\text{-}HT_{2A}$[46] receptor binding and mRNA,[47] and facilitate imipramine-induced down-regulation of $5\text{-}HT_2$ receptors in the rat frontal cortex, an action seen to accompany antidepressant administration.[48] $5HT_{1A}$ receptor binding, which is decreased in depression, is modulated by both estradiol[14,49–53] and progesterone.[54–57] Similarly, SERT message, protein, and binding have been reported to be changed by ovarian steroids in preclinical studies.[42,43,57–60]

In humans there are patterns of effects of ovarian steroids on the serotonin system similar to those observed in animals. Menstrual cycle phase effects on the concomitants of serotonergic stimulation include an increased prolactin secretion during the luteal phase after *m*-chlorophenylpiperazine (*m*-CPP)[61] and buspirone[62] administration compared to the early follicular phase, and a decreased prolactin response following L-tryptophan[63] or d-fenfluramine[64] compared to mid-cycle. Indeed, prolactin secretion is increased after progesterone administration in women with gonadotropin-releasing hormone (GnRH) agonist-induced hypogonadism.[65] Finally, although the effect of estrogen on $5\text{-}HT_{1A}$ receptor binding has not been examined in humans, one uncontrolled study reported an increase in $5\text{-}HT_{2A}$ binding (^{18}F altanserin) in the anterior cingulate, dorsolateral prefrontal cortex, and lateral orbital frontal cortex during combined estrogen and progestin replacement (but not after estradiol alone).[66]

Finally, several non-classical neural signaling systems have been identified as potential mediators of the therapeutic actions of antidepressants and electroconvulsive therapy (ECT) (e.g. c-AMP response element-binding protein [CREB] and brain-derived neurotrophic factor [BDNF][67]) based on observations that these systems are modulated by a range of therapies effective in depression (e.g. serotonergic and noradrenergic agents and ECT) and exhibit a pattern of change consistent with the latency to therapeutic efficacy for most antidepressants.[68] For example, antidepressants increase the expression and activity of CREB in certain brain regions (e.g. hippocampus)[69] and regulate (in a brain region-specific manner) activity of genes with a cAMP response element.[68] Genes for BDNF and its receptor trkB have been proposed as potential targets for antidepressant-related changes in CREB activity.[68] Similarly, estradiol has been reported to influence many of these same neuroregulatory processes. Specifically, ovariectomy has been reported to decrease, and estradiol increase, BDNF levels in the forebrain and hippocampus.[70] Estrogen also increases CREB activity,[71] trkA,[72] and decreases GSK-3β activity (Wnt pathway)[73] in the rat brain, changes similar to those seen with mood stabilizer drugs. In contrast, an estradiol-induced decrease in BDNF has been reported to mediate estradiol's regulation of dendritic spine formation in hippocampal neurons.[74] Thus, the therapeutic potential of gonadal steroids in depression is suggested not only by their widespread actions on neurotransmitter systems but also by certain neuroregulatory actions shared by both ovarian steroids and traditional therapies for depression (i.e. antidepressants, ECT).

Neurocircuitry

Several studies have employed neuroimaging techniques (i.e. positron emission tomography [PET] or functional magnetic resonance imaging [fMRI]) to examine the effects of ovarian steroids or the normal menstrual cycle on regional cerebral blood flow under conditions of cognitive activation. For example, using PET ($H_2^{15}O$) Berman et al[75] employed the Wisconsin Card Sort Test, a measure of executive function and cognitive set shifting, and observed that both estradiol and progesterone regulated cortical activity in brain regions (prefrontal cortex, parietal and temporal cortex, and hippocampus) also reported to be involved in the regulation of mood. Similarly, Shaywitz et al[76] reported, in a randomized, double-blind, placebo-controlled crossover trial, that postmenopausal women did not perform differently on estrogen therapy (ET) compared with placebo, but fMRI during ET showed significantly increased activation in the inferior parietal lobule and right superior frontal gyrus during verbal encoding, with significant decreases in the inferior parietal lobule during non-verbal coding. More recently, fMRI studies have documented menstrual cycle phase-related changes in the activities of several brain regions involved in the neurocircuitry of both arousal and reward processing, including the amygdala, orbitofrontal cortex, and striatum.[77,78,209] Although the brain regions potentially regulated by estrogen are inadequately characterized, the activities in the frontal cortex and hippocampus, areas subserving memory and the regulation of affect, appear to be regulated by ovarian steroids.

Stress axis

Extensive studies in animals demonstrate that both sex and reproductive steroids regulate basal and stimulated HPA axis function. In general, low-dose, short-term administration of estradiol inhibits HPA axis responses in ovariectomized animals,[79–82] whereas higher doses and longer treatment regimens enhance HPA axis reactivity to stressors.[83–85] The regulatory effects of changes in reproductive steroids or menstrual cycle phase on the HPA axis in women are less well studied. Although some studies using psychological stressors identified increased stimulated cortisol in the luteal phase,[86,87] others using psychological[88,89] or physiological (e.g. insulin-induced hypoglycemia, exercise)[90,91] stressors failed to find a luteal phase increase in HPA axis activity.

Altemus et al[92] recently demonstrated that exercise-stimulated HPA responses were increased in the mid-luteal compared with the follicular phase. However, in contrast to a large animal literature documenting the ability of estradiol to increase HPA axis secretion, Roca et al[93] found that progesterone, but not estradiol, significantly increased exercise-stimulated arginine vasopressin (AVP), adrenocorticotropic hormone (ACTH), and cortisol secretion compared with a leuprolide-induced hypogonadal condition or estradiol replacement. The mechanism by which progesterone augments stimulated HPA axis activity is currently unknown but could include the following: modulation of cortisol feedback restraint of the axis;[79,94–97] neurosteroid-related down-regulation of GABA receptors;[98] and up-regulation of AVP (consistent with luteal phase reductions in the threshold for AVP release).[99] Alternatively, Ochedalski et al suggest that progesterone enhances oxytocin-induced corticotropin-releasing hormone (CRH).[210]

ENDOCRINE STUDIES IN PREMENSTRUAL SYNDROME

Effects of hormone 'replacement' therapies

Despite the lack of evidence of ovarian dysfunction in women with PMS, the view that an abnormality of corpus luteum function caused PMS endured, largely because of the temporal association of PMS symptoms with the luteal phase of the menstrual cycle. Thus, multiple trials were conducted involving the administration of progesterone or progestin in women with PMS.[100] The widespread use of progesterone in women with PMS was considerably diminished, however, by the results of several recent studies. First, two large double-blind, placebo-controlled trials of natural progesterone (both suppository and oral forms) definitively demonstrated the lack of efficacy of progesterone compared with placebo in PMS.[101,102] Secondly, a study employing a progesterone receptor antagonist, RU-486, with or without human chorionic gonadotropin demonstrated that the normal symptoms of PMS could occur independent of the luteal phase of the menstrual cycle[103]

and, therefore, a luteal phase abnormality as a cause of PMS was no longer tenable.

The belief that PMS reflected a disturbance in ovarian function led to several trials of oral contraceptives (OCs) to suppress or regulate ovarian function in this condition. Earlier cross-sectional studies suggested that women using OCs experienced fewer PMS symptoms than non-users,[104–106] although opposite results were also reported.[107] Most studies demonstrated that women on OCs reported fewer physical symptoms (i.e. breast pain, bloating) but did not report fewer or less severe mood symptoms than non-users.[108–110] In fact, similar prevalence rates of cyclic mood symptoms, regardless of OC use, were prospectively documented by Sveindottir and Backstrom,[111] with 2–6% of women meeting criteria for severe PMS in both OC users and non-users. Despite similar prevalence rates of negative mood symptoms in OC users and non-users, some clinic-based studies suggested that a subgroup of women with PMS reported an improvement in mood symptoms while on OCs.[112–117] Results of recent controlled trials of OCs in PMS parallel those of the cross-sectional studies.[118–120] Significant reductions in symptom severity on OCs compared with placebo were observed, however, for some physical and behavioral symptoms, including loss of libido,[119] breast pain, and bloating,[118] and increased appetite and food cravings.[120] Thus, with one recent exception,[121] neither cross-sectional studies nor controlled trials support a role for any formulation of OCs (tested to date) in the treatment of PMS.

The efficacy in PMS of estradiol (without the progestin contained in OCs) and testosterone have also been tested. Trials of supraphysiological doses of estradiol with or without testosterone have documented beneficial effects compared with placebo in women with PMS.[122–124] Preliminary reports suggest that lower (more physiological) doses of testosterone alone may also be effective in the treatment of PMS.[125–127] Lower doses of estrogen, however, are not more effective than placebo[128] and, therefore, it is possible that the therapeutic benefits of the higher-dose estrogens are secondary to the suppression of ovulation.[124] Nevertheless, one cannot infer the efficacy of these compounds to be secondary to ovarian suppression alone, given the lack of efficacy of OCs which also inhibit ovulation, and the reported efficacy of compounds such as danazol[129] when administered after ovulation in at least one study.[130]

Basal hormone studies

As noted above, the temporal coincidence of symptoms and the luteal phase in women with PMS led to the presumption that reproductive endocrine function was disturbed in these patients. Comparisons of basal plasma hormone levels in women with PMS and controls, however, have revealed no consistent diagnosis-related differences. Specifically, we observed no diagnosis-related differences in the plasma levels, areas under the curve (AUCs), or patterns of hormone secretion for estradiol, progesterone, follicle-stimulating hormone (FSH), or luteinizing hormone (LH),[131] findings consistent with those of Backstrom et al[132] comparing patients with high and low degrees of cyclical mood change. In subsequent additions to the conflicting literature, Wang et al[133] observed increased estradiol and decreased progesterone levels in women with PMS, Redei and Freeman[134] reported non-significant increases in both estradiol and progesterone, and Facchinetti et al[135] found no differences from controls in integrated progesterone levels. Results for studies of androgen levels have been similarly inconsistent, demonstrating both normal and decreased testosterone levels[136–138] and elevated and decreased free testosterone levels.[137,138] Abnormalities of gonadotropin secretion have been observed (albeit inconsistently) in several studies, with reports of both higher[139] and lower[140] mid-luteal plasma FSH levels, delayed follicular development and prolonged follicular phase after corpus lute-ectomy[140] suggestive of decreased FSH or increased inhibin secretion, and no diagnosis-related differences in plasma LH[133,139–141] but a correlation in women with PMS between higher LH levels and more severe symptoms. In summation, then, there is no consistent or convincing evidence that PMS is characterized by abnormal circulating plasma levels of gonadal steroids or gonadotropins or by hypothalamic–pituitary–ovarian (HPO) axis dysfunction. Several studies do, however, suggest that levels of estrogen, progesterone, or neurosteroids (e.g. pregnenolone sulfate) may be correlated with symptom severity in women with PMS (see below).[133,142,143]

Recent speculations about the etiology of PMS have focused on putative abnormal neurosteroid levels. Observations central to these speculations include the following:

1. The GABA receptor (the presumed mediator of anxiolysis) is positively modulated by the 5a- and 5b-reduced metabolites of progesterone (allopregnanolone and pregnanolone, respectively).10
2. Withdrawal of progesterone in rats produces anxiety and insensitivity to benzodiazepines due to withdrawal of allopregnanolone, with consequent induction of $GABA_A$ α_4 subunit levels and inhibition of GABA currents.[98,144]
3. Allopregnanolone displays anxiolytic effects in several animal anxiety models[145–147] and may be involved in the stress response.[148]

4. Decreased plasma allopregnanolone levels are seen in major depressive disorder and in depression associated with alcohol withdrawal, with an increase in levels seen in plasma and cerebrospinal fluid (CSF) following successful antidepressant treatment.[149–152]
5. Antidepressants may promote the reductive activity of one of the neurosteroid synthetic enzymes (3α-HSOR), thus favoring the formation of allopregnanolone.[153]
6. PMS patients show differences in pregnanolone-modulated saccadic eye velocity (SEV) and sedation in the luteal phase compared with controls[154] (although the reported differences seem attributable to an SEV response to vehicle in those with PMS and a blunted sedation response in the follicular phase in controls).
7. High-severity PMS patients show blunted SEV and sedation responses to $GABA_A$ receptor agonists – pregnanolone[154] or midazolam[155] – compared with low-severity PMS patients.

Whereas one investigator observed decreased serum allopregnanolone levels in women with PMS compared with controls on menstrual cycle day 26,[156] other studies showed no diagnosis-related differences in allopregnanolone or pregnanolone,[133,157] nor any difference in allopregnanolone levels in women with PMS before and after successful treatment with citalopram.[158] Wang et al[133] did find that if two cycles differed in the AUC of a hormone by more than 10%, the cycle with the lower levels of allopregnanolone and higher levels of E_2, pregnanolone, and pregnenolone sulfate was accompanied by higher levels of symptom severity. Additionally, in a study in which progesterone was administered to women with leuprolide-suppressed ovarian function, women with PMS, but not comparison women, showed a significant relationship between symptom development and declining allopregnanolone levels during progesterone administration.

Studies of a variety of other endocrine factors in patients with PMS have been similarly unrevealing. In general, no differences have been observed in basal plasma cortisol levels, urinary free cortisol, the circadian pattern of plasma cortisol secretion, or basal plasma ACTH levels.[159] (Both decreased ACTH levels in PMS patients across the menstrual cycle and no differences from controls have been reported.[138,160,161]) Similarly, studies of other hormones have done little to elucidate the cause of PMS. Despite the appearance of abnormal baseline thyroid function in 10% of our subjects and abnormal (both blunted and exaggerated) thyroid-stimulating hormone (TSH) response to thyrotropin-releasing hormone (TRH) in 30% of our subjects, the vast majority of patients with PMS have normal hypothalamic–pituitary–thyroid axis function.[162] Luteal phase decreases in both plasma β-endorphin[163,164] and platelet serotonin uptake[165,166] have been reported in PMS; neither the diagnostic group-related decreases nor their confinement to the luteal phase are consistently observed.[138,167–170] Finally, in a study of CSF, Eriksson et al[171] observed no differences in CSF monoamine metabolites in PMS patients compared with controls, nor were there menstrual cycle-related differences in either group. Similarly, Parry et al[172] found no cycle-related differences (midcycle vs premenstrual) in CSF ACTH, β-endorphin, GABA, 5-hydroxyindoleacetic acid (5-HIAA), homovanillic acid (HVA), or norepinephrine; a slight but significant premenstrual increase in CSF 3-methoxy-4-hydroxyphenyl glycol (MHPG) was noted.

Even if these differences are confirmed, their persistence across the menstrual cycle would appear to argue against their direct role in the expression of a disorder confined to the luteal phase. Presently, then, there is no clearly demonstrated luteal phase-specific physiological abnormality in PMS.

Dynamic studies of hormone secretion

Several strategies have been employed to assess hypothalamic and pituitary function in women with PMS. First, basal plasma levels of gonadotropins have been measured across the menstrual cycle in women with and without PMS. Efforts to distinguish hypothalamic function from that of the pituitary led to studies of LH pulsatility (i.e. the frequency of LH pulses rather than mean LH levels). Additionally, evidence that endogenous opiate peptides modulated GnRH/LH secretion during the early- and mid-luteal phase of the menstrual cycle, when PMS symptoms appear, prompted the use of pharmacological challenges with opiate antagonists to indirectly evaluate the level of central opiate tone. (Alterations in the amount of disinhibition of LH secretion after the administration of an opiate antagonist could suggest differences in the secretion of endogenous opiates that may be relevant to the development of PMS symptoms.) Finally, acute GnRH challenge studies have been employed to evaluate stimulated gonadotropin secretion and, possibly, identify differences in hypothalamic or pituitary feedback mechanisms and pituitary gonadotropin reserve.[173]

The pattern of pulsatile secretion of LH has been characterized in women with and without PMS, employing serial blood sampling (e.g. every 10 minutes) during the luteal phase of the menstrual cycle. Facchinetti and coworkers[135,174] observed diagnostic differences in the pattern of pulsatile secretion of LH during the luteal phase: women with PMS had an increased frequency and a decreased amplitude and duration of both LH and

progesterone secretion compared with controls, suggesting a reduced level of opioid inhibition of LH (frequency) in PMS during the luteal phase as well as the possibility of decreased pituitary responsiveness (LH amplitude) compared with women without PMS. However, two subsequent studies could not confirm this finding.[175,176] Similarly, two studies[177,178] using single-dose administration of naloxone failed to identify differences between the pattern of secretion of LH after naloxone during the mid-luteal phase in women with PMS compared with controls, suggesting the absence of differences in the central opioid tone in these two groups of women. However, Rapkin et al[179] employed a continuous infusion of naloxone in the mid-luteal phase and observed a significantly blunted LH response to naloxone. These authors suggested that prolonged opiate antagonism was necessary to reveal the abnormal central opioid tone during the mid-luteal phase in women with PMS. If these findings are confirmed, it is, nonetheless, premature to suggest that the differences in naloxone-induced LH secretion reflect a deficiency of central opiate functions in PMS. Indeed, as suggested by Rapkin,[179] the regulatory effects of endogenous opiates, progesterone, and progesterone's neurosteroid metabolites on GnRH secretion are part of a complex physiological system[180,181] and not easily translated, at this point, into a pathophysiology of PMS.

Four studies have performed GnRH stimulation with 100 or 10 μg doses of GnRH in women with PMS and controls.[177,178,182,183] No differences have been reported in the pattern of gonadotropin secretion in single tests during either the luteal[178] or the follicular phase.[177] In one study in which GnRH stimulation tests were performed in both follicular and luteal phases, blunted progesterone and allopregnanolone secretion after 100 μg of GnRH were observed in women with PMS compared with a group of asymptomatic controls,[182] but gonadotropin levels were not reported, and hence the source of the blunted progesterone cannot be identified.

The above-noted study by Facchinetti et al[178] observed lower GnRH-stimulated LH secretion in five women with PMS than in four controls. Although the observed LH AUC was not significantly different across diagnostic groups, the calculated effect size (1.05) between groups was moderate and suggested that their findings could reflect a type II error. We used a supraphysiological dose of GnRH in a larger sample size and, similar to Facchinetti's results, women with PMS were not distinguished from controls by an abnormal LH or FSH response to GnRH stimulation. Our data and those of others, then, document no abnormalities of gonadotropin secretion in response to acute GnRH stimulation in women with PMS. These data also provide indirect evidence of normal HPO feedback during the follicular and mid-luteal phases of the menstrual cycle in this condition as well. Overall, extant data do not support a dynamic disturbance of the HPO axis in women with PMS.

Manipulations of menstrual cycle physiology

Given the absence of basal or stimulated reproductive endocrine abnormalities or luteal phase-specific biological abnormalities in PMS, one could reasonably ask whether the luteal phase is required for the expression of PMS. We[103] answered this question by blinding women with PMS to menstrual cycle phase with the progesterone antagonist mifepristone (RU-486) combined with either human chorionic gonadotropin (hCG) or placebo. Mifepristone administered alone 7 days after the mid-cycle LH surge precipitated menses and the premature termination of the luteal phase, while the addition of hCG preserved the luteal phase even after the mifepristone-induced menses. Consequently, following the mifepristone-induced menses, patients did not know whether they were in the follicular phase of a new cycle (mifepristone alone) or in the preserved luteal phase of the first cycle (mifepristone + hCG). We observed that women with PMS experienced their characteristic premenstrual mood state after the mifepristone-induced menses in both groups, despite the presence of an experimentally induced follicular phase in the women receiving mifepristone alone. The mid to late luteal phase, then, is clearly not required for the appearance of PMS symptoms. Nonetheless, it remained possible that symptoms could be triggered by hormonal events prior to the mid to late luteal phase, consistent with reports that the suppression of ovulation results in a remission of PMS symptoms.[184,185]

Studies employing different methods to suppress or eliminate ovarian function (e.g. GnRH agonists, the synthetic androgen danazol, or oophorectomy) have consistently demonstrated the therapeutic efficacy of ovarian suppression in PMS. As noted above, however, it is difficult to ascribe the efficacy of these treatments solely to ovarian suppression, given the lack of efficacy of oral contraceptives (which inhibit ovulation)[118] and the reported efficacy of danazol when administered after ovulation.[186] Administration of an OC does of course introduce a new estrogen/progestogen cycle, which could explain the persistence of symptoms despite ovulation suppression. Recently, we confirmed the efficacy shown by others of GnRH agonists (e.g. leuprolide acetate [Lupron]) in the treatment of PMS.[185,187–190] Consistent with Bancroft's[187] earlier observations, a therapeutic response was not observed in all patients despite the consistent reduction of gonadal steroids to hypogonadal levels. While the majority of study participants did show a therapeutic response (10/18), the mechanism of action remained unclear (e.g. low plasma gonadal steroid levels, consistent gonadal steroid levels, anovulation, suppression of follicular development). This uncertainty was in part addressed by the double-blind, placebo-controlled reintroduction of estradiol (0.1 mg Estraderm patch) or progesterone (200 mg bid by suppository) in the study participants in whom Lupron displayed efficacy. The results unequivocally demonstrated the precipitation of a wide range of characteristic symptoms of PMS during both estrogen and progesterone add-back but not during placebo add back (Figure 10.2). Both Muse[191] and Mortola et al[189] previously described the return of symptoms during 1-month trials of estrogen, progestin, or placebo, although symptom return was not seen by Mortola et al with the combination of estrogen and progestin. Despite the questions raised by Mortola's study – Why was placebo as able to induce the return of behavioral symptoms as were the gonadal steroids? Why did solitary gonadal steroids precipitate the return of symptoms but sequential administration fail to stimulate symptom return? – the combined results from our study and those of Muse[191] and Mortola[189] strongly suggest the role of gonadal steroids in the occurrence of PMS symptoms. Particularly striking, however, is the observation that control subjects lacking a history of PMS and going through the same protocol (i.e. Lupron-induced hypogonadism followed by gonadal steroid add-back) showed no perturbation of mood during hypogonadism and no mood disturbance during hormonal add-back (see Figure 10.2). It would appear, therefore, that women with a history of PMS are differentially sensitive to the mood-perturbing effects of gonadal steroids, as similar steroid manipulations in women without a history of PMS are without effect on mood. This differential sensitivity may also be consistent with the observations mentioned earlier that PMS symptoms are correlated with progesterone levels in women with PMS despite mean levels in patients that are not different from those in controls.

OTHER NEUROBIOLOGICAL SYSTEMS IMPLICATED IN THE PATHOPHYSIOLOGY OF PREMENSTRUAL SYNDROME

Hypothalamic–pituitary–adrenal axis

Observations of both numerous reciprocal regulatory interactions between the stress and reproductive axes and abnormal HPA axis activity in depression suggested that dysregulation of the stress response in women with PMS may contribute to their susceptibility

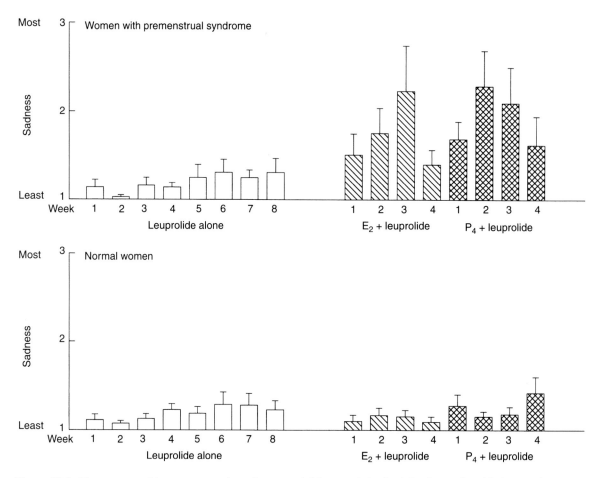

Figure 10.2 Ten women with premenstrual syndrome and 15 controls had minimal mood and behavioral symptoms during Lupron (leuprolide acetate). In contrast, women with premenstrual syndrome but not the controls had a significant increase in sadness during either estradiol (E_2) or progesterone (P_4) administration. Histograms represent the mean ($\pm$ SE) of the seven daily scores on the daily rating form sadness scale for each of the 8 weeks preceding hormone replacement (Lupron alone) and during the 4 weeks of Lupron + E_2 and Lupron + P_4 replacement. A score of 1 indicates that the symptom was not present and a score of 6 indicates that it was present in the extreme.

to affective disturbance. While studies of basal HPA axis function have been unrevealing, studies of stimulated HPA axis activity provide evidence of the involvement of this neuroendocrine axis in PMS. In a recent study, Roca et al[93] showed a differential HPA axis response to exercise stimulation in women with PMS compared with controls. Women with PMS fail to show the luteal phase increase in stimulated AVP, ACTH, and cortisol seen in normal women and additionally display adrenal hyporesponsivity. As it is progesterone rather than estradiol that enhances exercise-stimulated HPA activity,[93] women with PMS appear to display an abnormal response to progesterone. A variety of data

support these observations. In a prior study,[61] we showed that *m*-CPP-stimulated cortisol was significantly blunted in the luteal (but not the follicular) phase in women with PMS, consistent with the current findings as well as with data from Girdler et al[192] showing decreased luteal phase-stimulated cortisol in women with PMS. Additionally, blunted or absent cortisol response to CRH or naloxone, respectively, was observed in the luteal phase in women with PMS.[193] In a separate earlier study,[194] we showed that women with PMS display low evening cortisol levels across the menstrual cycle; this was also seen by Parry et al[195] and Odber et al[196] and is consistent with either adrenal hyposensitivity or altered circadian cortisol dynamics (although, see Parry et al[197] and Steiner et al[198]). Bancroft et al[63] identified blunted levels across the menstrual cycle of tryptophan-stimulated cortisol secretion in women with PMS. Finally, an abnormal response to (presumed) luteal phase progesterone in women with PMS was also seen in their failure to manifest the normal luteal phase alteration in the timing of the cortisol acrophase.[195] These data, then, suggest the following:

- stimulated cortisol (albeit paradigm specific) is decreased in women with PMS relative to controls during the luteal phase
- the adrenal response to ACTH may be blunted in women with PMS
- women with PMS manifest an abnormal HPA axis (and mood) response to progesterone
- women with PMS display disturbances of the HPA axis that are markedly different from those identified in major depression.

Although the determinants of these observations are unclear, they provide another compelling example of differential response to gonadal steroids in women with PMS and suggest an additional potential source of vulnerability to affective disturbance.

Serotonin

Serotonin (5-HT) plays a role in the regulation of mood,[199] impulsivity,[200] appetite,[201] sleep,[202] and sexual interest,[203] behaviors that vary during the menstrual cycle in women with PMS. Studies of serotonin measures and the efficacy of serotonergic agonists further suggest the relevance of the serotonin system for PMS and are reviewed in Chapters 3 and 9.

CONCLUSIONS

In order to identify what the study of PMS may contribute to our understanding of the effects of gonadal steroids on brain and behavior, several observations must be integrated. First, PMS does not reflect a disturbance of reproductive endocrine function. Secondly, estrogen and progesterone appear to be capable of triggering mood disturbances in a susceptible population; i.e. some pre-existing vulnerability must explain the capacity of the same biological stimulus (e.g. gonadal steroids) to elicit a differential behavioral response across groups of people. Thirdly, perturbations of non-reproductive endocrine systems may precipitate PMS. For example, PMS may appear in the context of hypothyroidism (with symptoms responsive to thyroid

hormone replacement),[204] and both provocative[61,205] and especially treatment studies[206] suggest the relevance of the serotonin system to PMS. PMS, then, may represent a behavioral state that is triggered by a reproductive endocrine stimulus in those who may be rendered susceptible to behavioral state changes by antecedent experiential events (e.g. history of major depression[207] or physical or sexual abuse[208]) or biological conditions (e.g. hypothyroidism).[204] Treatment can, therefore, be directed to either eliminating the trigger (e.g. ovarian suppression) or correcting the 'vulnerability' (e.g. serotonergic antidepressants).[206] Although the means by which alterations in gonadal steroids trigger changes in behavioral state in certain individuals are unclear, it is nonetheless striking that, in contrast to the pathological function of other endocrine systems (e.g. adrenal, thyroid) seen in association with mood disorders, gonadal steroids may precipitate mood disturbances in the context of *normal* ovarian function. This suggests that further study of the interactions between gonadal steroids and other neuroactive systems may help elucidate general mechanisms underlying affective regulation as well as the physiological substrate that predisposes certain people to experience reproductive endocrine-related mood disorders.

ACKNOWLEDGMENT

The research was supported by the Intramural Research Programs of the NIMH.

REFERENCES

1. Reid RL, Yen SSC. Premenstrual syndrome. Am J Obstet Gynecol 1981; 139:85–104.
2. Rubinow DR, Roy-Byrne PP. Premenstrual syndromes: overview from a methodologic perspective. Am J Psychiatry 1984; 141:163–72.
3. American Psychiatric Association. Diagnostic and Statistical Manual of Mental Disorders, 4th edn. Washington, DC: American Psychiatric Press; 1994.
4. NIMH. NIMH Premenstrual Syndrome Workshop Guidelines. Rockville, MD: National Institute of Mental Health (not published), 1983.
5. Miller WL. Steroid hormone biosynthesis and actions in the materno-feto-placental unit. Clin Perinatol 1998; 25:799–817.
6. Miller WL. Androgen biosynthesis from cholesterol to DHEA. Mol Cell Endocrinol 2002; 198:7–14.
7. Grino PB, Griffin JE, Wilson JD. Testosterone at high concentrations interacts with the human androgen receptor similarly to dihydrotestosterone. Endocrinology 1990; 126:1165–72.
8. Naftolin F, Garcia-Segura LM, Keefe D et al. Estrogen effects on the synaptology and neural membranes of the rat hypothalamic arcuate nucleus. Biol Reprod 1990; 42:21–8.
9. Mahendroo MS, Cala KM, Landrum DP et al. Fetal death in mice lacking 5alpha-reductase type 1 caused by estrogen excess. Mol Endocrinol 1997; 11:917–27.

10. Majewska MD, Harrison NL, Schwartz RD et al. Steroid hormone metabolites are barbiturate-like modulators of the GABA receptor. Science 1986; 232:1004–7.

11. Park-Chung M, Malayev A, Purdy RH et al. Sulfated and unsulfated steroids modulate γ-aminobutyric acid$_A$ receptor function through distinct sites. Brain Res 1999; 830:72–87.

12. Poletti A, Celotti F, Maggi R et al. Aspects of hormonal steroid metabolism in the nervous system. In: Baulieu E-E, Robel P, Schumacher M, eds. Contemporary Endocrinology: Neurosteroids: A New Regulatory Function in the Nervous System. Totowa, NJ: Humana Press Inc; 1999:97–123.

13. Uht RM, Anderson CM, Webb P et al. Transcriptional activities of estrogen and glucocorticoid receptors are functionally integrated at the AP-1 response element. Endocrinology 1997; 138:2900–8.

14. McEwen BS, Alves SE. Estrogen actions in the central nervous system. Endocr Rev 1999; 20:279–307.

15. McEwen BS. Steroid hormones: effect on brain development and function. Horm Res 1992; 37(Suppl 3):1–10.

16. Wong M, Moss RL. Long-term and short-term electrophysiological effects of estrogen on the synaptic properties of hippocampal CA1 neurons. J Neurosci 1992; 12:3217–25.

17. Valverde MA, Rojas P, Amigo J et al. Acute activation of Maxi-K channels (hSlo) by estradiol binding to the β subunit. Science 1999; 285:1929–31.

18. Aronica SM, Kraus WL, Katzenellenbogen BS. Estrogen action via the cAMP signaling pathway: stimulation of adenylate cyclase and cAMP-regulated gene transcription. Proc Natl Acad Sci USA 1994; 91:8517–21.

19. Ravindra R, Aronstam RS. Progesterone, testosterone and estradiol-17β inhibit gonadotropin-releasing hormone, stimulation of G protein GTPase activity in plasma membranes from rat anterior pituitary lobe. Acta Endocrinol (Copenh) 1992; 126:345–9.

20. Mermelstein PG, Becker JB, Surmeier DJ. Estradiol reduces calcium currents in rat neostriatal neurons via a membrane receptor. J Neurosci 1996; 16:595–604.

21. Migliaccio A, Piccolo D, Castoria G et al. Activation of the Src/p21ras/Erk pathway by progesterone receptor via cross-talk with estrogen receptor. EMBO J 1998; 17:2008–18.

22. Watters JJ, Campbell JS, Cunningham MJ et al. Rapid membrane effects of steroids in neuroblastoma cells: effects of estrogen on mitogen activated protein kinase signalling cascade and c-fos immediate early gene transcription. Endocrinology 1997; 138:4030–3.

23. Zhang L, Li B, Zhao W et al. Sex-related differences in MAPKs activation in rat astrocytes: effects of estrogen on cell death. Mol Brain Res 2002; 103:1–11.

24. Mani SK. Signaling mechanisms in progesterone–neurotransmitter interactions. Neuroscience 2006; 138:773–81.

25. Auger AP, Meredith JM, Snyder GL et al. Oestradiol increases phosphorylation of a dopamine- and cyclic AMP-regulated phosphoprotein (DARPP-32) in female rat brain. J Neuroendocrinol 2001; 13:761–8.

26. Greengard P. The neurobiology of slow synaptic transmission. Science 2001; 294:1024–30.

27. Brubaker KD, Gay CV. Evidence for plasma membrane-mediated effects of estrogen. Calcif Tissue Int 1999; 64:459–62.

28. Pilgrim C, Hutchison JB. Developmental regulation of sex differences in the brain: can the role of gonadal steroids be redefined? Neuroscience 1994; 60:843–55.

29. Ciocca DR, Vargas Roig LM. Estrogen receptors in human non-target tissues: biological and clinical implications. Endocr Rev 1995; 16:35–62.

30. Behl C, Skutella T, Lezoualc'h F et al. Neuroprotection against oxidative stress by estrogens: structure–activity relationship. Mol Pharmacol 1997; 51:535–41.

31. Mooradian AD. Antioxidant properties of steroids. J Steroid Biochem Mol Biol 1993; 45:509–11.

32. Singer CA, Rogers KL, Strickland TM et al. Estrogen protects primary cortical neurons from glutamate toxicity. Neurosci Lett 1996; 212:13–16.

33. Garcia-Segura LM, Cardona-Gomez P, Naftolin F et al. Estradiol upregulates Bcl-2 expression in adult brain neurons. NeuroReport 1998; 9:593–7.

34. Gouras GK, Xu H, Gross RS et al. Testosterone reduces neuronal secretion of Alzheimer's beta-amyloid peptides. Proc Natl Acad Sci USA 2000; 97:1202–5.

35. Toran-Allerand CD. Developmental interactions of estrogens with the neurotrophins and their receptors. In: Micevych P, Hammer RP, eds. Neurobiological Effects of Sex Steroid Hormones. Cambridge: Cambridge University Press; 1994:391–411.

36. Zhang L, Ma W, Barker JL et al. Sex differences in expression of serotonin receptors (subtypes 1A and 2A) in rat brain: a possible role of testosterone. Neuroscience 1999; 94:251–9.

37. Juraska JM. The structure of the rat cerebral cortex: effects of gender and the environment. In: Kolb B, Tees RC, eds. The Cerebral Cortex of the Rat. Cambridge, MA: MIT Press; 1990:483–505.

38. Moore CL, Dou H, Juraska JM. Maternal stimulation affects the number of motor neurons in a sexually dimorphic nucleus of the lumbar spinal cord. Brain Res 1992; 572:52–6.

39. Woolley CS, Schwartzkroin PA. Hormonal effects on the brain. Epilepsia 1998; 39:S2–8.

40. McEwen BS, Alves SE, Bulloch K et al. Ovarian steroids and the brain: implications for cognition and aging. Neurology 1997; 48(Suppl 7):S8–15.

41. Rachman IM, Unnerstall JR, Pfaff DW et al. Estrogen alters behavior and forebrain c-fos expression in ovariectomized rats subjected to the forced swim test. Proc Natl Acad Sci USA 1998; 95:13941–6.

42. Rubinow DR, Schmidt PJ, Roca CA. Estrogen–serotonin interactions: implications for affective regulation. Biol Psychiatry 1998; 44:839–50.

43. Pecins-Thompson M, Brown NA, Bethea CL. Regulation of serotonin re-uptake transporter mRNA expression by ovarian steroids in rhesus macaques. Brain Res Mol Brain Res 1998; 53:120–9.

44. Clarke WP, Maayani S. Estrogen effects on 5-HT$_{1A}$ receptors in hippocampal membranes from ovariectomized rats: functional and binding studies. Brain Res 1990; 518:287–91.

45. Thomas ML, Bland DA, Clarke CH et al. Estrogen regulation of serotonin (5-HT) transporter and 5-HT$_{1A}$ receptor mRNA in female rat brain. Abstr Soc Neurosci 1997; 23:1501.

46. Sumner BEH, Fink G. Estrogen increases the density of 5-hydroxytryptamine$_{2A}$ receptors in cerebral cortex and nucleus accumbens in the female rat. J Steroid Biochem Mol Biol 1995; 54:15–20.

47. Sumner BEH, Fink G. Effects of acute estradiol on 5-hydroxytryptamine and dopamine receptor subtype mRNA expression in female rat brain. Mol Cell Neurosci 1993; 4:83–92.

48. Kendall DA, Stancel GM, Enna SJ. Imipramine: effect of ovarian steroids on modifications in serotonin receptor binding. Science 1981; 211:1183–5.

49. Wissink S, van der Burg B, Katzenellenbogen BS et al. Synergistic activation of the serotonin-1A receptor by nuclear factor-kappa B and estrogen. Mol Endocrinol 2001; 15:543–52.

50. Bethea CL, Mirkes SJ, Su A et al. Effects of oral estrogen, raloxifene and arzoxifene on gene expression in serotonin neurons of macaques. Psychoneuroendocrinology 2002; 27:431–45.

51. Gundlah C, Pecins-Thompson M, Schutzer WE et al. Ovarian steroid effects on serotonin 1A, 2A and 2C receptor mRNA in macaque hypothalamus. Mol Brain Res 1999; 63:325–39.

52. Osterlund MK, Halldin C, Hurd YL. Effects of chronic 17β-estradiol treatment on the serotonin 5-HT1A receptor mRNA and binding levels in the rat brain. Synapse 2000; 35:39–44.

53. Krezel W, Dupont S, Krust A et al. Increased anxiety and synaptic plasticity in estrogen receptor beta-deficient mice. Proc Natl Acad Sci USA 2001; 98:12278–82.

54. Lu NZ, Bethea CL. Ovarian steroid regulation of 5-HT$_{1A}$ receptor binding and G protein activation in female monkeys. Neuropsychopharmacology 2002; 27:12–24.

55. Hery M, Becquet D, Francois-Bellan AM et al. Stimulatory effects of 5HT1A receptor agonists on luteinizing hormone-releasing hormone release from cultured fetal rat hypothalamic cells: interactions with progesterone. Neuroendocrinology 1995; 61:11–18.

56. Maswood S, Stewart G, Uphouse L. Gender and estrous cycle effects of the 5-HT$_{1A}$ agonist, 8-OH-DPAT, on hypothalamic serotonin. Pharmacol Biochem Behav 1995; 51:807–13.

57. Bethea CL, Lu NZ, Gundlah C et al. Diverse actions of ovarian steroids in the serotonin neural system. Front Neuroendocrinol 2002; 23:41–100.

58. Sumner BEH, Grant KE, Rosie R et al. Effects of tamoxifen on serotonin transporter and 5-hydroxytryptamine$_{2A}$ receptor binding sites and mRNA levels in the brain of ovariectomized rats with or without acute estradiol replacement. Mol Brain Res 1999; 73:119–28.

59. Fink G, Sumner BEH. Oestrogen and mental state. Nature 1996; 383:306.

60. McQueen JK, Wilson H, Dow RC et al. Oestradiol-17β increases serotonin transporter (SERT) binding sites and SERT mRNA expression in discrete regions of female rat brain. J Physiol 1996; 495.P:114P.

61. Su T-P, Schmidt PJ, Danaceau M et al. Effect of menstrual cycle phase on neuroendocrine and behavioral responses to the serotonin agonist m-chlorophenylpiperazine in women with premenstrual syndrome and controls. J Clin Endocrinol Metab 1997; 82:1220–8.

62. Dinan TG, Barry S, Yatham LN et al. The reproducibility of the prolactin response to buspirone: relationship to the menstrual cycle. Int Clin Psychopharmacol 1990; 5:119–23.

63. Bancroft J, Cook A, Davidson D et al. Blunting of neuroendocrine responses to infusion of L-tryptophan in women with perimenstrual mood change. Psychol Med 1991; 21:305–12.

64. O'Keane V, O'Hanlon M, Webb M et al. d-Fenfluramine/prolactin response throughout the menstrual cycle: evidence for an oestrogen-induced alteration. Clin Endocrinol 1991; 34:289–92.

65. Schmidt PJ, Raju J, Danaceau M et al. The effects of gender and gonadal steroids on the neuroendocrine and temperature response to m-chlorophenylpiperazine in leuprolide-induced hypogonadism in women and men. Neuropsychopharmacology 2002; 27:800–12.

66. Moses EL, Drevets WC, Smith G et al. Effects of estradiol and progesterone administration on human serotonin 2A receptor binding: a PET study. Biol Psychiatry 2000; 48:854–60.

67. Nestler EJ, Terwilliger RZ, Duman RS. Chronic antidepressant administration alters the subcellular distribution of cyclic AMP-dependent protein kinase in rat frontal cortex. J Neurochem 1989; 53:1644–7.

68. Duman RS, Heninger GR, Nestler EJ. A molecular and cellular theory of depression. Arch Gen Psychiatry 1997; 54:597–606.

69. Nibuya M, Nestler EJ, Duman RS. Chronic antidepressant administration increases the expression of cAMP response element-binding protein (CREB) in rat hippocampus. J Neurosci 1996; 16:2365–72.

70. Sohrabji F, Miranda RC, Toran-Allerand CD. Estrogen differentially regulates estrogen and nerve growth factor receptor mRNAs in adult sensory neurons. J Neurosci 1994; 14:459–71.

71. Zhou Y, Watters JJ, Dorsa DM. Estrogen rapidly induces the phosphorylation of the cAMP response element binding protein in rat brain. Endocrinology 1996; 137:2163–6.

72. Sohrabji F, Greene LA, Miranda RC et al. Reciprocal regulation of estrogen and NGF receptors by their ligands in PC12 cells. J Neurobiol 1994; 25:974–88.

73. Cardona-Gomez P, Perez M, Avila J et al. Estradiol inhibits GSK3 and regulates interaction of estrogen receptors, GSK3, and beta-catenin in the hippocampus. Mol Cell Neurosci 2004; 25:363–73.

74. Murphy DD, Cole NB, Segal M. Brain-derived neurotrophic factor mediates estradiol-induced dendritic spine formation in hippocampal neurons. Proc Natl Acad Sci USA 1998; 95:11412–17.

75. Berman KF, Schmidt PJ, Rubinow DR et al. Modulation of cognition-specific cortical activity by gonadal steroids: a positron-emission tomography study in women. Proc Natl Acad Sci USA 1997; 94:8836–41.

76. Shaywitz SE, Shaywitz BA, Pugh KR et al. Effect of estrogen on brain activation patterns in postmenopausal women during working memory tasks. JAMA 1999; 281:1197–202.

77. Protopopescu X, Pan H, Altemus M et al. Orbitofrontal cortex activity related to emotional processing changes across the menstrual cycle. Proc Natl Acad Sci USA 2005; 102:16060–5.

78. Goldstein JM, Jerram M, Poldrack R et al. Hormonal cycle modulates arousal circuitry in women using functional magnetic resonance imaging. J Neurosci 2005; 25:9309–16.

79. Redei E, Li L, Halasz I et al. Fast glucocorticoid feedback inhibition of ACTH secretion in the ovariectomized rat: effect of chronic estrogen and progesterone. Neuroendocrinology 1994; 60:113–23.

80. Young EA, Altemus M, Parkinson V et al. Effects of estrogen antagonists and agonists on the ACTH response to restraint stress in female rats. Neuropsychopharmacology 2001; 25:881–91.

81. Dayas CV, Xu Y, Buller KM et al. Effects of chronic oestrogen replacement on stress-induced activation of hypothalamic–pituitary–adrenal axis control pathways. J Neuroendocrinol 2000; 12:784–94.

82. Komesaroff PA, Esler M, Clarke IJ et al. Effects of estrogen and estrous cycle on glucocorticoid and catecholamine responses to stress in sheep. Am J Physiol 1998; 275:E671–8.

83. Burgess LH, Handa RJ. Chronic estrogen-induced alterations in adrenocorticotropin and corticosterone secretion, and glucocorticoid receptor-mediated functions in female rats. Endocrinology 1992; 131:1261–9.

84. Carey MP, Deterd CH, de Koning J et al. The influence of ovarian steroids on hypothalamic–pituitary–adrenal regulation in the female rat. J Endocrinol 1995; 144:311–21.

85. Viau V, Meaney MJ. Variations in the hypothalamic–pituitary–adrenal response to stress during the estrous cycle in the rat. Endocrinology 1991; 129:2503–11.

86. Marinari KT, Leschner AI, Doyle MP. Menstrual cycle status and adrenocortical reactivity to psychological stress. Psychoneuroendocrinology 1976; 1:213.

87. Kirschbaum C, Kudielka BM, Gaab J et al. Impact of gender, menstrual cycle phase, and oral contraceptives on the activity of the hypothalamic–pituitary–adrenal axis. Psychosom Med 1999; 61:154–62.

88. Collins A, Eneroth P, Landgren B. Psychoneuroendocrine stress responses and mood as related to the menstrual cycle. Psychosom Med 1985; 47:512–27.

89. Ablanalp JM, Livingston L, Rose RM et al. Cortisol and growth hormone responses to psychological stress during the menstrual cycle. Psychosom Med 1977; 39:158–77.

90. Long TD, Ellingrod VL, Kathol RG et al. Lack of menstrual cycle effects on hypothalamic–pituitary–adrenal axis response to

insulin-induced hypoglycaemia. Clin Endocrinol (Oxf) 2000; 52:781–7.

91. Galliven EA, Singh A, Michelson D et al. Hormonal and metabolic responses to exercise across time of day and menstrual cycle phase. J Appl Physiol 1997; 83:1822–31.

92. Altemus M, Roca C, Galliven E et al. Increased vasopressin and adrenocorticotropin responses to stress in the midluteal phase of the menstrual cycle. J Clin Endocrinol Metab 2001; 86:2525–30.

93. Roca CA, Schmidt PJ, Altemus M et al. Differential menstrual cycle regulation of hypothalamic–pituitary–adrenal axis in women with premenstrual syndrome and controls. J Clin Endocrinol Metab 2003; 88:3057–63.

94. Keller-Wood M, Silbiger J, Wood CE. Progesterone attenuates the inhibition of adrenocorticotropin responses by cortisol in nonpregnant ewes. Endocrinology 1988; 123:647–51.

95. Turner BB. Influence of gonadal steroids on brain corticosteriod receptors: a minireview. Neurochem Res 1997; 22:1375–85.

96. Patchev VK, Almeida OFX. Gonadal steroids exert facilitating and 'buffering' effects on glucocorticoid-mediated transcriptional regulation of corticotropin-releasing hormone and corticosteroid receptor genes in rat brain. J Neurosci 1996; 16:7077–84.

97. Young EA. The role of gonadal steroids in hypothalamic–pituitary–adrenal axis regulation. Crit Rev Neurobiol 1995; 9:371–81.

98. Smith SS, Gong QH, Hsu F-C et al. GABA$_A$ receptor alpha-4 subunit suppression prevents withdrawal properties of an endogenous steroid. Nature 1998; 392:926–30.

99. Spruce BA, Baylis PH, Burd J et al. Variation in osmoregulation of arginine vasopressin during the human menstrual cycle. Clin Endocrinol 1985; 22:37–42.

100. Wyatt K, Dimmock P, Jones P et al. Efficacy of progesterone and progestogens in management of premenstrual syndrome: systematic review. BMJ 2001; 323:776–80.

101. Freeman E, Rickels K, Sondheimer SJ et al. Ineffectiveness of progesterone suppository treatment for premenstrual syndrome. JAMA 1990; 264:349–53.

102. Freeman EW, Rickels K, Sondheimer SJ et al. A double-blind trial of oral progesterone, alprazolam, and placebo in treatment of severe premenstrual syndrome. JAMA 1995; 274:51–7.

103. Schmidt PJ, Nieman LK, Grover GN et al. Lack of effect of induced menses on symptoms in women with premenstrual syndrome. N Engl J Med 1991; 324:1174–9.

104. Cullberg J. Mood changes and menstrual symptoms with different gestagen/estrogen combinations: a double blind comparison with a placebo. Acta Psychiatr Scand 1972; 236(Suppl):1–86.

105. Kutner SJ, Brown WL. Types of oral contraceptives, depression and premenstrual symptoms. J Nerv Ment Dis 1972; 155:153–62.

106. Graham CA, Sherwin BB. The relationship between retrospective premenstrual symptom reporting and present oral contraceptive use. J Psychosom Res 1987; 31:45–53.

107. Lewis A, Hoghughi M. An evaluation of depression as a side effect of oral contraceptives. Br J Psychiatry 1969; 115:697–701.

108. Woods NF, Most A, Dery GK. Prevalence of perimenstrual symptoms. Am J Public Health 1982; 72:1257–64.

109. Marriott A, Faragher EB. An assessment of psychological state associated with the menstrual cycle in users of oral contraception. J Psychosom Res 1986; 30:41–7.

110. Slade P. Premenstrual emotional changes in normal women: fact or fiction? J Psychosom Res 1984; 28:1–7.

111. Sveindottir H, Backstrom T. Prevalence of menstrual cycle symptom cyclicity and premenstrual dysphoric disorder in a random sample of women using and not using oral contraceptives. Acta Obstet Gynecol Scand 2001; 79:405–13.

112. Andersch B, Hahn L. Premenstrual complaints. II. Influence of oral contraceptives. Acta Obstet Gynecol Scand 1981; 60:579–83.

113. Glick ID, Bennett SE. Psychiatric complications of progesterone and oral contraceptives. J Clin Psychopharmacol 1981; 1:350–67.

114. Herzberg BN, Johnson AL, Brown S. Depressive symptoms and oral contraceptives. Br Med J 1970; 4:142–5.

115. Kutner SJ, Phillips NR, Hoag EJ. Oral contraceptives, personality, and changes in depression. Contraception 1971; 4:327–36.

116. Moos RH. Psychological aspects of oral contraceptives. Arch Gen Psychiatry 1968; 19:87–94.

117. Freeman EW, Sondheimer S, Weinbaum PJ et al. Evaluating premenstrual symptoms in medical practice. Obstet Gynecol 1985; 65:500–5.

118. Graham CA, Sherwin BB. A prospective treatment study of premenstrual symptoms using a triphasic oral contraceptive. J Psychosom Res 1992; 36:257–66.

119. Graham CA, Sherwin BB. The relationship between mood and sexuality in women using an oral contraceptive as a treatment for premenstrual symptoms. Psychoneuroendocrinology 1993; 18:273–81.

120. Freeman EW, Kroll R, Rapkin A et al. Evaluation of a unique oral contraceptive in the treatment of premenstrual dysphoric disorder. J Womens Health Gend Based Med 2001; 10:561–9.

121. Yonkers KA, Brown C, Pearlstein TB et al. Efficacy of a new low-dose oral contraceptive with drospirenone in premenstrual dysphoric disorder. Obstet Gynecol 2005; 106:492–501.

122. Watson NR, Savvas M, Studd JWW et al. Treatment of severe premenstrual syndrome with oestradiol patches and cyclical oral norethisterone. Lancet 1989; 334:730–2.

123. Watson NR, Studd JWW, Savvas M et al. The long-term effects of estradiol implant therapy for the treatment of premenstrual syndrome. Gynecol Endocrinol 1990; 4:99–107.

124. Smith RNJ, Studd JWW, Zamblera D et al. A randomised comparison over 8 months of 100 mg and 200 mg twice weekly doses of transdermal oestradiol in the treatment of severe premenstrual syndrome. Br J Obstet Gynaecol 1995; 102:475–84.

125. Davis SR. Androgen treatment in women. Med J Aust 1999; 170:545–9.

126. Buckler HM, Misra R, Cantrill JA et al. The use of low dose (100 mg) testosterone implants in severe premenstrual syndrome (PMS). J Endocrinol 1989; 123:34.

127. Sheffield B, Buckler HM, Cantrill JA et al. Double-blind crossover trial of low dose testosterone implants in severe premenstrual syndrome (PMS). J Endocrinol 1989; 121:183.

128. Dhar V, Murphy BEP. Double-blind randomized crossover trial of luteal phase estrogens (Premarin) in the premenstrual syndrome (PMS). Psychoneuroendocrinology 1990; 15:489–93.

129. Halbreich U, Rojansky N, Palter S. Elimination of ovulation and menstrual cyclicity (with danazol) improves dysphoric premenstrual syndromes. Fertil Steril 1991; 56:1066–9.

130. Hahn PM, Van Vugt DA, Reid RL. A randomized, placebo-controlled, crossover trial of danazol for the treatment of premenstrual syndrome. Psychoneuroendocrinology 1995; 20:193–209.

131. Rubinow DR, Hoban MC, Grover GN et al. Changes in plasma hormones across the menstrual cycle in patients with menstrually related mood disorder and in control subjects. Am J Obstet Gynecol 1988; 158:5–11.

132. Backstrom T, Sanders D, Leask R et al. Mood, sexuality, hormones, and the menstrual cycle: II. Hormone levels and their relationship to the premenstrual syndrome. Psychosom Med 1983; 45:503–7.

133. Wang M, Seippel L, Purdy RH et al. Relationship between symptom severity and steroid variation in women with premenstrual syndrome: study on serum pregnenolone, pregnenolone sulfate, 5α-pregnane-3,20-dione and 3α-hydroxy-5α-pregnan-20-one. J Clin Endocrinol Metab 1996; 81:1076–82.

134. Redei E, Freeman EW. Daily plasma estradiol and progesterone levels over the menstrual cycle and their relation to premenstrual symptoms. Psychoneuroendocrinology 1995; 20:259–67.

135. Facchinetti F, Genazzani AD, Martignoni E et al. Neuroendocrine changes in luteal function in patients with premenstrual syndrome. J Clin Endocrinol Metab 1993; 76:1123–7.

136. Backstrom T, Aakvaag A. Plasma prolactin and testosterone during the luteal phase in women with premenstrual tension syndrome. Psychoneuroendocrinology 1981; 6:245–51.

137. Eriksson E, Sundblad C, Lisjo P et al. Serum levels of androgens are higher in women with premenstrual irritability and dysphoria than in controls. Psychoneuroendocrinology 1992; 17:195–204.

138. Bloch M, Schmidt PJ, Su T-P et al. Pituitary–adrenal hormones and testosterone across the menstrual cycle in women with premenstrual syndrome and controls. Biol Psychiatry 1998; 43:897–903.

139. Backstrom T, Wide L, Sodergard R et al. FSH, LH, TeBG-capacity, estrogen and progesterone in women with premenstrual tension during the luteal phase. J Steroid Biochem 1976; 7:473–6.

140. Backstrom T, Smith S, Lothian H et al. Prolonged follicular phase and depressed gonadotropins following hysterectomy and corpus lute-ectomy in women with premenstrual tension syndrome. Clin Endocrinol 1985; 22:723–32.

141. Hammarback S, Damber J-E, Backstrom T. Relationship between symptom severity and hormone changes in women with premenstrual syndrome. J Clin Endocrinol Metab 1989; 68:125–30.

142. Schechter D, Strasser TJ, Endicott J et al. Role of ovarian steroids in modulating mood in premenstrual syndrome. Abstr Soc Biol Psych 51st Annu Meeting 1996; 646.

143. Halbreich U, Endicott J, Goldstein S et al. Premenstrual changes and changes in gonadal hormones. Acta Psychiatr Scand 1986; 74:576–86.

144. Smith SS, Gong QH, Li X et al. Withdrawal from 3α-OH-5α-pregnan-20-one using a pseudopregnancy model alters the kinetics of hippocampal GABA_A-gated current and increases the GABA_A receptor α4 subunit in association with increased anxiety. J Neurosci 1998; 18:5275–84.

145. Bitran D, Purdy RH, Kellogg CK. Anxiolytic effect of progesterone is associated with increases in cortical allopregnanolone and GABA_A receptor function. Pharmacol Biochem Behav 1993; 45:423–8.

146. Bitran D, Hilvers RJ, Kellogg CK. Anxiolytic effects of 3α-hydroxy-5a[β]-pregnan-20-one: endogenous metabolites of progesterone that are active at the GABA_A receptor. Brain Res 1991; 561:157–61.

147. Wieland S, Lan NC, Mirasedeghi S et al. Anxiolytic activity of the progesterone metabolite 5α-pregnan-3α-ol-20-one. Brain Res 1991; 565:263–8.

148. Purdy RH, Morrow AL, Moore PH Jr et al. Stress-induced elevations of gamma-aminobutyric acid type A receptor-active steroids in the rat brain. Proc Natl Acad Sci USA 1991; 88:4553–7.

149. Ströhle A, Romeo E, Hermann B et al. Concentrations of 3α-reduced neuroactive steroids and their precursors in plasma of patients with major depression and after clinical recovery. Biol Psychiatry 1999; 45:274–7.

150. Romeo E, Brancati A, de Lorenzo A et al. Marked decrease of plasma neuroactive steroids during alcohol withdrawal. Clin Neuropharmacol 1996; 19:366–9.

151. Romeo E, Strohle A, Spalletta G et al. Effects of antidepressant treatment on neuroactive steroids in major depression. Am J Psychiatry 1998; 155:910–13.

152. Uzunova V, Sheline Y, Davis JM et al. Increase in the cerebrospinal fluid content of neurosteroids in patients with unipolar major depression who are receiving fluoxetine or fluvoxamine. Proc Natl Acad Sci USA 1998; 95:3239–44.

153. Griffin LD, Mellon SH. Selective serotonin reuptake inhibitors directly alter activity of neurosteroidogenic enzymes. Proc Natl Acad Sci USA 1999; 96:13512–17.

154. Sundstrom I, Andersson A, Nyberg S et al. Patients with premenstrual syndrome have a different sensitivity to a neuroactive steroid during the menstrual cycle compared to control subjects. Neuroendocrinology 1998; 67:126–38.

155. Sundstrom I, Nyberg S, Backstrom T. Patients with premenstrual syndrome have reduced sensitivity to midazolam compared to control subjects. Neuropsychopharmacology 1997; 17:370–81.

156. Rapkin AJ, Morgan M, Goldman L et al. Progesterone metabolite allopregnanolone in women with premenstrual syndrome. Obstet Gynecol 1997; 90:709–14.

157. Schmidt PJ, Purdy RH, Moore PH Jr et al. Circulating levels of anxiolytic steroids in the luteal phase in women with premenstrual syndrome and in control subjects. J Clin Endocrinol Metab 1994; 79:1256–60.

158. Sundstrom I, Backstrom T. Citalopram increases pregnanolone sensitivity in patients with premenstrual syndrome: an open trial. Psychoneuroendocrinology 1998; 23:73–88.

159. Rubinow DR, Schmidt PJ. The neuroendocrinology of menstrual cycle mood disorders. Ann NY Acad Sci 1995; 771:648–59.

160. Redei E, Freeman EW. Preliminary evidence for plasma adrenocorticotropin levels as biological correlates of premenstrual symptoms. Acta Endocrinol 1993; 128:536–42.

161. Rosenstein DL, Kalogeras KT, Kalafut M et al. Peripheral measures of arginine vasopressin, atrial natriuretic peptide and adrenocorticotropic hormone in premenstrual syndrome. Psychoneuroendocrinology 1996; 21:347–59.

162. Schmidt PJ, Grover GN, Roy-Byrne PP et al. Thyroid function in women with premenstrual syndrome. J Clin Endocrinol Metab 1993; 76:671–4.

163. Facchinetti F, Martignoni E, Petraglia F et al. Premenstrual fall of plasma β-endorphin in patients with premenstrual syndrome. Fertil Steril 1987; 47:570–3.

164. Chuong CJ, Coulam CB, Kao PC et al. Neuropeptide levels in premenstrual syndrome. Fertil Steril 1985; 44:760–5.

165. Taylor DL, Mathew RJ, Ho BT et al. Serotonin levels and platelet uptake during premenstrual tension. Neuropsychobiology 1984; 12:16–18.

166. Ashby CR Jr, Carr LA, Cook CL et al. Alteration of platelet serotonergic mechanisms and monoamine oxidase activity in premenstrual syndrome. Biol Psychiatry 1988; 24:225–33.

167. Malmgren R, Collins A, Nilsson CG. Platelet serotonin uptake and effects of vitamin B_6-treatment in premenstrual tension. Neuropsychobiology 1987; 18:83–8.

168. Veeninga AT, Westenberg HGM. Serotonergic function and late luteal phase dysphoric disorder. Psychopharmacology 1992; 108:153–8.

169. Tulenheimo A, Laatikainen T, Salminen K. Plasma β-endorphin immunoreactivity in premenstrual tension. Br J Obstet Gynaecol 1987; 94:26–9.

170. Hamilton JA, Gallant S. Premenstrual symptom changes and plasma β-endorphin/β-lipotropin throughout the menstrual cycle. Psychoneuroendocrinology 1988; 13:505–14.

171. Eriksson E, Alling C, Andersch B et al. Cerebrospinal fluid levels of monoamine metabolites: a preliminary study of their relation to menstrual cycle phase, sex steroids, and pituitary hormones in healthy women and in women with premenstrual syndrome. Neuropsychopharmacology 1994; 11:201–13.

172. Parry BL, Gerner RH, Wilkins JN et al. CSF and endocrine studies of premenstrual syndrome. Neuropsychopharmacology 1991; 5:127–37.

173. McNeilly AS, Hagen C. Prolactin, TSH, LH and FSH responses to a combined LHRH/TRH test at different stages of the menstrual cycle. Clin Endocrinol 1974; 3:427–35.

174. Facchinetti F, Genazzani AD, Martignoni E et al. Neuroendocrine correlates of premenstrual syndrome: changes in the pulsatile pattern of plasma LH. Psychoneuroendocrinology 1990; 15:269–77.

175. Reame NE, Marshall JC, Kelch RP. Pulsatile LH secretion in women with premenstrual syndrome (PMS): evidence for normal

neuroregulation of the menstrual cycle. Psychoneuroendocrinology 1992; 17:205–13.

176. Lewis LL, Greenblatt EM, Rittenhouse CA et al. Pulsatile release patterns of luteinizing hormone and progesterone in relation to symptom onset in women with premenstrual syndrome. Fertil Steril 1995; 64:288–92.

177. Chuong CJ, Hsi BP. Effect of naloxone on luteinizing hormone secretion in premenstrual syndrome. Fertil Steril 1994; 61:1039–44.

178. Facchinetti F, Martignoni E, Sola D et al. Transient failure of central opioid tonus and premenstrual symptoms. J Reprod Med 1988; 33:633–8.

179. Rapkin AJ, Shoupe D, Reading A et al. Decreased central opioid activity in premenstrual syndrome: luteinizing hormone response to naloxone. J Soc Gynecol Invest 1996; 3:93–8.

180. Lacreuse A, Verreault M, Herndon JG. Fluctuations in spatial recognition memory across the menstrual cycle in female rhesus monkeys. Psychoneuroendocrinology 2001; 26:623–39.

181. Dhandapani KM, Mahesh VB, Brann DW. Astrocytes and brain function: implications for reproduction. Exp Biol Medl (Maywood) 2003; 228:253–60.

182. Monteleone P, Luisi S, Tonetti A et al. Allopregnanolone concentrations and premenstrual syndrome. Eur J Endocrinol 2000; 142:269–73.

183. Smith MJ, Schmidt PJ, Su T-P et al. Gonadotropin-releasing hormone-stimulated gonadotropin levels in women with premenstrual dysphoria. Gynecol Endocrinol 2004; 19:335–43.

184. Casson P, Hahn PM, VanVugt DA et al. Lasting response to ovariectomy in severe intractable premenstrual syndrome. Am J Obstet Gynecol 1990; 162:99–105.

185. Muse KN, Cetel NS, Futterman LA et al. The premenstrual syndrome: effects of 'medical ovariectomy'. N Engl J Med 1984; 311:1345–9.

186. Sarno AP, Miller EJ Jr, Lundblad EG. Premenstrual syndrome: beneficial effects of periodic, low-dose danazol. Obstet Gynecol 1987; 70:33–6.

187. Bancroft J, Boyle H, Warner P et al. The use of an LHRH agonist, buserelin, in the long-term management of premenstrual syndromes. Clin Endocrinol 1987; 27:171–82.

188. West CP, Hillier H. Ovarian suppression with the gonadotrophin-releasing hormone agonist goserelin (Zoladex) in management of the premenstrual tension syndrome. Hum Reprod 1994; 9:1058–63.

189. Mortola JF, Girton L, Fischer U. Successful treatment of severe premenstrual syndrome by combined use of gonadotropin-releasing hormone agonist and estrogen/progestin. J Clin Endocrinol Metab 1991; 71:252A–F.

190. Mezrow G, Shoupe D, Spicer D et al. Depot leuprolide acetate with estrogen and progestin add-back for long-term treatment of premenstrual syndrome. Fertil Steril 1994; 62:932–7.

191. Muse K. Gonadotropin-releasing hormone agonist-suppressed premenstrual syndrome (PMS): PMS symptom induction by estrogen, progestin, or both. Abst Soc Gynecol Invest 1989; 118.

192. Girdler SS, Straneva PA, Light KC et al. Allopregnanolone levels and reactivity to mental stress in premenstrual dysphoric disorder. Biol Psychiatry 2001; 49:788–97.

193. Facchinetti F, Fioroni L, Martignoni E et al. Changes of opioid modulation of the hypothalamo–pituitary–adrenal axis in patients with severe premenstrual syndrome. Psychosom Med 1994; 56:418–22.

194. Rabin DS, Schmidt PJ, Campbell G et al. Hypothalamic–pituitary–adrenal function in patients with the premenstrual syndrome. J Clin Endocrinol Metab 1990; 71:1158–62.

195. Parry BL, Javeed S, Laughlin GA et al. Cortisol circadian rhythms during the menstrual cycle and with sleep deprivation in premenstrual dysphoric disorder and normal control subjects. Biol Psychiatry 2000; 48:920–31.

196. Odber J, Cawood EHH, Bancroft J. Salivary cortisol in women with and without premenstrual mood changes. J Psychosom Res 1998; 45:557–68.

197. Parry BL, Hauger R, Lin E et al. Neuroendocrine effects of light therapy in late luteal phase dysphoric disorder. Biol Psychiatry 1994; 36:356–64.

198. Steiner M, Haskett RF, Carroll BJ. Circadian hormone secretory profiles in women with severe premenstrual tension syndrome. Br J Obstet Gynaecol 1984; 91:466–71.

199. Eriksson E, Humble M. Serotonin in psychiatric pathophysiology: a review of data from experimental and clinical research. In: Pohl R, Gershon S, eds. The Biological Basis of Psychiatric Treatment. Basel: Karger; 1990:66–119.

200. Linnoila M, Virkkunen M, George T et al. Impulse control disorders. Int Clin Psychopharmacol 1993; 8:53–6.

201. Wurtman JJ. Carbohydrate craving: relationships between carbohydrate intake and disorders of mood. Drugs 1990; 39:49–52.

202. Keck PE Jr, Hudson JI, Dorsey CM et al. Effect of fluoxetine on sleep: letter to the editor. Biol Psychiatry 1991; 29:618–25.

203. Gitlin MJ. Psychotropic medications and their effects on sexual function: diagnosis, biology, and treatment approaches. J Clin Psychiatry 1994; 55:406–13.

204. Schmidt PJ, Rosenfeld D, Muller KL et al. A case of autoimmune thyroiditis presenting as menstrual related mood disorder. J Clin Psychiatry 1990; 51:434–6.

205. Bancroft J. The premenstrual syndrome – a reappraisal of the concept and the evidence. Psychol Med 1993; Suppl 24:1–47.

206. Stone AB, Pearlstein TB, Brown WA. Fluoxetine in the treatment of premenstrual syndrome. Psychopharmacol Bull 1990; 26:331–5.

207. DeJong R, Rubinow DR, Roy-Byrne PP et al. Premenstrual mood disorder and psychiatric illness. Am J Psychiatry 1985; 142:1359–61.

208. Paddison PL, Gise LH, Lebovits A et al. Sexual abuse and premenstrual syndrome: comparison between a lower and higher socioeconomic group. Psychosomatics 1990; 31:265–72.

209. Dreher J, Schmidt PJ, Kohn P, et al. Menstrual cycle phase modulates reward-related neural function in women. Proc Natl Acad Sci USA 2007; 104:2465–70.

210. Ochedalski T, Subburaju S, Wynn PC et al. Interaction between oestrogen and oxytocin on hypothalamic-pituitary-adrenal axis activity. J Neuroendocrinol 2007; 19:189–97.

11

Pathophysiology II: neuroimaging, GABA, and the menstrual cycle

C Neill Epperson, Zenab Amin, and Graeme F Mason

INTRODUCTION

In the more than quarter of a century since the introduction of nuclear magnetic resonance (NMR) techniques to the armamentarium of the scientist exploring the inner workings of the human brain, relatively few neuroimaging studies have focused on the interplay between gonadal steroids, neurochemistry, and brain function. Nowhere is this void more obvious than when it comes to examining the role of hormonal fluctuations in disorders associated with reproductive function such as premenstrual syndrome (PMS)/premenstrual dysphoric disorder (PMDD), postpartum depression, or mood changes occurring during the menopause or with the use of steroid contraceptives. Indeed, the vast majority of studies utilizing NMR and other imaging techniques such as positron emission tomography (PET) and single-photon emission computed tomography (SPECT) to study women under various hormonal conditions, focus, not on the brain, but on the breast, uterus, and ovaries.

With the recent advancements in proton magnetic resonance spectroscopy (^{1}H-MRS), which allows the non-invasive quantification of important amino acid neurotransmitters such as γ-aminobutryic acid (GABA) and glutamate,[1] has come the opportunity to gain unprecedented access to brain chemistry in living human subjects. As reviewed by Backstrom and colleagues in Chapter 13 of this book, progesterone modulation of GABAergic function via its neurosteroid metabolite allopregnanolone (ALLO) is likely to be critical to the pathogenesis, and perhaps treatment, of PMS/PMDD. Additionally, Backstrom points out that estrogen, which has antidepressant effects in some populations, also contributes to mood deterioration when paired with certain doses of progesterone. Estrogen

enhances N-methyl-D-aspartate (NMDA) receptor function,[2] and alters glial morphology and function in a manner that may impact removal of glutamate from the synaptic cleft (reviewed by McEwen,[3] Garcia-Segura and McCarthy,[4] Pawlak et al,[5] and Mong and Blutstein[6]). That both ovarian hormones are likely to be powerful modulators in the balance between neuronal excitation and inhibition sets in bold relief the unique promise that MRS holds as a neuroimaging technique to further our understanding of the neuroendocrine milieu that leads to negative affect.

This present chapter provides a brief overview of neuroimaging studies that have examined menstrual cycle and/or hormonal modulation of brain chemistry and/or function. A particular emphasis will be placed on exploring the role of GABA and glutamate in PMS/PMDD and how neuroimaging techniques such as MRS can be further exploited to enhance our understanding of the neurosteroid–GABA interplay in neuropsychiatric disorders in women.

NEUROIMAGING STUDIES OF THE MENSTRUAL CYCLE

Although there are as yet few studies involving PMDD patients, there have been several neuroimaging studies focusing on changes across the menstrual cycle in healthy participants. One early PET study, for example, showed that regional cerebral blood flow (rCBF) during a prefrontal cortex-dependent task was attenuated by pharmacological ovarian suppression, but normalized with estrogen or progesterone replacement.[7] Neither behavioral response nor brain activation during a control task was affected by these manipulations, suggesting that ovarian steroids have a significant effect on prefrontal cortical activation during cognition.

Functional magnetic resonance imaging (fMRI) studies evaluating cognition have suggested little change in the location of activation across phases of the cycle, although some have found greater activation during high levels of estrogen or estrogen and progesterone. One study utilized a word-stem completion task, a mental rotation task, and a simple motor task (Table 11.1).[8] There were no differences between male and female subjects when females were scanned during the low estrogen phase, but during the periovulatory phase of high estrogen, women exhibited a marked increase in activation of cortical areas involved in the cognitive tasks, but not the motor task. Similarly, the luteal phase was marked by greater recruitment of brain regions involved in a semantic decision task than the early follicular phase.[9] Another study involving rhyme identification did not find differences in the regions that were activated during the follicular and luteal phases.[10] It is difficult in the absence of behavioral effects to determine whether increased activation during relatively high levels of estradiol and progesterone is the result of their direct effects on cognition or a result of other influences on the BOLD (blood oxygenation level dependent) signal, such as vascular effects.[11] Even when differences in activation exist in cognitive tasks of interest and not simple control tasks, it is possible that differences in cerebral vasculature in the regions activated by the control task may influence findings.[8] Thus, precise control conditions are required to evaluate changes in brain activation during cognition that coincide with changes in ovarian steroid levels.

Studies have also evaluated changes in affective processing across the menstrual cycle in healthy women by comparing activation to emotional vs neutral stimuli. These data may be useful in identifying abnormalities in women with PMDD. One study reported increased activation in several cortical and subcortical regions, including areas of the brainstem, hippocampus,

Table 11.1 Functional magnetic resonance imaging studies examining menstrual cycle effects on cognition and affective processing

Study	Sample	Findings/comments
Veltman et al[10]	8 healthy women scanned twice; early follicular and mid-luteal phases	No differences across phase in the regions activated during a rhyming task
Dietrich et al[8]	6 healthy women scanned twice; early and late follicular phases	Tasks: word-stem completion, mental rotation and simple motor. Activation areas larger during high estrogen, particularly during cognitive tasks
Fernandez et al[9]	12 healthy women scanned twice; early follicular and mid-luteal phases	Activation areas larger during high hormones for a semantic but not perceptual task
Goldstein et al[12]	12 healthy women scanned twice; early and late follicular phases	Increases activation in response to unpleasant visual stimuli during the early follicular phase (presumed low hormones) in several regions of interest; hormone levels were not obtained to verify phases of interest
Protopopescu et al[16]	12 healthy women scanned twice; follicular and late luteal phases	Increased medial orbitofrontal cortex (OFC) activation during response inhibition to negative words premenstrually, but increased lateral OFC activation postmenstrually; variation in hormone levels was not of interest
Amin et al[15]	14 healthy women scanned twice; early follicular and mid-luteal phases	Increased activation in regions of interest during response inhibition to positive words in the luteal phase. Activation correlating with luteal phase estradiol level was dissociated by valence

Derby Hospitals NHS Foundation Trust
Library and Knowledge Service

orbitofrontal cortex (OFC), and anterior cingulate cortex (ACC), in response to unpleasant images during low hormones compared to presumed high estrogen levels.[12] Thus, it is possible that high estrogen levels may decrease activation to negative stimuli, and possibly reduce their salience. However, hormone levels were not obtained, limiting inferences based on ovarian hormone effects. In addition, it was hypothesized that decreases in activation to aversive stimuli specifically related to the stress response,[12] but estrogen has also been associated with enhancing hypothalamic–pituitary–adrenal (HPA) axis function.[13,14] More research is necessary to investigate the pathway of estrogen's effects and to explore whether menstrual cycle phase may have influenced activation to unpleasant images through a mechanism not directly related to the stress response.

In a recent study from our laboratory, we utilized an emotional go/no-go task to evaluate menstrual cycle-related changes in response inhibition.[15] In each condition, participants were instructed to respond to one type of stimulus (e.g. positive words) but to ignore another type (e.g. neutral words). Compared with the follicular phase of low hormone levels, we found significantly increased activation in the ACC and dorsolateral prefrontal cortex (DLPFC) while inhibiting response to positive words (compared with when inhibiting response to neutral words) during the luteal phase of high estrogen and progesterone levels.[15] In addition, luteal phase DLPFC activation during response inhibition to positive words was significantly positively correlated with plasma estradiol level and activation in the caudate and inferior parietal gyrus during response inhibition to negative words was negatively correlated with estradiol. Thus, in healthy women, high estrogen levels during the latter half of the menstrual cycle may increase salience of positive stimuli and decrease salience of negative stimuli.

In order to begin evaluating differences in brain activation during emotional processing in healthy women compared to women with PMDD, one previous fMRI study assessed activation in healthy women during the late luteal phase (when PMDD symptoms are evinced) and mid-follicular (non-symptomatic) phase.[16] A variation of the emotional go/no-go task was used in which participants were instructed to inhibit response to italicized words, including positive, negative, and neutral stimuli. Anterior-medial OFC activation to negative stimuli, compared with neutral stimuli, was increased in the late luteal phase while lateral OFC activation increased in the follicular phase.[16] There were no differences in activation to positive stimuli. Because ovarian steroids are likely to be declining in the late luteal phase and may therefore not be very different from follicular phase levels, hormone effects were not the primary

focus of the experiment and levels were not obtained. Instead, these data serve to exemplify brain activation in healthy women at these timepoints in the menstrual cycle so that these patterns may be compared to those with PMDD. However, in an emotional processing task of this nature, mood is likely to have a significant impact on behavioral response and activation. Thus, it may be difficult to differentiate brain activation patterns resulting primarily from differences in mood between healthy women and those with PMDD and not the underlying disorder. Given that differences have been found between healthy women and women with PMDD even in the absence of symptoms (e.g. Epperson et al[17]), identification of differences in brain activation during the follicular (non-symptomatic) phase may be more valuable than identification of emotional processing-related differences during the late luteal phase.

In contrast to fMRI studies focusing on brain structures and cognitive processes that may be modulated by ovarian steroids, several PET, SPECT, and MRS studies have evaluated changes in neurotransmitter systems across the menstrual cycle in healthy women and in women with PMDD. For example, a recent SPECT study evaluated menstrual cycle-related changes in dopamine transporter (DAT) availability in the striatum and serotonin transporter availability in the brainstem-diencephalon (Table 11.2).[18] No differences were detected between the follicular and luteal phases, even after excluding two participants who experienced anovulatory cycles in which there was no progesterone increase in the luteal phase. However, it is possible that there was not sufficient power to detect small changes in transporter availability in the sample of eight participants.

Similarly, one PET study found no differences in D_2 dopamine receptor density, measured by putamen to cerebellum ratios, between follicular and luteal or periovulatory phases.[19] Although phase was verified by ovarian steroid levels, sample size for this study was small, with only four women completing tests in two different phases (three women in the follicular and luteal phases and one woman in early follicular and periovulatory phases). A more recent PET study investigated the serotonin hypothesis of PMDD.[20] Changes in daily prospective ratings of mood significantly correlated with changes in brain trapping of ^{11}C-labeled 5-hydroxytryptophan (^{11}C-5-HTP) in regions of interest across the menstrual cycle. While changes in irritability and depressed mood negatively correlated with changes in trapping of the labeled serotonin precursor, changes in happiness and energy in the follicular phase positively correlated with changes in brain ^{11}C-5-HTP trapping.[20] Thus, it appears that a more stable cycle, marked by little change in symptoms, is associated with an increase in ^{11}C-5-HTP trapping in the luteal phase, but

Table 11.2 Neuroimaging studies examining the impact of menstrual cycle phase on neurotransmitter systems

Study	Sample	Findings/comments
Positron emission tomography		
Nordstrom et al[19]	4 healthy women scanned; follicular and luteal/late follicular phases [^{11}C]raclopride tracer	Differences in putamen to cerebellum ratios of D$_2$ receptor density did not exceed those reported in test–retest analyses in men. Sample size extremely small
Eriksson et al[20]	8 women with PMDD scanned; follicular and late luteal phases; ^{11}C-labeled 5-hydroxytryptophan (5-HTP)	Changes in irritability and depressed mood negatively correlated with changes in brain ^{11}C-5-HTP trapping and changes in happiness and energy positively correlated with trapping. Hormone levels were not obtained to verify phases of interest
Single-photon emission computed tomography		
Best et al[18]	10 healthy women scanned twice; follicular and luteal phases	No menstrual cycle variation in striatal DAT or brainstem-diencephalon SERT availability. Hormone levels obtained, but Prog levels did not confirm luteal phase in two cases
Magnetic resonance spectroscopy		
Rasgon et al[21]	5 women with PMDD and 7 healthy women scanned; follicular and late luteal phases	Ratio of *N*-acetyl-aspartate to creatine in the medial prefrontal cortex was decreased in the luteal phase in both groups
Epperson et al[17]	14 healthy women and 9 women with PMDD scanned twice; follicular and mid-late luteal phases	Occipital cortex GABA concentrations fluctuate across the menstrual cycle in both healthy women and those with PMDD. Women with PMDD have signficantly reduced cortical GABA levels in the follicular phase compared with healthy controls
Epperson et al[56]	6 smoking women	Occipital cortex GABA concentrations were reduced in female smokers compared with non-smokers

PMDD, premenstrual dysphoric disorder; GABA, γ-aminobutyric acid; DAT, dopamine transporter; SERT, serotonin reuptake transporter.

an increase in symptoms in the luteal phase is associated with decrease in ^{11}C-5-HTP trapping. Although preliminary, these findings suggest a relationship between serotonin availability and PMDD symptoms.

Using ^{1}H-MRS to investigate the etiology of PMDD, Rasgon et al[21] found changes in neurochemistry across the menstrual cycle. While the ratio of *N*-acetyl-aspartate (NAA) to creatine in the medial prefrontal cortex was significantly lower in the luteal compared to follicular phase in all subjects, there was a non-significant trend toward higher myoinositol to creatine ratios in

women with PMDD in the luteal phase.[21] However, it is difficult to interpret the meaning of these changing ratios. With relatively recent advances in MRS techniques, our laboratory has been able to examine the role of GABA, the brain's major inhibitory neurotransmitter, in the pathogenesis of PMDD. Before we describe our findings, it is important for the reader to consider the preclinical and clinical evidence supporting the notion that altered GABAergic function contributes to the pathogenesis and perhaps treatment of PMDD.

EVIDENCE OF ALTERED GABAERGIC FUNCTION IN PMS/PMDD

Preclinical evidence

As reviewed in Chapter 9, estrogen and progesterone have numerous effects throughout the CNS, mediating/modulating reproductive as well as non-reproductive behaviors. As is true with all steroid hormones, estradiol and progesterone act through classic genomic mechanisms, binding to intracellular receptors and leading to gene transcription and protein synthesis over the course of several minutes to hours to days (reviewed by McEwen[3]). However, it is now well known that estrogen and progesterone (through its metabolites) can modulate glial and/or neuronal function within seconds via membrane-bound ion channels.[2,6,22] It is this latter action, which is likely to be most relevant to PMS/PMDD.

While estrogen acts directly on these membrane ion channels, particularly those of the NMDA receptor type,[2] the effects of progesterone are primarily, if not exclusively, mediated via its metabolites 3α-hydroxy-5α-pregnane-20-one (allopregnanolone; ALLO) and ALLO's β-stereoisomer 3α-hydroxy-5β-pregnane-20-one (pregnanolone; PREG) acting as potent $GABA_A$ receptor agonists.[23,24] Several studies indicate that estrogen binding to NMDA receptors on principal neurons in the CA1 region of the hippocampus leads to enhanced voltage-gated Ca^{2+} currents[2,25] and increased dendritic spine formation. Although it is somewhat controversial whether estrogen treatment in menopausal women enhances overall cognition,[26] the positive effects of estrogen on hippocampal-mediated cognitive function have been well demonstrated in humans,[27,28] non-human primates,[29] and rodents.[30,31] In addition, estrogen appears to be critical to the maintenance of cholinergic and catecholaminergic input to the dorsal lateral prefrontal cortex in young adult monkeys,[32] although the exact mechanism has not been fully elucidated. Estrogen treatment (ET) increases the gene and protein expression of the astrocytic enzyme glutamine synthase, which is important for the conversion of glutamate to glutamine.[6] As glutamine is the predominant precursor for glutamate synthesis, estradiol may enhance overall glutamatergic function and cortical excitability.

In contrast, ALLO and PREG exert sedative, hypnotic, and anxiolytic properties by enhancing the duration and frequency of the opening of $GABA_A$ receptor chloride channels.[22] While the seizure threshold is lowered in proestrus when estrogen is elevated, animals are less likely to seizure during periods of high progesterone.[33] Across the estrus and menstrual cycles, ALLO and PREG levels are thought to mirror the rise in plasma progesterone, which occurs after ovulation. However, ALLO and PREG are neurosteroids and, as such, can be produced in glia and some neurons independent of peripheral progesterone sources. Rodent studies indicate that when under stress, the brain ratio of ALLO/progesterone is greater than that of plasma.[23,34] It is thought that adrenal production of ALLO, which is usually negligible, rises in concert with cortisol during stress states, presumably to counteract and/or supplement some of the stress-related effects of cortisol.[35]

Thus, what happens to the $GABA_A$ receptor during the estrus and menstrual cycle, as well as during pregnancy and lactation, has become the focus of a number of preclinical and clinical research laboratories. Ground-breaking work from Smith and colleagues[36,37] shows that acute and prolonged exposure as well as withdrawal from ALLO results in an increase in α_4 subunit-containing $GABA_A$ receptors, which leads to decreased benzodiazepine sensitivity and enhanced anxiety behaviors in rodents. In contrast, progesterone and PREG dampen the accentuation of the acoustic startle response (ASR) in rodents undergoing corticotropin-releasing hormone (CRH) infusion into the basal nucleus of the stria terminalis (BNST), an area of the brain thought to mediate the effects of anxiety/stress on the ASR.[38] These data suggest that length of neurosteroid administration may contribute to varied effects on GABAergic function. While prolonged exposure and withdrawal may accentuate anxiety, a brief exposure to neurosteroids during stress may serve to dampen anxiety and the stress response. Alternatively, as discussed by Backstrom and colleagues in Chapter 13, ALLO may exert a bimodal effect on anxiety/mood/irritability/aggression, with lower doses that result in blood levels similar to those seen during the luteal phase, leading to negative affect in vulnerable individuals, while higher doses, similar to those seen in late pregnancy, are noted to improve mood.

Why consider the relationship between glutamate and GABA?

These profound, and often opposing effects of estrogen and progesterone highlight the importance of 'striking a balance' in the neuroendocrine milieu in order to maintain cognitive and neurobehavioral health. Although this is likely to be true with multiple neurotransmitter systems, the intimate link between the glutamatergic and GABAergic systems with respect to their synthesis and actions in the CNS is unique and underscores their critical role in balancing neuronal excitation and inhibition. Furthermore, glutamate and

GABA constitute more than 90% of cortical neurons in the adult mammalian brain[39] and are highly sensitive to sex hormones and neurosteroids.

Before reviewing the literature demonstrating altered GABAergic function in women with PMS/PMDD, it is important to consider the synthetic relationship between glutamate and GABA. In addition, glial cells, which were once simply thought to support neuronal function, are also sensitive to sex hormones and play a critical role in glutamate and GABA uptake from the synapse. Figure 11.1 depicts what is considered to be the 'tripartite synapse', which is composed of a presynaptic glutmatergic neuron, a postsynaptic neuron (in this case a GABAergic neuron), with a glial cell in close proximity to the synaptic cleft (reviewed by Hyder et al[40]). Glutamate is released from the presynaptic neuron and taken into the GABAergic neuron; it is transported and converted to GABA by glutamic acid decarboxylase (GAD). The astrocyte rapidly removes glutamate from the cleft via glutamate transporters, converts glutamate, to glutamine, and then releases glutamine, which can be recycled to supply glutamate for further neuronal release.

Glutamatergic stimulation of brain glucose utilization (reviewed by Sibson[41]), and thus neuronal and glial energetics, is yet another means by which sex hormones may alter brain function and behavior at a fundamental level. One of the ways in which estrogen is thought to mediate its neuroprotective effects is by enhancing astrocyte uptake of glutamate from the synaptic cleft.[6,42] Glutamate uptake then triggers a cascade of intracellular events, which leads to vasodilatation.[43] Through this mechanism astrocytes provide the critical link between neuronal activity, glucose utilization, and the functional hyperemia underlying the BOLD effect measured in fMRI studies (reviewed by Hyder et al[40]). Furthermore, postmenopausal women have relatively lower CBF as measured using SPECT, than premenopausal women.[44,45] Postmenopausal ET improves CBF in postmenopausal women, even those with previous CBF impairments due to cerebral vascular disease.[44] Whether this effect of estrogen is solely mediated by estrogen's direct impact on vascular tone or whether estrogen modulation of astrocytic glutamate uptake is a contributing factor is not clear. However, a PET study suggests that estrogen is responsible for the relatively higher cerebral glucose utilization in women than in men.[46]

Clinical evidence

The temporal association between the symptoms of PMS/PMDD and postovulatory increases and decreases in progesterone and its neurosteroid derivatives has prompted much investigation. While findings from studies focusing on peripheral measures of estradiol, progesterone, ALLO, and PREG have been disappointingly inconsistent, taken as a whole, they suggest that peripheral abnormalities in steroid levels and/or ratios are unlikely to be a major factor in the pathogenesis of PMS/PMDD. Instead, it is generally held that negative affective states occurring during the premenstruum, pregnancy/postpartum, and perimenopause are due to an anomalous interaction between steroids and their CNS targets. Alternatively, altered brain production of neurosteroids has not been ruled out.

In an effort to glean information regarding the role of GABAergic function in PMS/PMDD, Backstrom, Sundstrom, and colleagues from Sweden have conducted a number of seminal studies in which women with PMS/PMDD and healthy controls have been given a series of GABA$_A$ receptor agonists during the follicular and luteal phases of the menstrual cycle (described in Chapter 13 and reviewed in detail by Sundstrom Poromaa et al[47]). Using saccadic eye velocity (SEV) as an assay for GABA$_A$ receptor agonist activity, they found that healthy women are more sensitive to these agents during the mid-luteal phase when endogenous progesterone, estrogen, and neurosteroid levels are elevated than in the hypogonadal follicular phase. However, women with PMS/PMDD did not show this luteal phase sensitivity, a finding that is consistent with

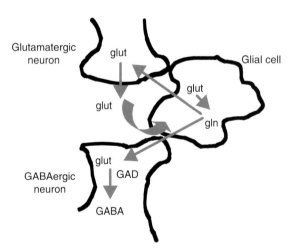

Figure 11.1 Normal glutamate–GABA–glutamine cycling. Glutamate (glut) is released from glutamatergic neurons. A portion of glut is taken up by glial cells and converted to glutamine (gln), which can then be released and taken up by glutamatergic neurons and converted back to glut. Alternatively, gln can be taken up by γ-aminobutyric acid (GABA) neurons, converted to glutamate and then to GABA by glutamic acid decarboxylase (GAD).

the preclinical data indicating that chronic exposure to neurosteroids can lead to reduced benzodiazepine sensitivity. Although it is unclear why this did not happen to healthy women, as one would presume that animal models using healthy organisms would reflect what is meant to be occurring in healthy humans, it does provide evidence in the human laboratory that altered GABAergic function contributes to the pathogenesis of PMS/PMDD. Moreover, selective serotonin reuptake inhibitors (SSRIs), which are preferentially efficacious in the treatment of PMS/PMDD (reviewed by Wyatt et al[48]), are known to enhance brain and cerebrospinal fluid (CSF) levels of ALLO in rodents and humans, respectively.[49,50] When administered in concert with fluoxetine, ALLO has been shown to enhance the antidepressant effects of the SSRI in the forced swim test, an animal model for depression.[51] That SSRIs are effective with luteal phase[48] and possibly symptom-onset treatment[52] suggests that blockade of serotonin reuptake may not be critical for the clinical efficacy of these agents and opens the possibility that SSRI modulation of ALLO, and thus GABA, may be imperative.

Research from other laboratories using a diverse array of investigative techniques has also implicated GABAergic dysregulation in PMDD. Using transcranial magnetic stimulation (TMS), Smith and co-investigators[53] sought to examine the balance of neuronal excitation and inhibition in the motor cortex under different hormonal states. In healthy controls, the late follicular phase (elevated estradiol) was characterized by enhanced facilitation, which is thought to reflect an increase in glutamatergic function and overall cortical excitation. In the luteal phase, the pattern was more consistent with increased paired-pulse inhibition, which isn't surprising given this is the effect seen with benzodiazepine or barbiturate administration (reviewed by Ziemann et al[54]). In a later study, women with PMDD showed a follicular to luteal phase increase in facilitation[55] instead of the increase in inhibition seen in healthy controls. These findings provide further clinical evidence that the balance between cortical excitation and inhibition is altered in the luteal phase of women with PMDD. Whether this is due to an enhancement of glutamatergic function or a reduction in GABAergic function is not known. However, either could tip the scale towards excessive excitation during the luteal phase.

Coming full circle to the role of neuroimaging as a tool to study PMS/PMDD, we utilized ^{1}H-MRS to investigate how occipital cortex GABA concentrations change across the menstrual cycle in women with PMDD and healthy controls.[17] Although luteal phase levels did not differ between groups, women with PMDD appear to have a deficiency in cortical GABA in the non-symptomatic follicular phase. In healthy controls, GABA levels were highest during the follicular phase and decreased as plasma estradiol, progesterone, and ALLO increased in the luteal phase. In women with PMDD, however, GABA levels increased with neuroactive steroid levels. In addition, there was a significant correlation between GABA and ALLO in healthy controls, but not in women with PMDD, suggesting an abnormal relationship between GABA and ALLO in these women.[17] These findings are consistent with those of Sundstrom and Backstrom discussed previously: namely, that women with PMDD have an atypical GABAergic response to endogenous or exogenous $GABA_A$ receptor agonist exposure.

Because nicotine is known to interact with amino acid neurotransmitter systems and women smokers appear to be at heightened risk of negative affect during smoking cessation, we investigated the effects of short-term smoking abstinence on occipital cortex GABA concentrations across the menstrual cycle in healthy female smokers.[56] Although there were no significant effects of 48 hours of abstinence, female smokers showed a lack of cyclicity in baseline cortical GABA level compared with healthy non-smokers, which resulted in decreased follicular phase GABA levels. These findings suggest that substances such as nicotine, which chronically alter GABA or glutamate, are likely to alter the normal neuroendocrine milieu in women. Finally, a recent pilot study demonstrated that, unlike certain subtypes of major depressive disorder,[57] cortical GABA levels are not reduced in postpartum depressed women compared with postpartum healthy controls.[58] However, both groups had lower cortical GABA levels than follicular phase controls despite both groups being in a relatively hypogonadal state. While preliminary, these data suggest that reductions in cortical GABA concentration may be permissive but not causal for postpartum depression.

Although ^{1}H-MRS is a non-invasive way of measuring brain GABA concentrations, our work to date has been restricted to the occipital cortex, which is not typically implicated in the pathogenesis of affective disorders. One cannot rule out the possibility that GABAergic and glutamatergic systems in other brain regions will experience different effects of neurosteroids and their interactions with other neurotransmitter systems. However, as in much of the cortex, GABA and glutamate neurons in the occipital cortex are a target for neuroactive steroids. In addition, $GABA_A$ receptor regulation in the occipital cortex has been associated with other changes in limbic and cortical regions.[59]

Although ^{1}H-MRS provides the means to measure amino acid neurotransmitters in vivo, it is limited in its ability to infer the functional significance of menstrual cycle alterations in cortical GABA concentrations. In the future, ^{1}H-MRS studies could examine the effects of acute and/or chronic administration of GABA$_A$ receptor agonists with affinity for the different receptor subunits. Unfortunately, there is not yet a pharmacological probe specific for the α_4 receptor subunit. Nevertheless, menstrual cycle phase and/or diagnostic specific changes in GABA concentrations with various agonists could provide further information regarding the functional integrity of this neurotransmitter system.

In addition, more advanced MRS techniques such as 13-carbon MRS (^{13}C-MRS) would allow for a dynamic assessment of glutamate–glutamine and GABA–glutamine cycling under different hormonal conditions. These studies would enable investigators to examine the impact of neuroactive steroids on GABA and glutamate synthesis as well as brain energy consumption.

SUMMARY

We have reviewed in this chapter the extant data regarding PET, SPECT, fMRI, and ^{1}H-MRS studies across the menstrual cycle. Taken as a group, they provide considerable evidence that hormonal changes alter brain function and chemistry in humans in a manner that is relatively consistent with that seen in rodents and non-human primates. While the majority of neuroimaging studies focus on the role of estrogen in cognitive processes, functional studies are now addressing the impact of sex steroid/menstrual cycle phase on the neuronal processing of affective tasks. As each of these fMRI studies examined women at slightly different points in the menstrual cycle and two of the three did not confirm menstrual cycle phase with estrogen or progesterone levels, it is somewhat difficult to compare results. However, altogether, they seem to suggest that menstrual cycle phase and/or estrogen alters response to emotionally laden stimuli; whether this hormonal effect is specific to positive or negative stimuli is not yet clear.

Relatively new neuroimaging techniques such a ^{1}H-MRS and ^{13}C-MRS enable investigation of the impact of ovarian hormones and neurosteroids on amino acid neurotransmitter concentration and flux, respectively. Present data provide additional, more direct evidence that GABAergic dysregulation contributes to the pathogenesis of PMDD. Future studies using MRS techniques should be designed to address functional efficacy of the GABAergic system. Finally, all neuroimaging studies should take into consideration the potential for the menstrual cycle to alter outcomes of interest. If the impact of sex steroids is not the focus of a particular neuroimaging paradigm, then studying women during the early to mid-follicular phase (days 1–8) will reduce the likelihood that hormonal variability will contribute significantly to the finding. When the impact of menstrual cycle and/or hormones is the outcome of interest, it is critical that hormone levels are obtained to confirm endocrine status on each test day.

REFERENCES

1. Rothman DL, Petroff OAC, Behar KL, Mattson RH. Localized ^{1}H NMR measurements of gamma-aminobutyric acid in human brain in vivo. Proc Natl Acad Sci USA 1993; 90:5662–6.
2. Woolley CS, Weiland NG, McEwen BS. Schwartzkroin PA. Estradiol increases the sensitivity of hippocampal CA1 pyramidal cells to NMDA receptor-mediated synaptic input: correlation with dendritic spine density. J Neurosci 1997; 17(5):1848–59.
3. McEwen B. Estrogen actions throughout the brain. Rec Prog Hormone Res 2002; 57:357–84.
4. Garcia-Segura LM, McCarthy MM. Minireview: role of glia in neuroendocrine function. Endocrinology 2004; 145(3):1082–6.
5. Pawlak J, Brito V, Kuppers E, Beyer C. Regulation of glutamate transporter GLAST and GLT1 expression in astrocytes by estrogen. Brain Res Mol Brain Res 2005; 138:1–7.
6. Mong JA, Blutstein T. Estradiol modulation of astrocytic form and function: implications for hormonal control of synaptic communication. Neuroscience 2006; 138:967–75.
7. Berman KF, Schmidt PJ, Rubinow DR et al. Modulation of cognition-specific cortical activity by gonadal steroids: a positron-emission tomography study in women. Proc Natl Acad Sci USA 1997; 94:8836–41.
8. Dietrich T, Krings T, Neulen J et al. Effects of blood estrogen level on cortical activation patterns during cognitive activation as measured by functional MRI. Neuroimage 2001; 13:425–32.
9. Fernandez G, Weis S, Stoffel-Wagner B et al. Menstrual cycle-dependent neural plasticity in the adult human brain is hormone, task, and region specific. J Neurosci 2003; 23:3790–5.
10. Veltman DJ, Friston KJ, Sanders G, Price CJ. Regionally specific sensitivity differences in fMRI and PET: where do they come from? Neuroimage 2000; 11:575–88.
11. Pelligrino DA, Galea E. Estrogen and cerebrovascular physiology and pathophysiology. Jpn J Pharmacol 2001; 86:137–58.
12. Goldstein JM, Jerram M, Poldrack R et al. Hormonal cycle modulates arousal circuitry in women using functional magnetic resonance imaging. J Neurosci 2005; 25:9309–16.
13. Magiakou MA, Mastorakos G, Webster E, Chrousos GP. The hypothalamic–pituitary–adrenal axis and the female reproductive system. Ann NY Acad Sci 1997; 816:42–56.
14. Viau V, Meaney MJ. Variations in the hypothalamic-pituitary–adrenal response to stress during the estrous cycle in the rat. Endocrinology 1991; 129:2503–11.
15. Amin Z, Epperson CN, Constable RT, Canli T. Effects of estrogen variation on neural correlates of emotional response inhibition. Neuroimage 2006; 32:457–64.
16. Protopopescu X, Pan H, Altemus M et al. Orbitofrontal cortex activity related to emotional processing changes across the menstrual cycle. Proc Natl Acad Sci USA 2005; 102:16060–5.
17. Epperson CN, Haga K, Mason GF et al. Cortical gamma-aminobutyric acid levels across the menstrual cycle in healthy women and those with premenstrual dysphoric disorder: a proton magnetic resonance spectroscopy study. Arch Gen Psychiatry 2002; 59:851–8.
18. Best SE, Sarrel PM, Malison RT et al. Striatal dopamine transporter availability with [123I]beta-CIT SPECT is unrelated to gender or menstrual cycle. Psychopharmacology (Berl) 2005; 183:181–9.

19. Nordstrom AL, Olsson H, Halldin C. A PET study of D_2 dopamine receptor density at different phases of the menstrual cycle. Psychiatry Res 1998; 83:1–6.

20. Eriksson O, Wall A, Marteinsdottir I et al. Mood changes correlate to changes in brain serotonin precursor trapping in women with premenstrual dysphoria. Psychiatry Res 2006; 146:107–16.

21. Rasgon NL, Thomas MA, Guze BH et al. Menstrual cycle-related brain metabolite changes using ^{1}H magnetic resonance spectroscopy in premenopausal women: a pilot study. Psychiatry Res 2001; 106:47–57.

22. Majewski MD, Harrison NL, Schwartz RD, Baker JL, Paul SM. Steroid hormone metabolites are barbiturate-like modulators of the GABA receptor. Science 1986; 232:1004–7.

23. Paul SM, Purdy RH. Neuroactive steroids. FASEB J 1992; 6:2311–22.

24. N-Wihlback AC, Sundstrom-Poromaa I, Backstrom T. Action by and sensitivity to neuroactive steroids in menstrual cycle related CNS disorders. Psychopharmacology 2006; 186:388–401.

25. Wong M, Moss RL. Long-term and short-term electrophysiological effects of estrogen on the synaptic properties of hippocampal CA1 neurons. J Neurosci 1992; 12(8):3217–25.

26. Epperson CN, Wisner KL, Yamamoto B. Gonadal steroids in the treatment of mood disorders. Psychosom Med 1999; 65:676–97.

27. Sherwin BB. Estrogen and cognitive aging in women. Neuroscience 2006; 138(3):1021–6.

28. LeBlanc ES, Janowsky J, Chan BK, Nelson HD. Hormone replacement therapy and cognition: systematic review and meta-analysis. JAMA 2001; 285:1489–99.

29. Rapp PR, Morrison JH, Roberts JA. Cyclic estrogen replacement improves cognitive function in aged ovariectomized rhesus monkeys. J Neurosci 2003; 23(13):5708–14.

30. Sandstrom NJ, Williams CL. Memory retention is modulated by acute estradiol and progesterone replacement. Behav Neurosci 2001; 115(2):384–93.

31. Fernandez SM, Frick KM. Chronic oral estrogen affects memory and neurochemistry in middle-aged female mice. Behav Neurosci 2004; 118:1340–51.

32. Kritzer MF, Kohama SG. Ovarian hormones differentially influence immunoreactivity for dopamine beta-hydroxylase, choline acetyltransferase, and serotonin in the dorsolateral prefrontal cortex of adult rhesus monkeys. J Comp Neurol 1999; 409(3):438–51.

33. Moran MH, Smith SS. Progesterone withdrawal I: pro-convulsant effects. Brain Res 1998; 807(1–2):84–90.

34. Purdy RH, Morrow AL, Moore PH Jr, Paul SM. Stress-induced elevations of gamma-aminobutyric acid type A receptor-active steroids in the rat brain. Proc Natl Acad Sci USA 1991; 88(10):4553–7.

35. Droogleever Fortuyn HA, van Broekhoven F, Span PN et al. Effects of PhD examination stress on allopregnanolone and cortisol plasma levels and peripheral benzodiazepine receptor density. Psychoneuroendocrinology 2004; 29(10):1341–4.

36. Smith SS, Gong QH, Hsu F et al. $GABA_A$ receptor alpha–4 subunit suppression prevents withdrawal properties of an endogenous steroid. Nature 1998; 392:926–9.

37. Gulinello M, Gong QH, Li X, Smith SS. Short-term exposure to a neuroactive steroid increases α4 $GABA_A$ receptor subunit levels in association with increased anxiety in the female rat. Brain Res 2001; 910:55–66.

38. Toufexis DJ, Davis C, Hammond A, Davis M. Progesterone attenuates corticotropin-releasing factor-enhanced but not fear-potentiated startle via the activity of its neuroactive metabolite, allopregnanolone. J Neurosci 2004; 24(45):10280–7.

39. Nicholls DG. The glutamatergic nerve terminal. Eur J Biochem 1993; 212:613–31.

40. Hyder F, Patel AB, Gjedde A et al. Neuronal-glial glucose oxidation and glutamatergic-GABAergic function. J Cereb Blood Flow Metab 2006; 26(7):865–77.

41. Sibson NR. Cerebral energetics and neurotransmitter fluxes. In: Shulman RG, Rothman DL, eds. Brain Energetics and Neuronal Activity. Chichester: John Wiley & Sons; 2004:75–97.

42. Liang Z, Valla M, Sefidvash-Hockley S et al. Effects of estrogen treatment on glutamate uptake in cultured human astrocytes derived from cortex of Alzheimer's disease patients. J Neurochem 2002; 80:807–14.

43. Rossi DJ. Another BOLD role for astrocytes: coupling blood flow to neural activity. Nat Neurosci 2006; 9(2):159–61.

44. Slopien R, Junik R, Meczekalski B, Halerz-Nowakowska B et al. Influence of hormonal replacement therapy on the regional cerebral blood flow in postmenpausal women. Maturitas 2003; 46:255–62.

45. Greene RA. Estrogen and cerebral blood flow: a mechanism to explain the impact of estrogen on the incidence and treatment of Alzheimer's disease. Int J Fertil Womens Med 2000; 45(4):253–7.

46. Baxter LR, Mazziotta JC, Phelps ME et al. Cerebral glucose metabolic rates in normal human females versus normal males. Psychiatry Res 1987; 21:237–45.

47. Sundstrom Poromaa I, Smith S, Gulinello M. GABA receptors, progesterone and premenstrual dysphoric disorder. Arch Womens Ment Health 2003; 6:23–41.

48. Wyatt KM, Dimmock PW, O'Brien PMS. Selective serotonin reuptake inhibitors for premenstrual syndrome. Cochrane Database Syst Rev 2002; (4):CD 001396.

49. Uzunov DP, Cooper TB, Costa E, Guidotti A. Fluoxetine-elicited changes in brain neurosteroid content measured by negative ion mass fragmentography. Proc Natl Acad Sci USA 1996; 93:12599–604.

50. Uzunova V, Sheline Y, Davis JM et al. Increase in the cerebrospinal fluid content of neurosteroids in patients with unipolar major depression who are receiving fluoxetine or fluvoxamine. Proc Natl Acad Sci USA 1998; 95:3239–44.

51. Khisti RT, Chopde CT. Serotonergic agents modulate antidepressant-like effect of the neurosteroid 3α-hydroxy-5α-pregnan-20-one in mice. Brain Res 2000; 865:291–300.

52. Yonkers KA, Holthausen GA, Poschman K, Howell HB. Symptom-onset treatment for women with premenstrual dysphoric disorder. J Clin Psychopharmacol 2006; 26:198–202.

53. Smith MJ, Adams LF, Schmidt PJ, Rubinow DR, Wassermann EM. Effects of ovarian hormones on human cortical excitability. Ann Neurol 2002; 51(5): 599–603.

54. Ziemann U, Steinhoff BJ, Tengan F, Paulus W. Transcranial Magnetic stimulation: its current role in epilepsy research Epilepsy Res 1998; 30(1):11–30.

55. Smith MJ, Adams LF, Schmidt PJ, Rubinow DR, Wassermann EM. Abnormal luteal phase excitability of the motor cortex in women with premenstrual syndrome. Biol Psychiatry 2003; 54(7):757–62.

56. Epperson CN, O'Malley S, Czarkowski KA et al. Sex, GABA, and nicotine: the impact of smoking on cortical GABA levels across the menstrual cycle as measured with proton magnetic resonance spectroscopy. Biol Psychiatry 2005; 57:44–8.

57. Sanacora G, Gueorguieva R, Epperson CN et al. Subtype specific alterations of gamma-aminobutyric acid and glutamate in patients with major depression. Arch Gen Psychiatry 2004; 61(7):705–13.

58. Epperson CN, Gueorguieva R, Czarkowski KA et al. Preliminary evidence of reduced occipital GABA concentrations in puerperal women: a ^{1}H-MRS study. Psychopharmacology (Berl) 2006; 186(3):425–33.

59. Abi-Dargham A, Krystal JH, Anjilvel S et al. Alterations of benzodiazepine receptors in type II alcoholic subjects measured with SPECT and [^{123}I]iomazenil. Am J Psychiatry 1998; 155:1550–5.

12

Hormonal therapies overview

Candace Brown and Frank Ling

INTRODUCTION

The importance of PMS/PMDD has been summarized in previous chapters and we will begin by briefly summarizing this. Premenstrual syndrome (PMS) is a condition of recurrent physical and psychological symptoms that occurs in a cyclic fashion during the 1- to 2-week period preceding a woman's menstrual period. Most surveys have found that as many as 85% of menstruating women report one or more mild premenstrual symptoms. Severe symptoms that meet the criteria for PMS, however, are much less common, with only 10% of women reporting significant impairment in their lifestyles.[1] Premenstrual dysphoric disorder (PMDD), a variant of PMS that entails more severe psychological symptoms and impairment of functioning, occurs in 2–9% of women of reproductive age.[2] This chapter will focus on hormonal treatments that have been used in both PMS and PMDD, since only recent studies have examined the latter.

Although the etiology of PMDD is incompletely understood, the leading hormonal theory is related to fluctuating sex steroid levels. Although there is a temporal relationship between symptoms of PMDD, female sex hormones, and phases of the menstrual cycle, women with PMDD show no consistent diagnosis-related differences in basal levels of ovarian hormones.[3] We have already seen that the likely etiology of PMS/ PMDD is the effect of postovulatory progesterone in sensitive women. This progesterone sensitivity is probably due to abnormal neurotransmitter function. Thus, in general terms, treatment can be achieved by means of correction of the neurotransmitter status, for example, by use of selective serotonin reuptake inhibitors (SSRIs) or by suppression of ovulation. Chapter 14 deals with the concept of treatment by ovarian suppression. In this chapter we outline the role of hormone therapy.

There is inevitably some overlap and differences of opinion.

Suppression of ovarian function with pharmacotherapy[4–6] or through surgical menopause[7,8] eliminates the symptoms of PMDD. Moreover, symptoms are eliminated during pregnancy and are absent during nonovulatory cycles and after menopause.[9] The most likely explanation is that women with PMDD are in some way vulnerable to the normal physiological changes associated with the menstrual cycle.[3] This hypothesis was supported in one study where women with PMDD developed depressed mood in response to challenge with physiological levels of estrogen and progesterone compared with controls.[10]

Androgens have also been suggested in the etiology of PMS/PMDD because of the prominence of irritability in the symptom profile. Elevated testosterone levels have been reported in women with severe premenstrual irritability,[11] and a positive correlation has been observed between free testosterone concentrations and irritability.[12] Moreover, some success has been reported in treating PMDD with androgen antagonists.[11] There are other studies where complex interactions with serotonin and even lower testosterone levels have been shown, leading to the use of testosterone for treatment.

Finally, metabolites of progesterone, allopregnanolone and pregnanolone, may be decreased in women with PMDD. These metabolites may have a positive effect on the central nervous system similar to that of GABA (γ-aminobutyric acid), and deficiencies may give rise to premenstrual symptoms.[13]

ORAL CONTRACEPTIVES

Combined oral contraceptive pills (OCPs) prevent ovulation and replace endogenous fluctuations of ovarian steroids with a stable endogenous hormonal environment. For this reason, combined OCPs have been used to treat premenstrual symptoms.[14] Unfortunately, unless given continuously, the OCPs introduce a new exogenous hormone cyclicity that results in a confusing picture when treatment studies are analyzed.

The major trend in the formulation of OCs over the last 40 years has been a reduction in the doses of both the estrogen and the progestin components, and, more recently, chemical alterations of the progestins to provide less androgenic compounds.[9] Estradiol (ethinyl estradiol) doses have decreased from 100 μg to 20–30 μg. The dose of the progestin component has also decreased. All but one currently prescribed OC still contains a progestin derived from 19-nortestosterone. Table 12.1 summarizes the pharmacological profile of progesterone, 19-nortestosterone, and a new progestin drospirenone derived from spironolactone.[15]

The palliative effect of OCPs, particularly for physical premenstrual symptoms, has been suggested by previous epidemiological and non-placebo-controlled research.[14,16–18] There have been three randomized, placebo-controlled trials investigating OCPs in treating premenstrual symptoms, one evaluating PMS[19] and two evaluating PMDD.[20,21]

In the first randomized trial, a triphasic formulation reduced physical symptoms but not mood alterations.[19] The study enrolled 82 women with PMS, and the active treatment was a triphasic OCP (ethinyl estradiol 35 μg + norethindrone 0.5 mg days 1–7 and 17–21 and 1.0 mg days 8–16).[19] Differences between the OCP and placebo were minimal, although mood worsened in the active-treatment group during the hormone-free, postmenstrual period.

The other two trials evaluated a new progestin, drospirenone, which possesses spironolactone-like antimineralocorticoid and antiandrogenic activity.[15] Previous studies of the diuretic spironolactone in PMS have demonstrated its efficacy in relieving the physical symptoms (bloating, breast tenderness) and the psychological symptoms (mood change, irritability) of this condition.[22–24] The antiandrogenic activity of drospirenone may improve premenstrual irritability and acne,[25] which may be due to elevated plasma testosterone in women with PMS.[26,27]

Freeman et al compared placebo to an OCP with drospirenone 3 mg and ethinyl estradiol 30 μg in a 21/7 platform to 82 women who met PMDD criteria.[20] The active treatment was associated with significantly greater improvement in appetite, acne, and food cravings, but there were no differences between groups in mood symptoms. The lack of between-group differences in mood symptoms may have been due to the modest sample size in the setting of a considerable placebo response rate (43%).

The more positive findings in the Freeman[20] compared with the Graham[19] study may be due to the use of a progestin that has antimineralocorticoid and antiandrogenic properties not observed in the progestins derived from 19-nortestosterone, such as norethindrone.[15]

Recently, a controlled study conducted by Yonkers et al[21] showed that the drospirenone-containing OCP formulation administered for 24 of 28 days in a cycle ameliorated symptoms associated with PMDD compared

Table 12.1 Pharmacological profile of progestins (in animal models)[a]

Progestins	Pharmacological activity			
	[a]Progestogenic	Antiandrogenic	Antimineralocorticoid	Androgenic
Progesterone	+	(+)	+	−
Drospirenone	+	+	+	−
Norgestimate[b]	+	−	−	(+)
Levonorgestrel	+	−	−	(+)
Desogestrel	+	−	−	(+)
Norethindrone	+	−	−	(+)
Cyproterone acetate[c]	+	+	−	−

[a]+ = distinct effect, (+) = negligible effect at therapeutic doses, − = no effect.
[b]Metabolized to levonorgestrel-3-oxime and levonorgestrel.
[c]Not available in the USA.
Adapted from Fuhrmann et al.[15]

with placebo in 450 women.[21] Mood symptoms (e.g. depression, anxiety, mood swings, irritability), behavioral symptoms (difficulty concentrating, sleep disturbance), and physical symptoms (e.g. fatigue, increased appetite, breast tenderness, headaches) were all significantly reduced with the OCP compared with placebo. It is particularly significant that active treatment was associated with a 49% reduction in premenstrual depression, as OCPs have been thought by some to worsen or cause symptoms of depression.[28,29]

The differences in estrogen dose and shortened drug-free interval between the Yonkers[21] and the Freeman[20] studies may explain the more favorable results in the former study. The Freeman study[20] used a higher dose of estradiol than the Yonkers study[21] (e.g. 30 μg rather than 20 μg), and the active drug was given for 21 rather than 24 days in a 28-day cycle.

In addition to their effect on premenstrual symptoms, there are numerous health advantages afforded by intake of OCPs. They provide effective, reversible contraception but also have other known benefits, including prevention of bone loss, decreased risks for ovarian and endometrial cancer, anemia, abnormal uterine bleeding, uterine myomata, endometriosis, pelvic inflammatory disease, as well as complications of unplanned pregnancy, such as ectopic pregnancy and molar gestation.[9,18] The most bothersome physical side effects of OCPs are bloating and breast tenderness, and these symptoms are, at least in part, attributable to water retention, probably related to their estrogenic component.[9,18]

Currently, the evidence suggests that OCPs should be considered if premenstrual symptoms are primarily physical, and the newer OCPs containing antiandrogenic progestins may be effective in treating mood symptoms as well. More controlled studies are needed to confirm the efficacy of continuous vs cyclical oral contraceptives in ameliorating premenstrual symptoms.[30] The newer OCPs with lower-dose estrogen and drospirenone may have a unique role in women who both desire contraception and suffer from symptoms of PMDD.

Table 12.2 lists the evidence supporting the efficacy and safety of OCPs as well as the other hormonal therapies to be discussed in this chapter.

Table 12.2 Evidence-based guidelines on the use of hormonal treatments in PMS/PMDD				
Treatment	Strength of recommendation[a]	Quality of evidence[b]	Efficacy[c]	Adverse events[d]
Oral contraceptives	A	Ib	A	A
Estradiol patches and implants	B	IIb	C	C
Progesterone suppositories and micronized tablets	A	Ia	D	A
Danazol	A	Ib	A	C
GnRH agonists	A	Ia	A	C
Ovariectomy	B	IIb	C	C
Chasteberry (*Vitex agnus-castus*)	A	Ib	C	D
Black cohosh (*Cimicifuga racemosa*)	C	IV	C	D

[a]*Strength of recommendation*   A = At least one randomized controlled trial as part of a body of literature of overall good quality and consistency addressing the specific recommendation. B = Well-controlled clinical studies available but no randomized clinical trials on the topic of recommendations. C = Evidence obtained from expert committee reports or opinions and/or clinical experiences of respected authorities. Indicates an absence of directly applicable clinical studies of good quality.
[b]*Quality of evidence*   Ia = Evidence obtained from a meta-analysis of randomized controlled trials. Ib = Evidence obtained from at least one randomized controlled trial. IIb = Evidence obtained from at least one other type of well-designed quasi-experimental study. III = Evidence obtained from well-designed non-experimental descriptive studies, such as comparative studies, correlation studies, and case studies. IV = Evidence obtained from expert committee reports or opinions and/or clinical experience of respected authorities.
[c]*Efficacy*   A = Effective. B = Conflicting data. C = Insufficient data. D = Ineffective.
[d]*Adverse effects*   A = Minimal/mild. B = Moderate. C = Major. D = Unknown.

ESTRADIOL

A high dosage of estradiol in the form of transdermal estradiol patches or subcutaneous implants has been given to suppress ovulation in controlled studies.[31–35] To hinder endometrial hyperplasia, cyclical progestogens are given to ensure a regular withdrawal bleed. Both routes of administering estradiol have shown positive effects for treating mental and physical symptoms in two non-controlled studies.

A randomized, prospective trial comparing estradiol patches in dosages of 100 and 200 μg twice weekly, combined with cyclical progestogens, showed no difference in the effectiveness of these two dosages. However, a greater dropout rate and a greater incidence of adverse effects attributed to estrogen was noted in the higher-dosage group.[34]

A long-term follow-up study of 50 patients who had used estradiol implants for PMS for a mean of 5.6 years (range 2–8 years) was conducted.[35] There was a continued beneficial response to treatment for all symptoms, varying from 74% for bloating to 96% for depression. Cyclical progestogenic symptoms occurred in 58% of patients. These were partially relieved by alteration in dose, type, and duration of progestogen treatment, but in seven patients the symptoms remained severe. Attempts to reduce the dose of progestogen led to cystic hyperplasia in four patients. There were no complications from venous thrombosis, pulmonary embolus, or breast disease of atypical endometrial hyperplasia. Based on insufficient data on efficacy and potentially significant adverse events, high-dose estrogen is not recommended for treating PMS/PMDD.

PROGESTERONE

The rationale for the use of progesterone and progestogens in the management of premenstrual symptoms was based on the premise that progesterone deficiency is the cause.[36] Historically, natural progesterone has been one of the most commonly employed therapies in women with PMS, but careful scientific scrutiny has not supported an overall benefit of this hormone when compared with placebo, whether administered as a vaginal suppository[37] or as oral micronized progesterone.[13]

Recently, a meta-analysis was conducted and included only those controlled trials that required a diagnosis of PMS.[9] Ten trials of progesterone therapy (531 women) and four trials of progestogen therapy (378 women) met criteria. None of the eight trials of progesterone suppositories were shown to have a positive effect. Micronized oral progesterone was found to have some benefit in a study of 23 patients[38] but a larger study of 106 patients found no difference between active treatment and placebo. There have been no controlled studies on topical progesterone cream, despite the fact that it has been popularized throughout the media and the Internet.

Four of 15 progestogen studies were included in the meta-analysis. Of those studies, two used dydrogesterone, one used norethisterone, and one used medroxyprogesterone. Medroxyprogesterone was found to be significantly more effective than placebo in improving both psychological symptoms and breast symptoms in 19 patients,[39] whereas norethisterone showed significantly greater improvement than placebo in treating breast symptoms only in 16 women.[39] However, didrogesterone was found to be no more effective than placebo in one study of 24 women[40] and in a larger study of 260 patients.[41] The low numbers of participants did not permit a comparative analysis of individual progestogens to be undertaken. The author concluded from the meta-analysis that exogenous administration of either progestogens or progesterone does not improve symptoms.

DANAZOL

Danazol, a progestogen with some androgen properties, given for the treatment of endometriosis, has also been used in the treatment of PMS. The dosages used in PMS treatment – 100 mg twice a day or 200 mg once a day – are lower than the dosages used for endometriosis. At these dosages, ovulation inhibition occurs in the majority of cases.[18] Five placebo-controlled, double-blind studies and one open-label study evaluated the efficacy of danazol 200 mg/day.[42–46] In each study, danazol had a beneficial effect on PMS symptoms compared with placebo in cycles where anovulaton was obtained, despite the relatively small sample sizes of the studies. Danazol is known to have androgenic adverse effects on lipids and to cause acne, vocal changes, and negative mood at dosages used for endometriosis. However, these symptoms were not observed with the dosages used in the six aforementioned studies. Despite this, the study withdrawal rates were higher in these studies (32.5%) than those seen in other PMS studies (11.5%).[44] Although studies have consistently shown danazol to effectively treat premenstrual symptoms, its side effect profile suggests its use only in patients who have failed more conservative treatments. Attempts to reduce side effects have been made by administering danazol in the luteal phase only. Whilst Sarno has demonstrated a beneficial effect on the general symptoms of PMS as well as for cyclical mastalgia, when patients are stratified, only breast-related symptoms are improved. Luteal phase danazol is a very effective treatment for breast symptoms and with virtual elimination of symptomatic side effects.

GONADOTROPIN-RELEASING HORMONE AGONISTS

Gonadotropin-releasing hormone (GnRH) agonists are an example of a group of drugs that suppress ovarian function, which is believed to be the trigger for PMDD.[47] GnRH agonists down-regulate the gonadotropin receptors in the pituitary gland to create a hypogonadotropic state whereby ovarian function is suppressed to menopausal levels and amenorrhea is induced.[47] Due to the low serum estradiol concentrations induced by GnRH agonists, side effects are common and, because of potential bone demineralization,[48] treatment with these compounds is usually restricted to 6 months.[49] In order to lengthen the period that GnRH agonists can be administered, several studies have used concomitant 'add-back' hormone replacement therapy. GnRH agonists are not frequently prescribed in primary care because of cost and side effects.

Recently, a meta-analysis of published randomized placebo-controlled trials was conducted to evaluate the efficacy of GnRH agonists with and without 'add-back' therapy in women with a diagnosis of PMS.[47] Five trials without add-back therapy (71 women on active treatment) met inclusion criteria. The equivalent odds ratio (OR) was 8.66 in favor of GnRH agonists. GnRH agonists were more efficacious for physical than behavioral symptoms, although the difference was not statistically significant. Women were three times more likely to experience side effects on treatment compared with placebo, which included hot flashes, aches, night sweats, and nausea. Of the five included trials, three used depot GnRH agonists,[4,6,50] one used daily injection,[51] and another gave GnRH agonists as a nasal spray.[52] However, the efficacy of individual GnRH types and routes of administration could not be assessed in the meta-analysis, owing to the small number of trials and participants.

Three randomized controlled trials (64 patients in total) compared the efficacy of add-back therapy and GnRH agonists + placebo in the management of PMS.[5,50,53] There was no significant reduction in effectiveness of GnRH agonists with the addition of add-back therapy. These finding were confirmed in a subsequent study of leuprolide acetate with and without add-back.[54] However, women were more likely to drop out of the trial while on add-back therapy.

Future studies on GnRH agonists in PMDD should include those which assess the safety of long-term combined therapy particularly in relation to lipid profiles and bone mineral densities. Additionally, cost and the need for long-term repeated injections needs consideration. Nevertheless, in patients unresponsive to successive trials of OCPs, GnRH agonists + add-back therapy should be considered second-line treatment.

DIETARY SUPPLEMENTATION

Some dietary supplements are thought to interact with steroid activity and are therefore considered here.

Chasteberry

Chasteberry, the fruit of the chaste tree (*Vitex agnus-castus*), is commonly used for treating premenstrual symptoms. Active constituents in chasteberries are the essential oils, iridoid glycosides, and the flavonoids.[55] The mechanism of action is unclear, but it may involve decreasing estrogen, and increasing progesterone, prolactin, and dopamine levels.[56] A 3-month, randomized double-blind placebo-controlled study of 217 PMS/PMDD subjects found chasteberry (600 mg three times daily) only alleviated restlessness.[57] Another study showed that chasteberry and vitamin B_6 had similar reductions in PMS scores (77% and 66%, respectively).[58] In general, the data show conflicting results but appear promising.

Black cohosh

The majority of studies looking at black cohosh (*Cimicifuga racemosa*) have been in the treatment of menopausal symptoms. The mechanism of action remains somewhat unclear, but may involve suppressing luteinizing hormone secretion.[56] A number of studies using Remifemin, a proprietary extract of black cohosh, show efficacy in treating menopausal symptoms (hot flashes, profuse sweating, sleep disturbance, and depressive moods).[59] Because these symptoms often present in women with PMDD, many clinicians have recommended the use of black cohosh in this population. Further clinical studies are needed to determine the efficacy of black cohosh in PMDD. The recommended dose is 40–80 mg of a standardized extract twice daily, providing 4–8 mg of triterpine glycosides.[59]

CONCLUSIONS

The ideal choice of a hormonal treatment in PMS/PMDD would be based on randomized, placebo-controlled trials consistently demonstrating efficacy in the treatment of emotional and physical symptoms with minimal side effects. Figure 12.1 provides an algorithm for hormonal treatments for PMS/PMDD. Oral contraceptives are the agents of first choice because they most closely approximately this goal. They do, however, introduce a new progestogen cyclicity that may negate its effect. Their efficacy in treating physical premenstrual symptoms has been demonstrated in controlled trials and they produce minimal to mild side effects. Moreover, they provide additional benefits such as contraception, control of abnormal uterine bleeding, and management of other pelvic conditions. Contraceptives containing drospirenone show potential. Recent data suggest that low-dose estrogen and antiandrogenic/antimineralocorticoid progestins, such as drospirenone,

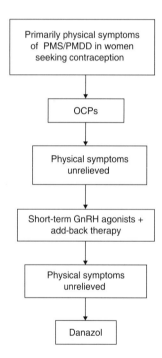

Figure 12.1 Algorithm for hormonal treatment of PMS/PMDD. OCPs = oral contraceptive pills; GnRH agonists = gonadotropin-releasing hormone agonists. Avoid estradiol patches and implants due to insufficient evidence of efficacy and potentially significant side effects from high-dose estrogen. Avoid progesterone suppositories and micronized tablets because of lack of efficacy. Avoid ovariectomy because of insufficient efficacy data and major side effects. Chasteberry and black cohosh may be suggested, but presently there is insufficient data to suggest their efficacy and/or potential side effects.

may also ameliorate emotional premenstrual symptoms, but further study is needed.

A recent meta-analysis of GnRH agonists demonstrated their efficacy in treating symptoms of PMS/PMDD. Their side effect profile and cost precludes long-term use, although there is some evidence to suggest that side effects can be reduced by add-back therapy with no detrimental effect on efficacy. Short-term therapy with GnRH agonists + add-back therapy is recommended when other treatment has failed and the woman demonstrates significant functional impairment from physical symptoms.

Like GnRH agonists, danazol has consistently shown efficacy in treating physical symptoms of PMS/PMDD in controlled studies. However, its practical use is limited by the need for concurrent administration of a reliable contraceptive method, weight gain, mood changes, acne, and possible virilization of the fetus. Thus, danazol is a suggested treatment for PMS/PMDD only when OCPs and GnRH agonists have failed, and premenstrual symptoms are significantly impairing daily functioning. It is a useful drug used in the luteal phase only in treating breast symptoms, and this is associated with minimal side effects.

High-dose estradiol has been investigated in a number of trials. No incidents of venous thrombosis, pulmonary embolus, or atypical endometrial hyperplasia occurred, but risks remain high. Estradiol patches and implants are not recommended for treating PMS/PMDD by the authors of this chapter, but there are differing views based on the same evidence (see Chapter 14).

Historically, natural progesterone has been one of the most commonly employed therapies in women with PMS/PMDD, but controlled trials have consistently shown no benefit of this hormone when compared with placebo, whether administered as a vaginal suppository or as oral micronized progesterone. Therefore, it is not recommended as treatment.

Data regarding use of dietary supplements which affect endocrine function is scant and conflicting. Clinical experience has shown no significant side effects of either chasteberry or cohosh, and there is anecdotal evidence to suggest a benefit.

REFERENCES

1. American College of Obstetricians and Gynecologists: Premenstrual syndrome. ACOG Practice Bulletin No. 15, April 2000.
2. American Psychiatric Association. Diagnostic and Statistical Manual of Mental Disorders, 4th edn, text revision. Washington, DC: American Psychiatric Association; 2000.
3. Roca CA, Schmidt PJ, Bloch M et al. Implications of endocrine studies of premenstrual syndrome. Psychiatr Ann 1996; 26:577–80.

4. Freeman EW, Sondheimer SJ, Rickels K. Gonadotropin-releasing hormone agonist in treatment of premenstrual symptoms with and without ongoing dysphoria: a controlled study. Psychopharmacol Bull 1997; 33:303–9.

5. Mortola AJF, Girton L, Fischer U. A successful treatment of severe premenstrual syndrome by combined use of gonadotropin-releasing hormone agonist and estrogen/progestin. J Clin Endocrinol Metab 1991; 72:252A–F.

6. Brown CS, Ling FW, Andersen RN et al. Efficacy of depot leprolide in premenstrual syndrome: effect of symptom severity and type in a controlled trial. Obstet Gynecol 1994; 84:779–86.

7. Casper RF, Heart MT. The effect of hysterectomy and bilateral oophorectomy in women with severe premenstrual syndrome. Am J Obstet Gynecol 1990; 162:105–9.

8. Casson P, Hahn PM, Van Vugt DA et al. Lasting response to ovariectomy in severe intractable premenstrual syndrome. Am J Obstet Gynecol 1990; 162:99–105.

9. Wyatt K, Dimmock P, Jones P et al. Efficacy of progesterone and progestogens in management of premenstrual syndrome: systematic review. BMJ 2001; 323:776–80.

10. Rapkin AJ. A review of treatment of premenstrual syndrome and premenstrual dysphoric disorder. Psychoneuroendocrinology 2003; 28(Suppl 3):39–53.

11. Eriksson E, Sundblad C, Landen M et al. Behavioral effects of androgens in women. In: Steiner M, Yonkers KA, Ericksson E, eds. Mood Disorders in Women. London: Martin Dunitz; 2000:233–46.

12. Steiner M, Dunn EJ, MacDougall M et al. Serotonin transporter gene polymorphism, free testosterone, and symptoms associated with premenstrual dysphoric disorder. Biol Psychiatry 2002; 51:91S.

13. Freeman EW, Rickels K, Sondheimer SJ et al. A double-blind trial of oral progesterone, alprazolam, and placebo in treatment of severe premenstrual syndrome. JAMA 1995; 274:51–7.

14. Hylan TR, Sundell K, Judge R. The impact of premenstrual symptomatology on functioning and treatment-seeking behavior: experience from the United States, United Kingdom, and France. J Womens Health Gend Based Med 1999; 8:1043–52.

15. Fuhrmann U, Krattenmacher R, Slater EP et al. The novel progestin drospirenone and its natural counterpart progesterone: biochemical profile and antiandrogenic potential. Contraception 1996; 54:243–51.

16. Walker A, Bancroft J. Relationship between premenstrual symptoms and oral contraceptive use: a controlled study. Psychosom Med 1990; 52:86–96.

17. Backstrom T, Hansson-Malmstrom Y, Lindhe BA et al. Oral contraceptives in premenstrual syndrome: a randomized comparison of triphasic and monophasic preparations. Contraception 1992; 36:257–66.

18. Backstrom T, Andreen I, Birzniece V et al. The role of hormones and hormonal treatments in premenstrual syndrome. CNS Drugs 2003; 17:325–42.

19. Graham CA, Sherwin BB A prospective treatment study of premenstrual symptoms using a triphasic oral contraceptive. Psychosom Res 1992; 36:257–66.

20. Freeman EW, Kroll R, Rapkin A et al. Evaluation of a unique oral contraceptive in the treatment of premenstrual dysphoric disorder. J Womens Health Gend Based Med 2001; 10:561–9.

21. Yonkers KA, Brown C, Pearlstein RB et al. Efficacy of a new low-dose oral contraceptive with drospirenone in premenstrual dysphoric disorder. Obstet Gynecol 2005; 106:492–501.

22. Vellacott ID, O'Brien PM. Effect of spironolactone on premenstrual syndrome symptoms. J Reprod Med 1987; 32:429–54.

23. Hellberg D, Claesson B, Nilsson S. Premenstrual tension: a placebo-controlled efficacy study with spironolactone and medroxyprogesterone acetate. Int J Gynaecol Obstet 1991; 34:243–7.

24. Aslaksen K, Falk V. Spironolactone in the treatment of premenstrual tension: a double-blind study of spironolactone versus bendroflumethiazide and placebo. Cur Ther Res Clin Exp 1991; 49:120–5.

25. Schmidt JB, Spona J. The levels of androgen in serum in female acne patients. Endocrinol Exp 1985; 19:17–21.

26. Dougherty DM, Bjork JM, Moeller PG et al. The influence of menstrual cycle phase on the relationship between testosterone and aggression. Physiol Behav 1997; 62:431–6.

27. Eriksson E, Sundblad C, Lisjo P et al. Serum levels of androgens are higher in women with premenstrual irritability and dysphoria than in controls. Psychoneuroendocrinology 1992; 17:195–204.

28. Slap GB. Oral contraceptives and depression: impact, prevalence and cause. J Adolesc Health Care 1981; 2:53–64.

29. Kahn LS, Halbreich U. Oral contraceptives and mood. Expert Opin Pharmacother 2001; 2:1367–82.

30. Sulak PJ, Scow RD, Preece D et al. Hormone withdrawal symptoms in oral contraceptive users, continuous use. Obstet Gynecol 2000; 95:261–6.

31. Magos AL, Brincat M, Studd JW. Treatment of the premenstrual syndrome by subcutaneous estradiol implants and cyclical oral norethisterone: placebo-controlled study. Br Med J (Clin Res Ed) 1986; 292:1629–34.

32. Magos AL, Collins WP, Studd JW. Management of the premenstrual syndrome by subcutaneous implants of oestradiol. J Psychosom Obstet Gynecol 1984; 3:93–9.

33. Watson NR, Studd JWW, Savvas M et al. Treatment of severe premenstrual syndrome with oestradiol patches and cyclical oral norethisterone. Lancet 1989; 2:730–2.

34. Smith RN, Studd JW, Zamblera D et al. A randomized comparison over 8 months of 100 micrograms and 200 micrograms twice weekly doses of transdermal oestradiol in the treatment of severe premenstrual syndrome. Br J Obstet Gynaecol 1995; 102:475–84.

35. Watson NR, Studd JW, Savvas M et al. The long-term effects of estradiol implant therapy for the treatment of premenstrual syndrome. Gynecol Endocrinol 1990; 4:99–107.

36. Dalton K. The Premenstrual Syndrome and Progesterone Therapy, 2nd edn. Chicago, IL: Year Book Medical Publishers; 1984.

37. Freeman E, Rickels K, Sondheimer SJ et al. Ineffectiveness of progesterone suppository treatment for premenstrual syndrome. JAMA 1990; 264:349–53.

38. Dennerstein L, Spencer-Gardner C, Gotts G et al. Progesterone and the premenstrual syndrome: a double-blind crossover trial. BMJ 1985; 290:1617–21.

39. West CP. Inhibition of ovulation with oral progestins – effectiveness in premenstrual syndrome. Eur J Obstet Gynecol Reprod Biol 1990; 34:119–28.

40. Dennerstein L, Morse C, Gotts G et al. Treatment of premenstrual syndrome: a double-blind trial of dydrogesterone. J Affect Disord 1986; 11:199–205.

41. Williams JGC, Martin AJ, Hulkenberg-Tromp A. Premenstrual syndrome in four European countries. Part 2. A double-blind controlled study of dydrogesterone. Br J Sex Med 1983; 10:8–18.

42. Hahn PM, Van Vugt, DA, Reid RL. A randomized, placebo-controlled, crossover trial of danazol for the treatment of premenstrual syndrome. Psychoneuroendocrinology 1995; 20:193–209.

43. Gilmore DH, Hawthorn RJ, Hart DM. Danazol for premenstrual syndrome: a preliminary report of a placebo-controlled double-blind study. J Int Med Res 1985; 13:129–30.

44. Watts JF, Edwards RL, Butt WR. Treatment of premenstrual syndrome using danazol: preliminary report of a placebo-controlled, double-blind dose ranging study. J Int Med Res 1985; 13:127–8.

45. Deeny M, Hawthorn R, McKay Hart D. Low dose danazol in the treatment of the premenstrual syndrome. Postgrad Med J 1991; 67:450–4.

46. Halbreich U, Rojansky N, Palter S. Elimination of ovulation and menstrual cyclicity (with danazol) improves dysphoric premenstrual syndromes. Fertil Steril 1991; 56:1066–9.

47. Wyatt K, Dimmock PW, Ismail KMK et al. The effectiveness of GnRHa with and without 'add-back' therapy in treating premenstrual syndrome: a meta analysis. BJOG 2004; 111:585–93.

48. Dodin S, Lemay A, Maheux R et al. Bone mass in endometriosis patients treated with GnRH implant or danazol. Obstet Gynaecol 1991; 7:410–15.

49. Studd J, Leather AT. The need for addback with gonadotrophin-releasing hormone agonist therapy. Br Obstet Gynaecol 1996; 103(Suppl 14):1–4.

50. Leather AT, Studd JW, Watson NR et al. The treatment of severe premenstrual syndrome with goserelin with and without 'add-back' estrogen therapy: a placebo-controlled study. Gynecol Endocrinol 1999; 13:48–55.

51. Muse KN, Cetel NS, Futterman LA, Yen SSC. The premenstrual syndrome: effects of 'medical ovariectomy'. N Engl J Med 1984; 311:1345–9.

52. Sundstrom I, Nyberg S, Bixo M et al. Treatment of premenstrual syndrome with gonadotrophin releasing hormone agonist in a low dose regimen. Acta Obstet Scand 1999; 78:891–9.

53. DiCarlo C, Palomba S, Tommaselli GA et al. Use of leuprolide acetate plus tibolone in the treatment of severe premenstrual syndrome. Fertil Steril 2001; 75(2):380–4.

54. Schmidt PJ, Nieman LK, Danaceau MA, Adams LF, Rubinow DR. Differential behavioral effects of gonadal steroids in women with and in those without premenstrual syndrome. N Engl J Med 1998; 338(4): 209–16.

55. Blumenthal M, Busse WR, Goldberg A et al. The complete German Commission E Monographs: Therapeutic Guide to Herbal Medicines. Austin, TX: American Botanical Council; 1998: 1694.

56. Girman A, Lee R, Kligler B. An integrative medicine approach to premenstrual syndrome (Editorial). Am J Obstet Gynecol 2003; 188(5, part 2) Suppl:S56–65.

57. Dittmar G, Bohnert K. Premenstrual syndrome: treatment with a phytopharmaceutical. TW Gynakol 1992; 5:60–8.

58. Schellenberg R. Treatment for the premenstrual syndrome with agnus castus fruit extract: prospective, randomized, placebo-controlled study. BMJ 2001; 322:134–7.

59. Williams JW, Mulrow CD, Chiquette E et al. A systematic review of newer pharmacotherapies for depression in adults: evidence report summary. Ann Intern Med 2000; 132:743–56.

60. O'Brien PM, Abukhalil IE. Randomised controlled trial of the management of premenstrual syndrome and premenstrual mastalgia using luteal phase-only danazol. Am J Obstet Gynecol 1999; 180:18–23.

13

The role of progesterone and GABA in PMS/PMDD

Torbjörn Bäckström, Lotta Andréen, Inger Björn, Inga-Maj Johansson, and Magnus Löfgren

TEMPORAL SYMPTOM – HORMONE RELATION

The relationship between the luteal phase of the menstrual cycle and symptom development in premenstrual dysphoric disorder/premenstrual syndrome (PMDD/PMS) is self-evident. Symptoms starts after ovulation and then increase in parallel with the rise in serum progesterone during the luteal phase. The symptom severity reaches a peak during the last five premenstrual days or the first day of menstruation. Thereafter, the symptoms decline and disappear 3–4 days after the onset of menstrual bleeding. During the postmenstrual phase there is a period of well-being, closely following estrogen production, to the estradiol peak. This suggests that there is a symptom-provoking factor produced by the corpus luteum of the ovary.[1] This is further supported by the fact that in anovulatory cycles, spontaneous or induced, when a corpus luteum is not formed, no symptom cyclicity occurs.[2–4]

NATURE OF THE SYMPTOM-INDUCING FACTOR PRODUCED BY THE CORPUS LUTEUM OF THE OVARY

Further evidence that progesterone and progestogens induce negative mood symptoms similar to those in PMDD/PMS is seen in postmenopausal women receiving estrogen/progesterone hormone therapy.[5–7] As discussed above, there are strong indications that steroids from the corpus luteum are the symptom-provoking factor in the central nervous system (CNS). But the classical hormonal receptor for progesterone seems not to be involved in the pathophysiology of PMS/PMDD; treatment with the progesterone receptor antagonist

mifepristone (RU-486) fails to reduce the physical or behavioral manifestations of PMS.[8]

THE DIRECT EFFECTS OF NEUROACTIVE PROGESTERONE METABOLITES ON THE GABA-A RECEPTOR

To understand progesterone-induced adverse mood effects, it is important to note that progesterone is to high degree metabolized to allopregnanolone (3α-OH-5α-pregnan-20-one) and pregnanolone (3α-OH-5β-pregnan-20-one), both of which act as agonists on the γ-aminobutyric acid A ($GABA_A$) receptor complex in the brain.[9] The GABA transmitter system is the major inhibitory system in the CNS. When GABA binds to the $GABA_A$ receptor, the influx of chloride ions increases, hyperpolarizing the postsynaptic membrane and making the postsynaptic cell less prone to excitation. Allopregnanolone is a $GABA_A$ receptor positive modulator and enhances the effect of GABA on the receptor. The behavioral and pharmacological characteristics are similar to ethanol, barbiturates, and benzodiazepines. Neurosteroids, benzodiazepines, barbiturates, alcohol, and most anesthetic agents bind to the $GABA_A$ receptor and increase the GABA-induced chloride ion influx by interacting with allosteric binding sites.[10,11]

NEUROACTIVE PROGESTERONE METABOLITES AS PMDD/PMS SYMPTOM-PROVOKING FACTOR

Thus far, studies have shown disparity regarding behavioral effects of these neuroactive progesterone metabolites. Studies in animals and humans have reported typical

GABA$_A$ receptor agonistic effects such as sedation/anesthesia,[12,13] anti epileptic effects,[14] anxiolytic effects[15] of high doses of allopregnanolone and pregnanolone. Studies have also reported the negative effects of allopregnanolone, which has been shown to increase irritability/aggression[16] and inhibit learning.[17] Treatment with progesterone in a rat model of PMDD induces anxiety, related to an increased α_4 subunit of the GABA$_A$ receptor in hippocampus, which in turn is attributed to an allopregnanolone effect.[18] Similar results, with a place aversion as a measure of anxiety in rats, were noted with a low dosage of allopregnanolone.[19]

Besides the neuroactive progesterone metabolites, benzodiazepines, barbiturates, and alcohol also act as positive modulators of the GABA$_A$ receptor. Recent reports from human and animal studies indicate that in certain individuals all GABA$_A$ receptor agonists can induce negative symptoms with anxiety and irritability/aggression. Strong irritability/aggression is induced in 3–6% of individuals; moderate symptoms are induced in 20–30%. Interestingly, the frequency parallels the 3–8% prevalence of PMDD among women in reproductive age and the 25–35% prevalence of milder symptoms, as in PMS.[20–22]

THE GABA ACTIVE AGONIST PARADOX

The GABA$_A$ receptor agonists are known to be anxiolytic, sedative, and antiepileptic. Why an increase in allopregnanolone is related to development of negative mood is puzzling. It appears that benzodiazepines, barbiturates, alcohol, and allopregnanolone possess bimodal action on mood symptoms. In both animals and humans, GABA$_A$ receptor agonists in high doses are anxiolytic, antiaggressive, sedative/anesthetic, and antiepileptic.[23,24] However, in low concentrations or doses, severe adverse emotional reactions are induced in a subset of individuals (2–3%) and moderate reactions in up to 20%. This paradoxical effect is induced by allopregnanolone,[16,19] benzodiazepines,[25,26] barbiturates,[20,27] and ethanol.[16,28] The symptoms induced by these GABA$_A$ receptor active drugs include depressed mood, irritability, aggression, and other typical symptoms of PMS/PMDD. A similar bimodal effect has also been noted for different doses of medroxyprogesterone (MPA) and natural progesterone in postmenopausal women taking hormone replacement therapy (HRT). These women feel worse on a lower dosage of MPA or progesterone than they do on higher doses or placebo.[29,30]

Thus, allopregnanolone seems to have a bimodal effect on mood with an inverted U-shaped relationship between concentration and effect. In postmenopausal women receiving vaginal or oral progesterone, a biphasic relation between the negative mood symptoms and the allopregnanolone concentrations in blood is noted. Negative mood increases with the rise in serum concentration of allopregnanolone up to a maximum, but then further increase in allopregnanolone concentration is associated with a decrease in the severity.[5,31] The increase in negative mood occurs at serum concentrations within the range seen during the luteal phase. With concentrations seen during late pregnancy, the symptoms decrease.[32,33] In late pregnancy when allopregnanolone concentrations are at their highest, PMDD patients often feel better. A similar inverted U-shaped relationship between allopregnanolone dose and irritability/aggression has also been noted in rats.[16]

Benzodiazepines also induce paradoxical reactions in certain individuals, with irritability, aggression, depression, confusion, violent behavior, and loss of impulse control compared with placebo.[25,26] Weinbroum et al reported a 10.2% incidence of paradoxical events to midazolam in patients who underwent surgery during a 3-month period and showed that the treatment with flumazenil (a benzodiazepine receptor antagonist) effectively reversed midazolam-induced paradoxical behavior.[22] Several reports from animal studies on benzodiazepine-heightened aggression show similar antagonistic effects of benzodiazepine antagonists, as seen in humans.[34]

ROLE OF ESTRADIOL IN PROGESTERONE-INDUCED MOOD SYMPTOMS

Estradiol concentration is also of importance in relation to the mood-inducing effect of progesterone. Higher estradiol doses in HRT during the progestogen period gave more severe symptoms compared with lower estradiol dosage in the same women but only during the period when the progestogen was given. During the period of unopposed estrogen, no difference in mood severity was noted in relation to the estrogen dose.[35] Similar results were seen in women with PMS/PMDD (but not controls) with, interrupted ovarian function where both estradiol and progesterone induced symptoms.[36] Increased plasma levels of estradiol and progesterone during the luteal phase in patients with PMS are related to more severe symptoms compared to cycles in the same individuals with lower levels.[37] Moreover, estradiol treatment during the luteal phase induced more negative symptoms than placebo in PMS/PMDD patients.[38] Estradiol and progesterone acting together seem to induce differing responses in the CNS than when they act separately.

SENSITIVITY IN THE GABA SYSTEM IN PMDD/PMS PATIENTS

It appears that a subset of individuals are very sensitive to low doses or concentrations of allopregnanolone and have severe adverse emotional reactions when provoked. There is evidence that steroid sensitivity in the brain differs between PMS/PMDD patients and controls. Negative effects of oral contraceptives on mood were found mainly in women with PMS/PMDD.[39] Add-back estradiol or progesterone, in women with PMS/PMDD and inhibited ovarian hormone production, gave rise to recurrence of symptoms. This did not happen either in normal women or in PMS/PMDD women during placebo treatment.[36] Postmenopausal women with a history of PMS/PMDD respond with more negative symptoms on progestogens than women without a PMS/PMDD history.[6] In PMS/PMDD patients but not controls, the sedative response to intravenous pregnanolone, diazepam, and alcohol is reduced in the luteal phase compared with the follicular phase.[40–42] In addition, patients with severe symptoms were less sensitive to the given pregnanolone or benzodiazepines compared to patients with more moderate symptoms.[36,38] The findings suggest that patients with PMS/PMDD develop tolerance to the administration of $GABA_A$ receptor allosteric agonists during the luteal phase. In an animal model of PMS/PMDD, the allopregnanolone effect occurs in parallel with an upregulation of the hippocampal α_4 subunit of the $GABA_A$ receptor and decreased benzodiazepine sensitivity.[18] This is in line with the decreased benzodiazepine sensitivity in women with PMDD.[41] Animals with high risk-taking behavior develop withdrawal symptoms on progesterone treatment.[43] The decreased sensitivity is an indication of the development of tolerance to allopregnanolone. Tolerance to allopregnanolone in rats after 90 minutes of anesthesia has already been noted.[44] There is also a relationship between tolerance development and change in the $GABA_A$ receptor subunit α_4 in thalamus.[45]

CONCLUSION

In conclusion, ovarian steroid hormones are of fundamental importance in inducing negative mood in PMS/PMDD. We are beginning to develop an understanding of a mechanism where $GABA_A$ receptor sensitivity seems to differ in women with PMS/PMDD and sensitive individuals appear to react to $GABA_A$ receptor agonists in a bimodal inverted U-shaped manner.

ACKNOWLEDGMENTS

This work is supported by EU structural fund objective 1, Swedish Research Council Medicine (proj. 4X-11198), Västerbottens County, Umeå Municipal, Northern Sweden health region, Norrlands University Hospital, Umeå University foundations.

REFERENCES

1. Bäckström T, Sanders D, Leask RM et al. Mood, sexuality, hormones and the menstrual cycle. II. Hormone levels and their relationship to premenstrual syndrome. Psychosom Med 1983; 45:503–7.
2. Hamarbäck S, Bäckström T. Induced anovulation as treatment of premenstrual tension syndrome. A double-blind cross-over study with GnRH-agonist versus placebo. Acta Obstet Gynecol Scand 1988; 67:159–66.
3. Hammarbäck S, Ekholm UB, Bäckström T. Spontaneous anovulation causing disappearance of cyclical symptoms in women with the premenstrual syndrome. Acta Endocrinol 1991; 125:132–7.
4. Mortola JF. Applications of gonadotropin-releasing hormone analogues in the treatment of premenstrual syndrome. Clin Obstet Gynecol 1993; 36:753–63.
5. Andréen L, Sundström-Poromaa I, Bixo M et al. Relationship between allopregnanolone and negative mood in postmenopausal women taking sequential hormone replacement therapy with vaginal progesterone. Psychoneuroendocrinology 2005; 30:212–24.
6. Björn I, Bixo M, Strandberg-Nöjd K et al. Negative mood changes during hormone replacement therapy: a comparison between two progestogens. Am J Obstet Gynecol 2000; 183: 1419–26.
7. Hammarbäck S, Bäckström T, Holst J et al. Cyclical mood changes as in the premenstrual tension syndrome during sequential estrogen-progestagen postmenopausal replacement treatment. Acta Obstet Gynecol Scand 1985; 64:393–7.
8. Chan AF, Mortola JF, Wood SH, Yen SS. Persistence of premenstrual syndrome during low-dose administration of the progesterone antagonist RU 486. Obstet Gynecol 1994; 84(6):1001–5.
9. Majewska MD, Harrison NL, Schwartz RD, Barker JL, Paul SM. Steroid hormone metabolites are barbiturate-like modulators of the GABA receptor. Science 1986; 232(4753):1004–7.
10. Bäckström T, Andersson A, Andree L et al. Pathogenesis in menstrual cycle-linked CNS disorders. Ann NY Acad Sci 2003; 1007:42–53.
11. Sieghart W. Structure and pharmacology of gamma-aminobutyric acidA receptor subtypes. Pharmacol Rev 1995; 47(2):181–234.
12. Carl P, Hogskilde S, Nielsen JW et al. Pregnanolone emulsion. A preliminary pharmacokinetic and pharmacodynamic study of a new intravenous anaesthetic agent. Anaesthesia 1990; 45(3): 189–97.
13. Timby E, Balgard M, Nyberg S et al. Pharmacokinetic and behavioral effects of allopregnanolone in healthy women. Psychopharmacology (Berl) 2006; 186(3):414–24.
14. Landgren S, Aasly J, Backstrom T, Dubrovsky B, Danielsson E. The effect of progesterone and its metabolites on the interictal epileptiform discharge in the cat's cerebral cortex. Acta Physiol Scand 1987; 131(1):33–42.
15. Wieland S, Lan NC, Mirasedeghi S, Gee KW. Anxiolytic activity of the progesterone metabolite 5 alpha-pregnan-3 alpha-ol-20-one. Brain Res 1991; 565: 263–8.
16. Miczek KA, Fish EW, De Bold JF. Neurosteroids, GABAA receptors, and escalated aggressive behavior. Horm Behav 2003; 44:242–57.

17. Johansson IM, Birzniece V, Lindblad C, Olsson T, Backotsom T. Allopregnanolone inhibits learning in the Morris water maze. Brain Res 2002; 934: 125–31.

18. Gulinello M, Gong QH, Li X et al. Short-term exposure to a neuroactive steroid increases alpha4 GABA(A) receptor subunit levels in association with increased anxiety in the female rat. Brain Res 2001; 910:55–66.

19. Beauchamp MH, Ormerod BK, Jhamandas K, Boegman RJ, Beninger RJ. Neurosteroids and reward: allopregnanolone produces a conditioned place aversion in rats. Pharmacol Biochem Behav 2000; 67:29–35.

20. Masia SL, Perrine K, Westbrook L, Alpor K, Devensky O. Emotional outbursts and post-traumatic stress disorder during intracarotid amobarbital procedure. Neurology 2000; 54(8):1691–3.

21. Sveindottir H, Backstrom T. Prevalence of menstrual cycle symptom cyclicity and premenstrual dysphoric disorder in a random sample of women using and not using oral contraceptives. Acta Obstet Gynecol Scand 2000; 79(5):405–13.

22. Weinbroum AA, Szold O, Ogorek D, Flaishon R. The midazolam-induced paradox phenomenon is reversible by flumazenil. Epidemiology, patient characteristics and review of the literature. Eur J Anaesthesiol 2001; 18(12):789–97.

23. Paul SM, Purdy RH. Neuroactive steriods. FASEB J 1992; 6: 2311–22.

24. Wang M, Bäckström T, Sundström I et al. Neuroactive steroids and central nervous system disorders. Int Rev Neurobiol 2001; 46:421–59.

25. Ben-Porath DD, Taylor SP. The effects of diazepam (valium) and aggressive disposition on human aggression: an experimental investigation. Addict Behav 2002; 27:167–77.

26. Wenzel RR, Bartel T, Eggebrecht H, Philipp T, Erbel R. Central-nervous side effects of midazolam during transesophageal echocardiography. J Am Soc Echocardiogr 2002; 15:1297–1300.

27. Kurthen M, Linke DB, Reuter BM, Hufnagel A, Elger CE. Severe negative emotional reactions in intracarotid sodium amytal procedures: further evidence for hemispheric asymmetries? Cortex 1991; 27:333–7.

28. Dougherty DM, Cherek DR, Bennett RH. The effects of alcohol on the aggressive responding of women. J Stud Alcohol 1996; 57:178–86.

29. Andreen L, Bixo M, Nyberg S, Sundström-Poromaa I, Bäckström T. Progesterone effects during sequential hormone replacement therapy. Eur J Endocrinol 2003; 148:571–7.

30. Björn I, Bixo M, Nöjd K et al. The impact of different doses of medroxyprogesterone acetate on mood symptoms in sequential hormonal therapy. Gynecol Endocrinol 2002; 16:1–8.

31. Andréen L, Sundström-Poromaa I, Bixo M, Nyberg S, Bäckström T. Allopregnanolone concentration and mood – a bimodal association in postmenopausal women treated with oral progesterone. Psychopharmacology 2006; 187(2):209–21.

32. Luisi S, Petraglia F, Benedetto C et al. Serum allopregnanolone levels in pregnant women: changes during pregnancy, at delivery, and in hypertensive patients. J Clin Endocrinol Metab 2000; 85: 2429–33.

33. Wang M, Seippel L, Purdy RH, Bäckström T. Relationship between symptom severity and steroid variation in women with premenstrual syndrome: study on serum pregnenolone, pregnenolone sulfate, 5 alpha-pregnane-3,20-dione and 3 alpha-hydroxy-5 alpha-pregnan-20-one. J Clin Endocrinol Metab 1996; 81:1076–82.

34. Gourley SL, Debold JF, Yin W, Cook J, Miczek KA. Benzodiazepines and heightened aggressive behavior in rats: reduction by GABA(A)/alpha(1) receptor antagonists. Psychopharmacology (Berl) 2005; 178(2–3): 232–40.

35. Bjorn I, Sundstrom-Poromaa I, Bixo M et al. Increase of estrogen dose deteriorates mood during progestin phase in sequential hormonal therapy. J Clin Endocrinol Metab 2003; 88(5): 2026–30.

36. Schmidt PJ, Nieman LK, Danaceau MA et al. Differential behavioral effects of gonadal steroids in women with and in those without premenstrual syndrome. N Engl J Med 1998; 338:209–16.

37. Hammarbäck S, Damber JE, Bäckström T. Relationship between symptom severity and hormone changes in women with premenstrual syndrome. J Clin Endocrinol Metab 1989; 68:125–30.

38. Dhar V, Murphy BE. Double-blind randomized crossover trial of luteal phase estrogens (Premarin) in the premenstrual syndrome (PMS). Psychoneuroendocrinology 1990; 15:489–93.

39. Cullberg J. Mood changes and menstrual symptoms with different gestagen/estrogen combinations. A double blind comparison with placebo. Acta Psychiat Scand 1972; 236 (Suppl):1–84.

40. Sundström I, Andersson A, Nyberg S et al. Patients with premenstrual syndrome have a different sensitivity to a neuroactive steroid during the menstrual cycle compared to control subjects. Neuroendocrinology 1998; 67:126–38.

41. Sundström I, Ashbrook D, Bäckström T. Reduced benzodiazepine sensitivity in patients with premenstrual syndrome: a pilot study. Psychoneuroendocrinology 1997; 22:25–38.

42. Nyberg S, Wahlström G, Bäckström T, Sundström-Poromaa I. Altered sensitivity to alcohol in the late luteal phase among patients with premenstrual dysphoric disorder. Psychoneuroendocrinology 2004; 29:767–77.

43. Löfgren M, Johansson IM, Meyerson B, Lundgren P, Bäckström T. Progesterone withdrawal effects in the open field test can be predicted by elevated plus maze performance. Horm Behav 2006; 50(2):208–15.

44. Zhu D, Birzniece V, Bäckström T, Wahlström G. Dynamic aspects of acute tolerance to allopregnanolone evaluated using anaesthesia threshold in male rats. Br J Anaesth 2004; 93:560–7.

45. Birzniece V, Türkmen S, Lindblad C et al. GABA-A receptor mRNA changes in acute allopregnanolone tolerance. Eur J Pharmacol 2006; 535(1–3):125–34.

46. Sundström I, Nyberg S, Bäckström T. Patients with premenstrual syndrome have reduced sensitivity to midazolam compared to control subjects. Neuropsychopharmacology 1997; 17:370–81.

14

The management of PMS/PMDD through ovarian cycle suppression

Nick Panay and John WW Studd

INTRODUCTION

We have seen in previous chapters that the underlying cause of premenstrual syndrome/premenstrual dysphoric disorder (PMS/PMDD) remains unknown, although cyclical ovarian activity appears to be a key factor.[1] A logical treatment, therefore, is to suppress ovulation and thus prevent the neuroendocrine changes that cause the distressing symptoms. The current therapy for PMS/PMDD is varied and includes psychotherapeutic, cognitive, or hormonal. However, the cornerstone of hormonal treatment relies upon suppression of ovulation and removal of the hormonal changes that follow ovulation in the luteal phase. When there are no cyclical hormonal changes during pregnancy, not only are there no cyclical mood symptoms but also depression is uncommon. There then often follows an episode of postpartum depression when there is a fall of levels of placental hormones, with a recurrence of symptoms when the periods return.[2]

There are now many placebo-controlled studies showing that suppression of ovulation by increasing plasma estradiol levels or by down-regulation results in an improvement in PMS/PMDD. A number of drugs are capable of achieving this but they are not without their own side effects, and this may influence the efficacy of the treatment and the duration for which they may be given. The purpose of this chapter will be to review the evidence for the available therapies and offer some practical advice as to how these preparations can be incorporated into day-to-day clinical practice.

THE COMBINED ORAL CONTRACEPTIVE PILL

Although able to suppress ovulation and used commonly to improve PMS/PMDD symptoms, the combined oral contraceptive pill (COCP) was initially not shown to be of benefit in randomized prospective trials.[3] This is probably because the daily progestogen in the second-generation pills caused PMDD-type symptoms of its own accord. A new combined contraceptive pill (Yasmin, Schering Corporation) contains an antimineralocorticoid and antiandrogenic progestogen, drospirenone. This has shown considerable promise in the treatment of PMS/PMDD, as it is devoid of progestogenic side effects and provides additional benefits from the mild diuretic and antiandrogenic effect. There are now both observational and small randomized trial data supporting its efficacy; these data require confirmation with larger studies.[4]

More recently, a lower-dose version of this COCP (Yaz, Schering Corporation) with 20 µg ethinylestradiol and 3 mg drospirenone (24 active, 4 inactive tablets, per cycle) has been shown to be effective for treating PMDD in a moderately sized randomized controlled trial of 450 subjects over three treatment cycles.[5] There was a significantly greater improvement of the total Daily Record of Severity of Problems (DRSP) for active treatment compared with placebo (-37.49 vs -29.99, $p < 0.001$). Specifically, mood symptoms improved significantly (-19.2 vs -15.3, $p = 0.003$). There was a reduction in daily symptoms of 48% for active vs 36% for placebo (RR = 1.7, $p = 0.015$).

Practical aspects

If the COCP is used to treat PMS/PMDD, pill packets should be used back to back (bicycling/tricycling or continuously) and a break only introduced if erratic bleeding occurs. Recognizing the benefits of longer cycle regimens, a four bleed per year COCP has already been licensed and a no-bleed regimen is planned. Data are required to confirm the superiority of these regimens in comparison to traditional regimens.

PERCUTANEOUS ESTRADIOL (PATCHES AND IMPLANTS)

The only ovulation suppressant treatment of proven efficacy in placebo-controlled trials which appears suitable for long-term usage is continuous percutaneous 17β-estradiol combined with cyclical progestogen. Oral preparations in the standard estradiol doses found in hormone replacement therapy (HRT) are not sufficient to suppress ovarian activity. The use of estradiol patches was first reported in a study in which a 100 mg subcutaneous implant of estradiol was administered, achieving serum estradiol levels of around 800 pmol/L; this proved to be highly effective in every Moos Menstrual Distress Questionnaire (MDQ) cluster of symptoms compared with placebo.[6]

Estradiol implants are long-lasting and transdermal estradiol patches were subsequently used so that treatment could be administered more simply (avoiding a minor surgical procedure) and be discontinued at short notice if required. Initially it was found that, 200 μg estradiol patches suppressed ovulation; they were tested against placebo in a cross-over trial and found to be highly effective (Figure 14.1).[7] The study was a randomized, double-blind, placebo-controlled trial with cross-over at 3 months; 20 patients in the active treatment group received 200 μg (two × 100 μg) estradiol patches followed by placebo and 20 patients were treated in reverse order. Patients completed the MDQ and Premenstrual Distress Questionnaire (PDQ) daily throughout the study. After 3 months, both groups showed improvements in MDQ and PDQ scores. In general, patients who switched from active treatment to placebo had deteriorating scores, whereas patients who switched from placebo to active treatment maintained or improved upon their initial gains. Significant improvements occurred after changing to active treatment in 5 of 6 negative MDQ symptom clusters and in 6 of 10 PDQ symptoms.

However, there was concern that estradiol 200 μg twice weekly was too high a dose to be used as long-term therapy. A subsequent observational study[8] showed that 100 μg estradiol patches twice weekly were as effective as 200 μg twice weekly in reducing symptom levels in severe premenstrual syndrome. This dosage was better tolerated in that there was a lower incidence of nausea and breast tenderness at initiation of treatment. The most recent randomized controlled study using 100 μg estradiol patches showed efficacy over a longer time period. This was an 8-month placebo-controlled randomized trial with cross-over at 4 months and a 6-month extension phase (Figure 14.2).[9] What was particularly interesting about the findings of this trial was that not only was there a significant improvement in symptoms over the initial 8 months but also these improvements continued through the extension phase of the trial.

Although the authors of this chapter believe that ovulation suppression by transdermal estrogens can be a first-line therapy for PMS/PMDD, they are surprised that the original Lancet paper[7] of a randomized trial published 18 years ago has not been replicated. Either the study is considered perfect or there are other possibly commercial reasons why manufacturers of estradiol implants and patches have been less enthusiastic about pursuing a licensed indication for PMS/PMDD than those producing selective serotonin reuptake inhibitors (SSRIs).

Practical aspects

Transdermal estradiol patches can be used effectively as a first-line therapy for PMS/PMDD to treat both psychological and physical symptoms. Although there have

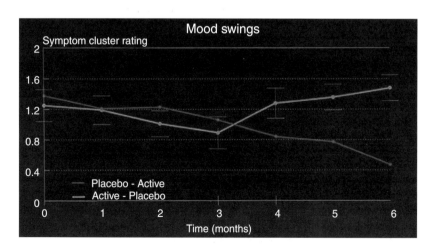

Figure 14.1 A trial of 200 μg transdermal estradiol vs placebo for PMDD – a 6-month randomized placebo-controlled study with cross-over at 3 months. (Adapted from Watson et al,[7] with permission.)

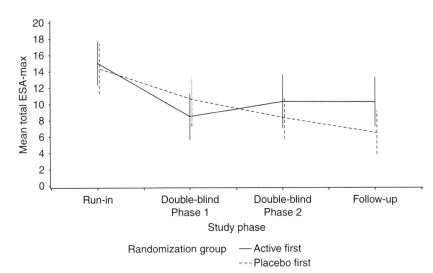

Figure 14.2 ESA-max (exponentially smoothed average maximum scores) scores for depression of women randomized to receive E_2 100 µg patches or placebo – (an 8-month study with cross-over at 4 months and a 6-month extension) – new data from the authors' unit. Mean values with 95% CI.

been no clinical studies on the use of estradiol gel in PMDD, it is clear that adequate estradiol levels can be achieved and thus a beneficial clinical response would be expected if patients prefer to use this rather than patches. Treatment with estradiol should be continued for a minimum of 1 year, as efficacy may improve even after the initial 6–8 months. As this is not a cure for PMS/PMDD, patients should be warned that symptoms can return when treatment is discontinued.

Mild adverse effects occur in 15–20% of users. These include nausea, breast tenderness, fluid retention, increased appetite, and patch site skin reactions. Skin reactions are less common with the newer matrix patch systems and with estradiol gel. Patients should be counseled that any adverse effects usually wear off after the first 6 weeks of use.

Concerns regarding breast and endometrial cancer risks (as found in menopausal patients) are unfounded in this age group. The area under the curve (AUC) for estradiol levels is unchanged (compared with that in spontaneous cycles), as it is the distribution which is altered. Note that 100 µg patches produce mid-follicular estradiol levels (250–350 pmol/L) that are entirely normal in premenopausal women. Clinical observation shows no evidence of an increased risk of endometrial or breast carcinoma in premenopausal women using percutaneous patches and either cyclical progestogen or a levonorgestrel-releasing intrauterine system (LNG IUS). However, hard randomized placebo-controlled trial data in large populations looking at these major outcome measures over a long period of time are lacking. There is no evidence that the risk of venous thromboembolism is increased by this treatment and recent data in menopausal women support this finding.[10]

Contraception

The observation that estradiol 100 µg, producing physiological levels of serum estradiol, was equally as effective as estradiol 200 µg in treating PMS, strongly suggested that the principal mechanism of action was ovarian suppression. Data have shown that luteal phase progesterone levels were suppressed to anovulatory levels by this treatment. However, there are insufficient data in large enough numbers over a long enough period of time to recommend estradiol patches as a reliable ovulation suppression method. Thus, additional contraception should be used with estradiol therapy, except when LNG IUS is being used for progestogenic opposition.

Progestogen intolerance

One of the limitations of continuous estrogen therapy for PMS/PMDD is that the endometrium requires protection from possible hyperplasia and carcinoma by the administration of progestogen or progesterone. Unfortunately, this progestogenic opposition can lead to a resurgence of PMDD-like symptoms (not usually as severe as the original symptoms being treated). A previous study showed that PMDD could be recreated in postmenopausal women administered cyclical norethisterone.[11]

Attempts to avoid this (see Chapter 18) include reduction of the duration or dosage of progestogen, but this must be counterbalanced by the small increased risk of hyperplasia with progestogen restriction. Sturdee and colleagues showed that 12 days of progestogen avoids hyperplasia altogether, but a shorter duration

(10 or 7 days) was associated with a 2–4% risk of hyperplasia.[11] These were data from a study of estrogen therapy in postmenopausal women and so not directly relevant. However, a study of PMS/PMDD from the authors' unit (unpublished data)[9] of longer-term treatment with the 100 μg estradiol dosage using a lower dose of cyclical norethisterone acetate (1 mg) for only 10 days each cycle has shown benefit over placebo for eight cycles, with continued improvement in a 6-month extension. Not surprisingly, the incidence of progestogen intolerance was reduced with this regimen. There were no reported cases of endometrial thickening (a surrogate for endometrial hyperplasia assessed by transvaginal ultrasound) in this study, despite the lower dose and shorter duration of progestogen.[13]

Work is now ongoing in the authors' unit to show if use of a natural progesterone or LNG IUS (Mirena) as progestogenic opposition can maximize efficacy while minimizing PMDD-like side effects. In the interim, it is possible to use a LNG IUS, progesterone pessaries, or progesterone gel 8% in the progestogen-intolerant woman.[13,14]

There is then clearcut evidence that estradiol can be used to manage PMS/PMDD by suppressing ovulation. There is also clear evidence that the LNG IUS protects from endometrial hyperplasia. Only limited evidence exists as yet to demonstrate efficacy of the combination (Domoney et al, unpublished data). No studies have been undertaken to directly compare hormonal therapy with drugs such as the SSRIs.

DANAZOL

Cycle suppression may also be achieved using danazol, an androgenic steroid. Mansel and Wisby first assessed the effect of danazol on PMS symptoms and showed benefit only for breast tenderness.[15] Other studies have shown greater benefit.[15,16] A relatively recent randomized, double-blind, cross-over study compared three successive cycles of danazol at a dose of 200 mg bd to three cycles of placebo:[17] 28 of 31 women completed at least one cycle of treatment while recording symptoms. From this study, the authors demonstrated that danazol at a dose of 200 mg bd was superior to placebo for the relief of severe PMS during the premenstrual period for the main outcome measures. However, this superiority is muted or even reversed when the entire cycle is considered. This may be explained by the fact that danazol therapy does have some nuisance side effects that may interfere with the usual symptom-free late follicular phase of women with PMS. One solution suggested for this problem might be to limit treatment to the luteal phase only. It is clear that luteal phase only treatment with 200 mg danazol effectively reduces breast symptoms with minimal side effects.

Practical aspects

Danazol is an effective treatment for PMS and patients should be counseled that it is an option. However, the potential for masculinizing side effects usually acts as a deterrent in the majority of women. Thus, due to its masculinizing side effects, especially at higher, cycle-suppressing doses, danazol is not commonly used for treatment of premenstrual syndrome. High doses of danazol reliably suppress ovulation but are more likely to induce masculinization. Lower doses avoid such side effects but as ovulation suppression becomes less reliable the risk of pregnancy with the risk of masculinization of a female fetus becomes significant. All women taking danazol, whatever the dose, should use adequate contraception.

GONADOTROPIN-RELEASING HORMONE ANALOGUES

Gonadotropin-releasing hormone (GnRH) analogues have been successfully employed to suppress gonadal steroid production in conditions such as breast cancer, fibroids, and endometriosis. A recent meta-analysis of GnRH analogues has confirmed their efficacy compared with placebo (Figure 14.3).[18] Seventy-one patients on active treatment were identified in seven trials. The overall standardized mean difference (SMD) for all trials was −1.19 (CI −1.88 to −0.51) (Cohen criteria: 0.3 = small, 0.5 = medium, 1.0 = large effect). The odds ratio (OR) for benefit was 8.66 (95% CI 2.52–30.26). The SMD was −1.43 and OR = 13.38 (CI 3.9–46) if data were taken only from anovulation trials. Efficacy of symptom relief was greater for physical than for behavioral symptoms (physical SMD = −1.16 (CI −1.53 to −0.79); behavioral SMD = −0.68 (CI −1.11 to −0.25)) but difference was not significant $p = 0.484$. One trial used low-dose GnRH analogue to avoid ovulation suppression but did not show clinical significance over placebo.[19]

Thus, GnRH analogue therapy results in profound cycle suppression and elimination of premenstrual symptoms. In practice, lack of efficacy suggests that the diagnosis should be questioned rather than considered a limitation of therapy. GnRH analogues are usually recommended as second- or even third-line treatment due to their hypoestrogenic side effects, but in the opinion of the authors they are extremely valuable as first-line therapy in women with the most severe PMDD.

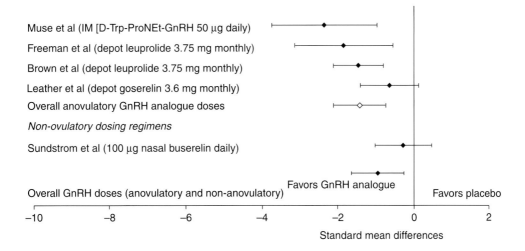

Figure 14.3 Meta-analysis of studies using GnRH analogue therapy for PMDD. (Adapted from Wyatt et al 2004,[18] with permission.)

Add-back hormone therapy

Menopausal symptoms and osteoporosis limit the use of GnRH analogues. The use of add-back hormonal therapy may reduce these side effects and prolong their use. There has been some debate as to what the best form of add-back hormone therapy is for women on long-term GnRH analogues, both from the point of view of maintaining efficacy and avoiding osteoporosis. Data show that bone mineral density can be maintained by use of standard preparations of both cyclical and continuous HRT. Continuous combined therapy or tibolone is preferable to sequential combined therapy if one is to minimize the risks of symptom resurgence during the progestogen phase from PMDD-like progestogenic side effects.[20,21] Overall, the meta-analysis favored neither GnRH alone or GnRH with add-back = 0.12 (CI −0.34 to 0.59),[18] which means that the highly beneficial effect of the analogues is not diminished by the addition of add-back therapy, particularly for tibolone.

Practical aspects

Because symptoms recur with the return of ovarian function, therapy may have to be continued indefinitely; this is precluded by significant trabecular bone loss, which can occur by 6 months' therapy. The use of GnRH analogues with add-back estrogen or tibolone can be protective to the skeleton, but bone density should be monitored in women using analogues for more than 6 months, as bone loss may still occur in some individuals.[22] There is little published evidence to guide management. It seems likely that bone density scanning is

unnecessary for short-term therapy. If therapy is prolonged, then it would seem safest to undertake bone density scans (ideally by dual energy X-ray absorptiometry) annually throughout therapy, even when add-back is used. Treatment should be stopped if bone density declines significantly in scans performed 1 year apart.

PROGESTERONE AND PROGESTOGENS

The efficacy of progestogens and progesterone in the treatment of PMS/PMDD remains questionable. Progestogens (synthetic progesterone) produce PMDD-like side effects due to competition for the mineralocorticoid, androgen, and central nervous system (CNS) receptors. It is therefore not surprising that the data for their efficacy is poor. On the other hand, progesterone is diuretic, natriuretic, and is a CNS anxiolytic. As such, there is some logic to using a progesterone preparation for treatment of PMD/PMDD.[13] However, we have seen that no evidence exists to demonstrate progesterone deficiency (see Chapter 10) and so if progesterone was effective it would be pharmacotherapeutic rather than replacement therapy.

Possible mechanism of action

One of the theories regarding the genesis of PMS/PMDD symptoms was that symptoms were due to a progesterone deficiency in the luteal phase. It is known that progesterone does produce CNS depression and in very large doses can be anesthetic. It follows that, in theory, women with symptoms of irritability and agitated depression may therefore respond favorably to progesterone. However, the most plausible mechanism of action is that at high doses, particularly when used through the whole cycle, progestogens and progesterone can have an ovulation suppressant effect which can improve symptoms. However, what often happens when preparations such as depot medroxyprogesterone acetate are used is that cyclical symptoms are replaced by lower-grade continuous PMDD-type side effects.

Most studies have shown no benefit. One prospective randomized study undertaken and published by a pharmaceutical company did show 'a benefit for both psychological and physical symptoms in the pre-menstruum with absence of symptoms in the post-menstruum'.[23] Patients were randomized to use either progesterone pessaries (400 mg twice a day) or matching placebo, by vaginal or rectal administration, from 14 days before the expected onset of menstruation until onset of vaginal bleeding for four consecutive cycles; 45 general practitioners identified a total of 281 patients. The main outcome variables were change in the severity of each patient's most severe symptoms and in the average score of all the patients' symptoms. The response to progesterone was greater than to placebo during each cycle; the difference was clinically and statistically significant. Adverse events of irregularity of menstruation, vaginal pruritus, and headache were reported more frequently by patients taking active therapy.

A recent meta-analysis of all published studies meeting strict methodological criteria for the treatment of PMS/PMDD failed to confirm benefit with either progesterone or progestogens in the management of PMS.[24] The objective of this meta-analysis was to evaluate the efficacy of progesterone and progestogens in the management of premenstrual syndrome. Ten trials of progestogen therapy (531 women) and four trials of progesterone therapy (378 women) were reviewed. The main outcome measure was a reduction in overall symptoms of PMS. All the trials of progesterone (by both routes of administration) showed no clinically significant difference between progesterone and placebo. For progestogens, the overall SMD for reduction in symptoms showed a slight non-significant difference in favor of progestogen with the mean difference being -0.036 (95% CI -0.059 to -0.014). The meta-analysis of this systematic review therefore suggested that there was no published evidence to support the use of either progesterone or progestogen therapy in the management of premenstrual syndrome.

The evidence for the use of progesterone and progestogens is poor and does not support their continued use for PMS. There is some justification for undertaking better-designed studies in patients with well-defined PMDD for the established progestogens and progesterone and for looking at the newer progestogens: for instance, etonorgestrel, as found in some modern ovulation suppressant progestogen-only contraceptives (e.g. Cerazette, Organon Laboratories). Whether study of the so-called natural progesterone preparations should be undertaken is more debatable and should not be conducted before there are formulations which give rise to consistent elevation of blood progesterone levels.

HYSTERECTOMY AND BILATERAL SALPINGO-OOPHORECTOMY

A historical perspective

Henry Maudlsey was the first to recognize the association of physical and emotional symptoms with the woman's cycle and with great prescience noted the association of behavioral changes with ovarian cycles:

'the monthly activity of the ovaries which marks the advent of puberty in women has a notable effect upon the mind and body wherefore it may become an important cause of mental and physical derangement.'

Thus it was clear that the cyclical symptoms of insanity or menstrual madness were believed to be due to ovarian function rather than menstruation, and treatment took the form of removal of ovaries. Thus evolved the original form of 'ovarian cycle suppression'.

It was not until 1872 that normal ovariotomy – i.e. removal of normal ovaries – was performed for a disorder or malady which was not essentially gynecological.[25] The first surgeon to perform this was Alfred Hegar of Freiberg, to be followed 7 days later by Lawson Tait of Birmingham and Robert Battey of Georgia, USA. At the latter's insistence, it became known as Battey's operation,[26] but in Britain, 'Tait's operation' was used, particularly by his enemies. Battey believed that insanity was, 'not infrequently caused by uterine and ovarian disease'. He describes how he had a Southern girl, of more than unusual beauty, as a patient with cyclical vomiting and hysteria. If we regard menstrual madness as severe PMDD, and ovarian ablation by GnRH analogues as a medical castration equivalent to oophorectomy, then there is ample evidence that removing the ovarian cycle in this way will improve all of the symptom groups of severe PMDD. These historical events have recently been reviewed by Studd and found to have great relevance to our current medical treatment of PMDD.

Although the procedure would have had the desired effect of curing cyclical monthly symptoms, if the surgeon had correctly selected his patients, the 19th century surgeons had no concept of menopausal symptoms or osteoporosis. Thus, this operation would ultimately be followed by severe medical problems. Misplaced overenthusiasm for the surgery removed any sense of good clinical judgment and usually more harm was done than good.

More recent data

Although total abdominal hysterectomy and bilateral salpingo-oophorectomy (TAH/BSO) is a common operation for many indications, there are very few data concerning PMDD. Casson et al[27] found it to be effective in 14 patients for physical and psychological symptoms as well as having a favorable effect on lifestyle, after first suppressing ovarian steroidogenesis with danazol. Casper and Hearn[28] also showed a dramatic improvement in mood, general affect, well-being, life satisfaction and quality of life in another small study of 14 women. Cronje et al (Figure 14.4)[29] subsequently published the results of 49 such women collected over 10 years from two busy PMDD clinics, with all but one being symptom-free and enthusiastic about the treatment. Such surgery is rarely required but is very effective and indeed curative. However, it is significant that some disapproving correspondence following the Cronje publication[29] referred to the 19th century scandal of Battey's operation. All but one of these women had tried various ineffective medical treatments for a mean of 3.6 years before referral to the specialist PMS clinic. They were treated with anovulatory doses of estradiol patches or implants for a mean of 3 years before problems with bleeding or progestogen intolerance made surgical treatment necessary. One patient, the one who refused any medical therapy, regretted the operation but all

others were very satisfied with a complete resolution of symptoms.

The importance of ovarian function in the causation and treatment of PMS should be a factor for discussion with a patient concerning prophylactic oophorectomy at the time of consenting for hysterectomy.[30] Conservation of ovaries does not cure the symptoms of PMDD, for the patient will still have cyclical symptoms of depression, irritability, irrational behavior, etc., as well as cyclical headaches that may be the equivalent of menstrual migraine before surgery. The psycho-protective value of estrogens compared with progesterone can be seen in the beneficial response of women with postnatal depression and perimenopausal depression, the other components of 'reproductive depression'.[31,32]

Practical aspects

Total abdominal hysterectomy and bilateral salpingo-oophorectomy is the ultimate form of ovulation suppression and the only true cure for PMS, as this operation removes the ovarian cycle completely. The procedure is not commonly performed for this indication, as a lesser alternative can usually be found. However, data suggest a highly beneficial effect in the selected women undergoing TAH/BSO, the majority of which are highly satisfied following this procedure and, as such, it should be offered as a therapeutic option. Preoperative GnRH analogues, although not mandatory, are a useful test of whether bilateral oophorectomy (with or without hysterectomy) would be successful in treating symptoms. This appears to be such a valuable approach in gynecological practice that it is disappointing that research has not been conducted to provide the evidence for the value of this 'GnRH test'. It is essential that adequate hormone therapy is given (including, possibly, testosterone replacement) to prevent simply replacing one set of symptoms with another. Women who have had a hysterectomy with ovarian conservation will often continue to have cyclical symptoms in the absence of menstruation (ovarian cycle syndrome).[30]

Women who undergo bilateral oophorectomy laparoscopically, with conservation of the uterus, can expect a much less-invasive procedure. But the persistence of the uterus and therefore, of course, the endometrium, entails protection of the endometrium and all that that entails regarding progestogenic restimulation of symptoms. There are no research studies in this area.

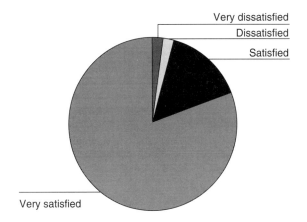

Figure 14.4 Total abdominal hysterectomy and bilateral salpingo-oophorectomy for premenstrual syndrome. (Adapted from Cronje et al,[29] with permission.)

CONCLUSIONS

Although the genesis of PMS/PMDD is probably multifactorial, it is likely that through polygenic inheritance and environmental factors certain women are vulnerable to the neuroendocrine fluctuations which occur in the ovulatory and premenstrual parts of the normal cycle.[33] The logical ways of treating PMS/PMDD would therefore seem to be the stabilization of the ovarian activity that triggers the symptoms or reducing the neuroendocrinological susceptibility (see Chapter 15). This can be achieved in a number of ways, as outlined in this chapter and in the Royal College of Obstetricians and Gynaecologists (RCOG) guidelines.[34] The least invasive and effective means of ovarian suppression is with transdermal estrogens used continuously, either with a low-dose cyclical oral progestogen or better still with a progestogen-releasing intrauterine system. Second-line therapy with GnRH analogues and add-back hormone therapy should be used where transdermal estradiol has not produced adequate symptom relief after a minimum trial of 3 months. GnRH analogue treatment can be used as a first-line therapy where the patient's symptoms are causing major disruption of her life. Assuming GnRH analogue treatment is successful, the patient can continue long-term if using adequate add-back hormone therapy, but bone density should be monitored annually. Where fertility is not an issue, hysterectomy and bilateral salpingo-oophorectomy should be offered as a third-line option, as long as the patient is willing to use hormone therapy at least until the average age of natural menopause. This is the only definitive cure for PMS/PMDD and is highly successful in a very small number of appropriately selected individuals.

Future work in this area should concentrate on maximizing the benefit of transdermal estrogens by minimizing PMDD-like side effects with local delivery of low-dose progestogen/progesterone and the use of selective progestogen receptor modulators. It is also imperative that licensing is sought for the treatment of PMDD with transdermal estrogens and GnRH analogues with add-back therapy, in order to facilitate the usage of these truly effective treatments amongst a greater body of gynecologists, psychiatrists, and interested primary care physicians.

REFERENCES

1. Studd JWW. Premenstrual tension syndrome. Br Med J 1979; 1:410.
2. Studd JWW. Ovariotomy for menstrual madness and premenstrual syndrome – 19th century history and lessons for current practice. Gynecol Endocrinol 2006; 22(8):411–15.
3. Graham CA, Sherwin BB. A prospective treatment study of premenstrual symptoms using a triphasic oral contraceptive. J Psychosom Res 1992; 36:257–66.
4. Freeman EW, Kroll R, Rapkin A et al. PMS/PMDD Research Group. Evaluation of a unique oral contraceptive in the treatment of premenstrual dysphoric disorder. J Womens Health Gend Based Med 2001; 10:561–9.
5. Perlstein TB, Bachmann GA, Zacur HA, Yonkers KA. Treatment of premenstrual dysphoric disorder with a new drospirenone-containing oral contraceptive formulation. Contraception 2005; 72(6):414–21.
6. Magos AL, Brincat M, Studd JWW. Treatment of the premenstrual syndrome by subcutaneous estradiol implants and cyclical oral norethisterone: placebo controlled study. Br Med J (Clin Res Ed) 1986; 292:1629–33.
7. Watson NR, Studd JWW, Savvas M, Garnett T, Baber RJ. Treatment of severe premenstrual syndrome with oestradiol patches and cyclical oral norethisterone. Lancet 1989; 2(8665):730–2.
8. Smith RNJ, Studd JWW, Zamblera D, Holland EF. A randomized comparison over 8 months of 100 μg and 200 μg twice weekly doses of transdermal oestradiol in the treatment of severe premenstrual syndrome. Br J Obstet Gynaecol 1995; 102:475–84.
9. Panay N, Rees M, Zakaria F, Guilford S, Studd JWW. Randomized, prospective, placebo controlled, multicentre study of women with severe PMS, treated with 100 μg transdermal oestradiol. BJOG (in preparation).
10. Scarabin PY, Olger E, Plu-Bureau G. Differential association of oral and transdermal oestrogen replacement therapy with venous thromboembolism risk. Lancet 2003; 362:428–32.
11. Magos AL, Brewster E, Singh R et al. The effects of norethisterone in postmenopausal women on oestrogen replacement therapy: a model for premenstrual syndrome. Br J Obstet Gynaecol 1986; 93:1290–6.
12. Sturdee DW, Wade-Evans T, Paterson ME, Thom M, Studd JW. Relations between bleeding pattern, endometrial history, and oestrogen treatment in menopausal women. Br Med J 1978; 1(6127):1575–7.
13. Panay N, Studd J. Progestogen intolerance and compliance with hormone replacement therapy in menopausal women. Hum Reprod Update 1997; 3:159–71.
14. Faculty of Family Planning and Reproductive Health Care Clinical Effectiveness Unit. FFPRHC Guidance (April 2004). The levonorgestrel-releasing intrauterine system (LNG-IUS) in contraception and reproductive health. J Fam Plann Reprod Health Care 2004; 30(22):99–109.
15. Mansel RE, Wisby J. The effect of gonadotrophin suppression by danazol on symptomatic breast disease. Br J Surg 1980; 67:827.
16. Watts JF, Butt WR, Logan Edwards R. A clinical trial using danazol for the treatment of premenstrual tension. Br J Obstet Gynaecol 1987; 94:30–4.
17. Hahn PM, Van Vugt DA, Reid RL. A randomized, placebo-controlled, crossover trial of danazol for the treatment of premenstrual syndrome. Psychoneuroendocrinology 1995; 20(2):193–209.
18. Wyatt KM, Dimmock PW, Ismail KM, Jones PW, O'Brien PM. The effectiveness of GnRHa with and without 'add-back' therapy in treating premenstrual syndrome: a meta analysis. Br J Obstet Gynaecol 2004; 111(6):585–93.
19. Sundstrom I, Nyberg S, Bixo M, Hammarback S, Backstrom T. Treatment of premenstrual syndrome with gonadotropin-releasing hormone agonist in a low dose regimen. Acta Obstet Gynecol Scand 1999; 78(10):891–9.
20. Leather AT, Studd JWW, Watson NR, Holland EF. The prevention of bone loss in young women treated with GnRH analogues with add back estrogen therapy. Obstet Gynaecol 1993; 81(1):104–7.
21. Di Carlo C, Palomba S, Tommaselli GA et al. Use of leuprolide acetate plus tibolone in the treatment of severe premenstrual syndrome. Fertil Steril 2001; 75:380–4.
22. Sagsveen M, Farmer J, Prentice A, Breeze A. Gonadotrophin-releasing analogues for endometriosis: bone mineral density. Cochrane Datbase Syst Rev 2003; (4):CD001297.
23. Magill PJ, Progesterone Study Group. Investigation of the efficacy of progesterone pessaries in the relief of symptoms of premenstrual syndrome. Br J Gen Pract 1995; 45:589–93.

24. Wyatt K, Dimmock P, Jones P, Obhrai M, O'Brien S. Efficacy of progesterone and progestogens in management of premenstrual syndrome: systematic review. Br Med J 2001; 323:1–8.

25. Dalley A. Women Under the Knife. London: Huchinson Radius; 1991.

26. Battey R. The history of Battey's operation. Atlanta Med Surg J 1886; 3:657–75.

27. Casson P, Hahn PM, Van Hugt DA, Reid RL. Lasting response to ovariectomy in severe intractable premenstrual syndrome. Am J Obstet Gynecol 1990; 162(1):99–105.

28. Casper RF, Hearn MT. The effect of hysterectomy and bilateral oophorectomy in women with severe premenstrual syndrome. Am J Obstet Gynecol 1990; 162(1):105–9.

29. Cronje WH, Vashisht A, Studd JW. Hysterectomy and bilateral oophorectomy for severe premenstrual syndrome. Hum Reprod 2004; 19(9):2152–5.

30. Studd JWW. Prophylactic oophorectomy. Br J Obstet Gynaecol 1989; 96:506–9.

31. Panay N, Studd JWW. The psychotherapeutic effects of estrogens. Gynecol Endocrinol 1998; 5:353–65.

32. Studd JWW, Panay N. Hormones and depression in women. Climacteric 2004; 7:338–46.

33. Huo L, Straub RE, Schmidt PJ et al. Risk for premenstrual dysphoric disorder with genetic variation in ESR1, the estrogen receptor alpha gene. Biol Psychiatry 2007; June; [Epub ahead of print].

34. Panay N. The Management of Premenstrual Syndrome Green Top Guidelines. RCOG Press 2007 (submitted).

15

Psychotropic therapies

Meir Steiner and Claudio N Soares

INTRODUCTION

We have seen in previous chapters that the current management of severe premenstrual syndrome (PMS) and premenstrual dysphoric disorder (PMDD) includes hormonal, alternative, and non-medication therapies as well as ovarian suppression (see Chapters 14, 15, and 17). Limited evidence supports the effectiveness of some of these treatment strategies, particularly the complementary and so-called 'natural remedies'; in addition, potential side effects and risks involving long-term use of hormone treatments may limit their use.

Evidence from numerous open-label as well as randomized placebo-controlled trials (RCTs) has clearly demonstrated the efficacy of the selective serotonin reuptake inhibitors (SSRIs) and, to a lesser degree, the serotonin/norepinephrine reuptake inhibitors (SNRIs), either when used continuously or intermittently. Overall, the use of these agents has shown excellent efficacy and minimal side effects. This chapter will summarize this evidence and will also discuss the potential use of anxiolytics in this population.

ANTIDEPRESSANTS

Of all the neurotransmitters studied to date, serotonin has been identified as the most plausible candidate to be relevant in the pathophysiology of PMS and PMDD (see Chapter XX). It has been suggested that women with severe PMS or PMDD are more sensitive to the premenstrual decrease in circulating progesterone metabolites. It has been suggested that serotonergic agents have the potential for enhancing the production of these metabolites and thus prevent the occurrence of premenstrual symptoms (see Chapters 7, 10, and 12). It should therefore come as no surprise that pharmacological interventions have focused primarily on such agents.

A Swedish group of researchers deserves the credit for being the first to show that a relatively small dose (25–50 mg) of clomipramine, a non-selective serotonin reuptake inhibitor, was effective in reducing symptoms of irritability and sadness in women with severe PMS.[1]

Subsequent open-label as well as RCTs have all confirmed the efficacy of clomipramine[2] as well as of the SSRIs[3–20] and the SNRIs.[21,22] Initially most of these trials reported on continuous daily dosing of the medication (Table 15.1).

It soon became evident that not only do women with severe PMS or PMDD respond to somewhat lower doses of these antidepressants as compared with the usual doses needed in depression or some of the anxiety disorders but also that the onset of action was much shorter (days rather than weeks). This observation, along with the fact that premenstrual symptoms are generally limited to the luteal phase of the cycle, led the same Swedish group to initiate the first ever study of intermittent (luteal phase only) administration of clomipramine.[23] Again, subsequent open-label as well as RCTs have confirmed the efficacy of SSRIs[24–37] and SNRIs[38] when administered intermittently (Table 15.2).

The form of intermittent dosing that has been evaluated is treatment enduring for the last 2 weeks of the menstrual cycle. With intermittent or luteal phase dosing, treatment is initiated around the time of ovulation and is discontinued 1 or 2 days after the onset of menstruation. Intermittent dosing should not be confused with symptom-onset therapy, in which treatment begins immediately after the first appearance of symptoms.[26,36] An intermittent dosing regimen is a reasonable choice for patients with regular menstrual cycles who are able to adhere to the on/off dosing regimen, for patients with no evidence of mood symptoms during the follicular phase (i.e. patients whose symptoms persist throughout the menstrual cycle), for patients concerned about long-term adverse effects (e.g. sexual dysfunction), and for patients who experience few side effects at treatment initiation.

Table 15.1 Continuous dosing of antidepressants

Treatment	Daily dose	Duration	N	Conclusion	References
Open label					
Clomipramine	25–50 mg	5 cycles	5	+	Eriksson et al 1990[1]
Fluoxetine	20 mg (cross-over)	3 cycles	16	+	Menkes et al 1992[3]
	20 mg	6 cycles	60	+	Hunter et al 2002[4]
Fluvoxamine	50–100 mg	2 cycles	10	+	Freeman et al 1996[5]
Paroxetine	10–30 mg	3 cycles	14	+	Yonkers et al 1996[6]
Venlafaxine	37.5–150 mg	2 cycles	20	+	Hsiao and Liu 2003[22]
RCTs					
Clomipramine	25–75 mg	3 cycles	20	+ +	Sundblad et al 1992[2]
Fluoxetine	20 mg	2 cycles	10	+ +	Stone et al 1991[7]
	20 mg	3 cycles	8	+ +	Wood et al 1992[8]
	20 or 60 mg	6 cycles	128	+ +	Steiner et al 1995[9]
	20–60 mg (cross-over)	3 cycles	17	+	Su et al 1997[10]
	20 mg	2 cycles	10	+ +	Pearlstein et al 1997[11]
	20 mg	3 cycles	15	+	Ozeren et al 1997[12]
	10 mg	3 cycles	30	+ +	Diegoli et al 1998[13]
	20–40 mg	2 cycles	19	+	Atmaca et al 2003[14]
Fluvoxamine	50–150 mg	2 cycles	10	–	Veeninga et al 1990[15]
Paroxetine	10–30 mg	3 cycles	22	+ +	Eriksson et al 1995[16]
Paroxetine CR	12.5 or 25 mg	3 cycles	142	+ +	Cohen et al 2004[17]
	12.5 or 25 mg	3 cycles	171	+ +	Pearlstein et al 2005[18]
Sertraline	50–150 mg	3 cycles	99	+ +	Yonkers et al 1997[19]
	50–150 mg	3 cycles	62	+ +	Freeman et al 1999[20]
Venlafaxine	50–200 mg	4 cycles	68	+ +	Freeman et al 2001[21]

N = the number of women who were on the active compound.
Conclusion: + +, statistically significant improvement vs placebo; +, quality of evidence limited but positive outcome; –, no statistically significant improvement vs placebo.

Table 15.2 Intermittent dosing (luteal phase only) of antidepressants

Treatment	Daily dose	Duration	N	Conclusion	References
Open label					
Escitalopram	10–20 mg	3 cycles	27	+	Freeman et al 2005[24]
Nefazodone	100–150 mg	1 cycle	3	+	Kodesh et al 2001[25]
Paroxetine CR	25 mg (cross-over)	2 cycles	20	+	Yonkers et al 2006[26]
Venlafaxine	75–112.5 mg	2 cycles	11	+	Cohen et al 2004[38]
RCTs					
Clomipramine	25–75 mg	3 cycles	15	+ +	Sundblad et al 1993[23]
Fluoxetine	90 mg (weekly)	3 cycles	167	+ +	Miner et al 2002[27]
	10 or 20 mg	3 cycles	141	+ +	Cohen et al 2002[28]
Nefazodone	100–400 mg	4 cycles	22	–	Landen et al 2001[29]
Paroxetine	10 or 20 mg	4 cycles	48	+	Steiner et al 2006[30]
Paroxetine CR	12.5 or 25 mg	3 cycles	191	+ +	Steiner et al 2005[31]
Sertraline	100 mg (cross-over)	2 cycles	8	+	Halbreich and Smoller 1997[32]
	50 mg	2 cycles	11	+	Young et al 1998[33]
	50–100 mg (cross-over)	2 cycles	57	+	Jermain et al 1999[34]
	50–100 mg	3 cycles	115	+ +	Halbreich et al 2002[35]
	25–50 mg	2 cycles	151	+ +	Kornstein et al 2006[36]
L-tryptophan	6 g	3 cycles	37	+ +	Steinberg et al 1999[37]

N = the number of women who were on the active compound.

Conclusion: + +, statistically significant improvement vs placebo; +, quality of evidence limited but positive outcome; –, no statistically significant improvement vs placebo.

Weekly luteal phase dosing with enteric-coated fluoxetine 90 mg tablets has been reported to be efficacious in one RCT,[27] but to our knowledge this dosage regimen has not been widely disseminated into clinical practice.

Semi-intermittent dosing is a more complicated regimen and involves continuous administration of the SSRI throughout the menstrual cycle, with increased doses during the luteal phase. Although intuitive, particularly for patients who experience premenstrual worsening of underlying mood and/or anxiety disorders, this intervention has not been widely assessed in controlled trials. To date, only one randomized, placebo-controlled study has examined the efficacy of semi-intermittent treatment.[39]

Several studies have also compared intermittent vs continuous dosing and found either no differences or advantage of the intermittent dosing[39–44] (Table 15.3). The extent to which different subgroups of women who suffer from severe PMS/PMDD could preferably benefit from either continuous or intermittent dosing remains to be investigated.

So far, clinicians and patients have opted for intermittent vs continuous dosing primarily based on the patient's symptom profile and treatment tolerability. Good candidates for intermittent therapy are patients who wish to limit the amount of medication they take, are not able to adhere properly to the continuous regimen, have no mood symptoms during the follicular phase, or are concerned about long-term adverse effects (e.g. sexual dysfunction).[45] Treatment cost may also play a role in the option for intermittent treatment. Other alternatives for patients who are treated intermittently and do not achieve a robust clinical response include increasing the dose of the intermittently administered SSRI or switching to continuous SSRI treatment. If mood or anxiety symptoms emerge during the follicular phase of the menstrual cycle, strong consideration should be given to switching to continuous SSRI therapy. Finally, intolerable adverse effects that occur during intermittent SSRI therapy may be addressed in one of two ways: by watchful waiting to determine if they resolve over time or by a reduction in dose. For patients treated with continuous SSRIs and who only achieve suboptimal clinical response, the dose should be increased after the second menstrual cycle. Adverse effects are managed by watchful waiting; if this approach is not effective or if the adverse effect is intolerable, the dose should be reduced. When dosage reduction is not successful, consideration should be given to switching to intermittent SSRI administration.

The specificity of the serotonergic antidepressants in the treatment of PMS/PMDD has been demonstrated in several comparative RCTs. Sertraline has been compared to desipramine,[20] fluoxetine to bupropion,[11] and paroxetine to maprotiline,[16] all clearly demonstrating the lack of efficacy of the non-SSRIs. Preliminary results have also shown that L-tryptophan, a serotonergic precursor, is an effective treatment for PMS,[37] whereas lithium is not. Treatment with nefazodone, a serotonin modulator, has been shown initially to have some beneficial effect[25] but in a subsequent RCT, nefazodone was not more effective than placebo.[29] The effectiveness of milnacipran, a presynaptic SNRI, has recently been demonstrated in three women with PMDD who were intolerant to SSRIs.[46] Overall, the response rate in most RCTs for clomipramine, the SSRIs and the SNRIs is ≥60% with a standardized mean difference in favor of the active drug (for reviews see also References 45, 47–49). To date, no evidence supports a differential treatment response to either SSRIs or SNRIs for patients with PMDD.

Several of the larger RCTs have also clearly demonstrated that the improvement is not only in the behavioral/psychological symptoms of PMS/PMDD (in particular irritability) but also in the physical symptoms (breast tenderness and bloating) (e.g. References 16, 17, 19, 44, 49, and 50) as well as in the psychosocial domain.[44,51,52] Interestingly, premenstrual headaches do not appear to benefit from treatment with these agents. The side-effect profile and compliance reported in these studies do not differ significantly from those reported in studies using the same medications for other indications. Nonetheless, intermittent and low doses of clomipramine, SSRIs, and SNRIs, when used in the treatment of PMS/PMDD, seem to reduce the burden of side effects. The concern that intermittent dosing, especially of the antidepressants with a relatively short half-life, might cause withdrawal symptoms or the discontinuation syndrome has also been evaluated. The studies of intermittent dosing report neither a high frequency of initial side effects each time the medication is restarted nor any marked discontinuation symptoms.[53] The lack of significant withdrawal or discontinuation symptoms seen with intermittent dosing may be related to its unique mechanism of action (possibly GABA-a mediated), by which no prolonged exposure is needed to promote the therapeutic effect. In fact, subjects treated with intermittent dosing of SSRIs and SNRIs not only fail to experience discontinuation symptoms but also show improvement of symptoms that continues into the early follicular phase.[38,54]

Adverse drug–drug interactions, especially with drugs competing for the same microsomal systems in the liver, are nevertheless potentially dangerous during intermittent dosing, as much as when used continuously. Given that PMS/PMDD affects women during their reproductive years, it is important to note that there is no

Table 15.3 Intermittent vs continuous dosing of antidepressants

Treatment	Daily dose	Duration	N intermittent	N continuous	Conclusion	References
Open label						
Citalopram	20–40 mg	3 cycles	11	6	+ I = C	Freeman et al 2002[41]
Fluoxetine	20 mg	3 cycles	24	24	+ I = C	Steiner et al 1997[43]
RCTs						
Citalopram	10–30 mg	3 cycles	18	34	+ + I >C	Wikander et al 1998[39]
Paroxetine	20 mg	3 cycles	50	51	+ + I = C	Landen et al 2007[44]
Sertraline	50–150 mg	3 cycles	18	13	+ + I = C	Freeman et al 1999[40]
	50–100 mg	3 cycles	35	40	+ + I = C	Freeman et al 2004[42]

N = the number of women who were on the active compound.
Conclusion: + +, statistically significant improvement vs placebo; +, quality of evidence limited but positive outcome; −, no statistically significant improvement vs placebo; I ≥C: intermittent equal to or better than continuous.

Table 15.4 Anxiolytics

Treatment	Daily dose	Duration	N	Conclusion	References
RCTs					
Alprazolam	1–4 mg/continuous	3 cycles	8	–	Dennerstein et al 1986[60]
	0.25–4 mg (cross-over)/intermittent	4 cycles	14	+ +	Smith et al 1987[61]
	0.25 mg (cross-over)/intermittent	6 cycles	30	+ +	Harrison et al 1990[62]
	0.75–2.25 mg/intermittent	4 cycles	11	–	Schmidt et al 1993[63]
	0.25–2 mg/continuous	3 cycles	31	+	Berger and Presser 1994[64]
	0.25–2 mg/intermittent	3 cycles	56	+ +	Freeman et al 1995[65]
Buspirone	25–60 mg/intermittent	3 cycles	17	+	Rickels et al 1989[66]
	10–40 mg/intermittent	4 cycles	19	+ +	Landen et al 2001[29]

N = the number of women who were on the active compound.
Conclusion: + +, statistically significant improvement vs placebo; +, quality of evidence limited but positive outcome; –, no statistically significant improvement vs placebo.

Derby Hospitals NHS Foundation
Trust
Library and Knowledge Service

clinical evidence that concomitant use of oral contraceptives and antidepressants affects the safety or efficacy of either agent.[55] There is also no evidence of ovulation disturbance in women using SSRIs or SNRIs, although a dose-dependent change in cycle length in women with PMDD treated with continuous dosing of fluoxetine has been noted.[56]

Despite the chronicity, symptom severity, and burden of illness associated with severe PMS/PMDD, RCTs have focused only on acute phase therapy. Most studies report on improvement (not remission) of symptoms after 2–3 treatment cycles only and it is therefore not known whether women are able to stop medications after a period of time and remain well. It is also not known whether the efficacy of these interventions wanes over time, or whether the rapid remission of symptoms could result in better long-term treatment outcome. Studies are needed to identify whether or not some women develop tolerance to the SSRI over time that necessitates increases in dosage or switch to another medication, and whether or not some women stay in remission for a period of time following SSRI discontinuation. Nevertheless, preliminary data suggest that there is a recurrence of symptoms after the cessations of short-term (three cycles) treatment[57] and that long-term fluoxetine treatment is effective and well-tolerated.[58]

All the studies reported here have excluded the younger age group of adolescents (12–18 years of age), who are nevertheless known to suffer from PMS/PMDD.[59] Thus, there is no evidence-based information regarding the efficacy of these interventions for this age group, and regulatory agencies around the world have excluded them when granting the use of SSRIs for this indication.

ANXIOLYTICS

The anxiolytics alprazolam[60–65] and buspirone[29,66] have demonstrated efficacy in some but not all trials (Table 15.4); however, the magnitude of the therapeutic effect is not as high as for the SSRIs/SNRIs. The side-effect profile and the potential for dependence, especially with alprazolam, make them a less desirable option, to be used preferably as a third line of choice.

CONCLUSIONS

It is now more than 15 years since the first reports appeared in the literature on the effectiveness of serotonin-enhancing agents in treating women with severe premenstrual symptoms. Based on data to date on more than 3000 women who participated in more than 40 studies, both open-label and RCTs, using clomipramine, SSRIs, or SNRIs, there is now ample evidence that supports the beneficial role that these medications have in this condition. Both continuous and intermittent dosing are believed to be effective, but the decision as to which regimen to use has to be made on an individual basis. Continuous dosing should be reserved for women with a history of comorbid anxiety or depressive disorders or for women who experience concurrent subsyndromal (underlying) anxiety or mood symptoms throughout the entire cycle. These women may also benefit from semi-intermittent dosing, i.e. dose increase during the late luteal phase (e.g. Wikander et al[39]). Continuous dosing may also be the choice for women who may find it easier to adhere to the daily dosing regimen. Intermittent, or even symptom-onset dosing, may be more appropriate for women with 'pure' PMS/PMDD, i.e. those whose symptoms are limited to the late luteal phase only, with a definite 'on-off' presentation. This should also be the option for women who prefer not to take medication throughout the entire cycle or who experience bothersome side effects (especially sexual dysfunction), which can be minimized with intermittent dosing.

The choice of anxiolytics is limited, but both alprazolam and buspirone have been shown, primarily, to reduce premenstrual irritability. These medications, to be used intermittently or even for a couple of days, on a 'as-needed basis' (prn), should be reserved mostly for women who are intolerant to the serotonergic or noradrenergic agents and they should be used cautiously due to their addictive nature.

REFERENCES

1. Eriksson E, Lisjo P, Sundblad C et al. Effect of clomipramine on premenstrual syndrome. Acta Psychiatr Scand 1990; 81:87–8.
2. Sundblad C, Modigh K, Andersch B, Eriksson E. Clomipramine effectively reduces premenstrual irritability and dysphoria: a placebo-controlled trial. Acta Psychiatr Scand 1992; 85:39–47.
3. Menkes DB, Taghavi E, Mason PA, Spears GF, Howard RC. Fluoxetine treatment of severe premenstrual syndrome. BMJ 1992; 305:346–7.
4. Hunter MS, Ussher JM, Browne SJ et al. A randomized comparison of psychological (cognitive behavior therapy), medical (fluoxetine) and combined treatment for women with premenstrual dysphoric disorder. J Psychosom Obstet Gynaecol 2002; 23: 193–9.
5. Freeman EW, Rickels K, Sondheimer SJ. Fluvoxamine for premenstrual dysphoric disorder: a pilot study. J Clin Psychiatry 1996; 57(Suppl 8):56–9.
6. Yonkers KA, Guillion CA, Williams A, Novak K, Rush AJ. Paroxetine as a treatment for premenstrual dysphoric disorder. J Clin Psychopharmacol 1996; 16:3–8.
7. Stone AB, Pearlstein TB, Brown WA. Fluoxetine in the treatment of late luteal phase dysphoric disorder. J Clin Psychiatry 1991; 52:290–3.

8. Wood SH, Mortola JF, Chan YF, Moossazadeh F, Yen SS. Treatment of premenstrual syndrome with fluoxetine: a double-blind, placebo-controlled, crossover study. Obstet Gynecol 1992; 80:339–44.

9. Steiner M, Steinberg S, Stewart D et al. Fluoxetine in the treatment of premenstrual dysphoria. Canadian Fluoxetine/Premenstrual Dysphoria Collaborative Study Group. N Engl J Med 1995; 332:1529–34.

10. Su TP, Schmidt PJ, Danaceau MA et al. Fluoxetine in the treatment of premenstrual dysphoria. Neuropsychopharmacology 1997; 16:346–56.

11. Pearlstein T, Stone AB, Lund SA et al. Comparison of fluoxetine, bupropion, and placebo in the treatment of premenstrual dysphoric disorder. J Clin Psychopharmacol 1997; 17:261–6.

12. Ozeren S, Corrakci A, Yucesoy I, Mercan R, Erhan G. Fluoxetine in the treatment of premenstrual syndrome. Eur J Obstet Gynecol Reprod Biol 1997; 73:167–70.

13. Diegoli MS, da Fonseca AM, Diegoli CA, Pinotti JA. A double-blind trial of four medications to treat severe premenstrual syndrome. Int J Gynaecol Obstet 1998; 62:63–7.

14. Atmaca M, Kumru S, Tezcan E. Fluoxetine versus Vitex agnus castus extract in the treatment of premenstrual dysphoric disorder. Hum Psychopharmacol 2003; 18:191–5.

15. Veeninga AT, Westenberg GM, Weusten JT. Fluvoxamine in the treatment of menstrually related mood disorders. Psychopharmacology 1990; 102:414–16.

16. Eriksson E, Hedberg MA, Andersch B, Sundblad C. The serotonin reuptake inhibitor paroxetine is superior to the noradrenaline reuptake inhibitor maprotiline in the treatment of premenstrual syndrome. Neuropsychopharmacology 1995; 12:167–76.

17. Cohen LS, Soares CN, Yonkers KA et al. Paroxetine controlled release for premenstrual dysphoric disorder: a double-blind, placebo-controlled trial. Psychosom Med 2004; 66:707–13.

18. Pearlstein TB, Bellew KM, Endicott J, Steiner M. Paroxetine controlled release for premenstrual dysphoric disorder: remission analysis following a randomized, double-blind, placebo-controlled trial. Prim Care Companion J Clin Psychiatry 2005; 7:53–60.

19. Yonkers KA, Halbreich U, Freeman E et al. Symptomatic improvement of premenstrual dysphoric disorder with sertraline treatment. JAMA 1997; 278:983–8.

20. Freeman EW, Rickels K, Sondheimer SJ, Polansky M. Differential response to antidepressants in women with premenstrual syndrome/premenstrual dysphoric disorder. A randomized controlled trial. Arch Gen Psychiatry 1999; 56:932–9.

21. Freeman EW, Rickels K, Yonkers KA et al. Venlafaxine in the treatment of premenstrual dysphoric disorder. Obstet Gynecol 2001; 98:737–44.

22. Hsiao M-C, Liu C-Y. Effective open-label treatment of premenstrual dysphoric disorder with venlafaxine. Psychiatry Clin Neurosci 2003; 57:317–21.

23. Sundblad C, Hedberg MA, Eriksson E. Clomipramine administered during the luteal phase reduces the symptoms of premenstrual syndrome: a placebo-controlled trial. Neuropsychopharmacology 1993; 9:133–45.

24. Freeman EW, Sondheimer SJ, Sammel MD, Ferdousi T, Lin H. A preliminary study of luteal phase versus symptom-onset dosing with escitalopram for premenstrual dysphoric disorder. J Clin Psychiatry 2005; 66:769–73.

25. Kodesh A, Katz S, Lerner AG, Finkel B, Sigal M. Intermittent, luteal phase nefazodone treatment of premenstrual dysphoric disorder. J Psychopharmacol 2001; 15:58–60.

26. Yonkers KA, Holthausen GA, Poschman K, Howell HB. Symptom-onset treatment for women with premenstrual dysphoric disorder. J Clin Psychopharmacol 2006; 26:198–202.

27. Miner C, Brown E, McCray S, Gonzales J, Wohlreich M. Weekly luteal-phase dosing with enteric-coated fluoxetine 90 mg in premenstrual dysphoric disorder: a randomized, double-blind, placebo-controlled clinical trial. Clin Ther 2002; 24:417–33.

28. Cohen LS, Miner C, Brown EW et al. Premenstrual daily fluoxetine for premenstrual dysphoric disorder: a placebo-controlled, clinical trial using computerized diaries. Obstet Gynecol 2002; 100:435–44.

29. Landen M, Eriksson O, Sundblad C et al. Compounds with affinity for serotonergic receptors in the treatment of premenstrual dysphoria: a comparison of buspirone, nefazodone and placebo. Psychopharmacology (Berl) 2001; 155:292–8.

30. Steiner M, Ravindran A, LeMelledo JM et al. Luteal-phase administration of paroxetine for the treatment of premenstrual dysphoric disorder: a randomized, double-blind, placebo controlled trial in Canadian women. Can J Psychiatry 2006: (in press).

31. Steiner M, Hirschberg AL, Bergeron R et al. Luteal phase dosing with paroxetine controlled release (CR) in the treatment of premenstrual dysphoric disorder. Am J Obstet Gynecol 2005; 193: 352–60.

32. Halbreich U, Smoller JW. Intermittent luteal phase sertraline treatment of dysphoric premenstrual syndrome. J Clin Psychiatry 1997; 58:399–402.

33. Young SA, Hurt PH, Benedek DM, Howard RS. Treatment of premenstrual dysphoric disorder with sertraline during the luteal phase: a randomized, double-blind, placebo-controlled crossover trial. J Clin Psychiatry 1998; 59:76–80.

34. Jermain DM, Preece CK, Sykes RL, Kuehi TJ, Sulak PJ. Luteal phase sertraline treatment for premenstrual dysphoric disorder. Results of a double-blind, placebo-controlled, crossover study. Arch Fam Med 1999; 8:328–32.

35. Halbreich U, Bergeron R, Yonkers KA et al. Efficacy of intermittent, luteal phase sertraline treatment of premenstrual dysphoric disorder. Obstet Gynecol 2002; 100:1219–29.

36. Kornstein SG, Pearlstein TB, Fayyad R, Farfel GM, Gillespie JA. Low-dose sertraline in the treatment of moderate-to-severe premenstrual syndrome: efficacy of 3 dosing strategies. J Clin Psychiatry 2006; 67:1624–32.

37. Steinberg S, Annable L, Young SN, Liyanage N. A placebo-controlled clinical trial of L-tryptophan in premenstrual dysphoria. Biol Psychiatry 1999; 45:313–20.

38. Cohen LS, Soares CN, Lyster A et al. Efficacy and tolerability of premenstrual use of venlafaxine (flexible dose) in the treatment of premenstrual dysphoric disorder. J Clin Psychopharmacol 2004; 24:540–3.

39. Wikander I, Sundblad C, Andersch B et al. Citalopram in premenstrual dysphoria: is intermittent treatment during luteal phases more effective than continuous medication throughout the menstrual cycle? J Clin Psychopharmacol 1998; 18:390–8.

40. Freeman EW, Rickels K, Arredondo F et al. Full- or half-cycle treatment of severe premenstrual syndrome with a serotonergic antidepressant. J Clin Psychopharmacol 1999; 19:3–8.

41. Freeman EW, Jabara S, Sondheimer SJ, Auletto R. Citalopram in PMS patients with prior SSRI treatment failure: a preliminary study. J Womens Health Gend Based Med 2002; 11:459–64.

42. Freeman EW, Rickels K, Sondheimer SJ, Polansky M, Xiao S. Continuous or intermittent dosing with sertraline for patients with severe premenstrual syndrome or premenstrual dysphoric disorder. Am J Psychiatry 2004; 161:343–51.

43. Steiner M, Korzekwa M, Lamont J, Wilkins A. Intermittent fluoxetine dosing in the treatment of women with premenstrual dysphoria. Psychopharmacol Bull 1997; 33:771–4.

44. Landen M, Nissbrandt H, Allgulander C et al. Placebo-controlled trial comparing intermittent and continuous paroxetine in premenstrual dysphoric disorder. Neuropsychopharmacology 2007; 32:153–61.

45. Pearlstein T. Selective serotonin reuptake inhibitors for premenstrual dysphoric disorder: the emerging gold standard? Drugs 2002; 62:1869–85.

46. Yamada K, Kanba S. Effectiveness of milnacipran for SSRI-intolerant patients with premenstrual dysphoric disorder. J Clin Psychopharmacol 2005; 25:398–9.

47. Rapkin A. A review of treatment of premenstrual syndrome & premenstrual dysphoric disorder. Psychoneuroendocrinology 2003; 28:39–53.

48. Wyatt KM, Dimmock PW, O'Brien PMS. Selective serotonin reuptake inhibitors for premenstrual syndrome. Cochrane Database Syst Rev 2002; (4):CD001396.

49. Steiner M, Pearlstein T, Cohen LS et al. Expert guidelines for the treatment of severe PMS, PMDD, and comorbidities: the role of SSRIs. J Womens Health (Larchmt) 2006; 15:57–69.

50. Steiner M, Romano SJ, Babcock S et al. The efficacy of fluoxetine in improving physical symptoms associated with premenstrual dysphoric disorder. BJOG 2001; 108:462–8.

51. Pearlstein TB, Halbreich U, Batzar ED et al. Psychosocial functioning in women with premenstrual dysphoric disorder before and after treatment with sertraline or placebo. J Clin Psychiatry 2000; 61:101–9.

52. Steiner M, Brown E, Trzepacz P et al. Fluoxetine improves functional work capacity in women with premenstrual dysphoric disorder. Arch Womens Ment Health 2003; 6:71–7.

53. Macdougall M, Steiner M. Treatment of premenstrual dysphoria with selective serotonin re-uptake inhibitors: focus on safety. Expert Opin Drug Saf 2003; 2:1–6.

54. Yonkers KA, Pearlstein T, Fayyad R, Gillespie JA. Luteal phase treatment of premenstrual dysphoric disorder improves symptoms that continue into the postmenstrual phase. J Affect Disord 2005; 85:317–21.

55. Koke SC, Brown EB, Miner CM. Safety and efficacy of fluoxetine in patients who recieve oral contraceptive therapy. Am J Obstet Gynecol 2002; 187:551–5.

56. Steiner M, Lamont J, Steinberg S et al. Effect of fluoxetine on menstrual cycle length in women with premenstrual dysphoria. Obstet Gynecol 1997; 90:590–5.

57. Pearlstein T, Joliat MJ, Brown EB, Miner CM. Recurrence of symptoms of premenstrual dysphoric disorder after the cessation of luteal-phase fluoxetine treatment. Am J Obstet Gynecol 2003; 188:887–95.

58. Pearlstein TB, Stone AB. Long-term fluoxetine treatment of late luteal phase dysphoric disorder. J Clin Psychiatry 1994; 55:332–5.

59. Rapkin AJ, Mikacich JA. Premenstrual syndrome in adolescents: diagnosis and treatment. Pediatr Endocrinol Rev 2006; 3(Suppl 1):132–7.

60. Dennerstein l, Morse C, Burrows G, Brown J, Smith M. Alprazolam in the treatment of premenstrual syndrome. In: Dennerstein L, Fraser I, eds. Hormones and Behavior. New York: Elsevier Science Publishing; 1986:175–82.

61. Smith S, Rinehart JS, Ruddock VE, Schiff I. Treatment of premenstrual syndrome with alprazolam: results of a double-blind, placebo-controlled, randomized crossover clinical trial. Obstet Gynecol 1987; 70:37–43.

62. Harrison WM, Endicott J, Nee J. Treatment of premenstrual dysphoria with alprazolam. Arch Gen Psychiatry 1990; 47:270–5.

63. Schmidt PJ, Grover GN, Rubinow DR. Alprazolam in the treatment of premenstrual syndrome. A double-blind, placebo-controlled trial. Arch Gen Psychiatry 1993; 50:467–73.

64. Berger CP, Presser B. Alprazolam in the treatment of two subsamples of patients with late luteal phase dysphoric disorder: a double-blind, placebo-controlled crossover study. Obstet Gynecol 1994; 84:379–85.

65. Freeman EW, Rickels K, Sondheimer SJ, Polansky M. A double-blind trial of oral progesterone, alprazolam, and placebo in treatment of severe premenstrual syndrome. JAMA 1995; 274:51–7.

66. Rickels K, Freeman E, Sondheimer S. Buspirone in treatment of premenstrual syndrome. Lancet 1989; 1:777.

16

Complementary and alternative therapies

Edzard Ernst

INTRODUCTION

It is far from easy to define complementary and alternative medicine (CAM). Describing it by what it is not (e.g. scientifically plausible or tested, not taught in medical school) was always unsatisfactory and is becoming increasingly incorrect. Intuitively, we seem to know what CAM is (Table 16.1), but this is clearly not enough. One definition which is widely used describes CAM as:

> Diagnosis, treatment and/or prevention which complements mainstream medicine by contributing to a common whole, by satisfying a demand not met by orthodoxy or by diversifying the conceptual frameworks of medicine.[1]

Definitions of CAM are difficult and problematic, not least because CAM entails a bewildering array of therapeutic and diagnostic modalities (Table 16.2). Despite this heterogeneity, there are common features of CAM, which include:

- emphasis is on holism
- treatments are alleged to be natural
- treatments are often assumed to be harmless
- treatments are often individualized according to the characteristics of each patient
- there is much emphasis on the body's power to heal itself
- a long tradition of usage for most modalities
- by and large, CAM is private healthcare
- it may be administered by a practitioner or self-administered.

CAM has become increasingly important for healthcare professionals, simply because patients are voting with their feet and their wallets in favor of it.[2] Many healthcare professionals, however, remain sceptical about its value and few have sound knowledge of the subject.

But, because of its popularity, it seems desirable that all healthcare providers are aware of the basics of CAM: we may love or hate CAM, but if patients use it, we need to know about it.

PREVALENCE

About 65% of all US citizens seem to try at least one form of CAM within a year.[3] These figures can be even higher in patient populations, especially those suffering from chronic conditions. Virtually all surveys agree that women use CAM significantly more often than men. Women suffering from premenstrual dysphoric disorder (PMDD) frequently try CAM.[4,5] Popular choices include exercise (arguably not CAM), vitamins (arguably not CAM), other dietary supplements (including herbal medicine), meditation, yoga, acupuncture, massage, homeopathy, and chiropractic.[4,5]

REASONS FOR POPULARITY

Many conventional healthcare providers are puzzled by the current popularity and commercial success of CAM. Surely, conventional medicine is more effective than ever before – so why do people turn towards 'alternatives'?

The first important point to make here is that CAM is not normally employed as an alternative. In the vast majority of cases, it is used as an 'add on' to conventional healthcare. The term 'alternative medicine' is therefore inappropriate. The second important point is that no single reason or set of reasons for the popularity of CAM exist. Notwithstanding these caveats, research has identified numerous motivators for trying CAM. They can be categorized into positive (pull) and negative (push) factors (Table 16.3).[6] Depending on the precise circumstances, the relative importance of these factors varies.

Table 16.1 'Tongue in cheek' definitions of CAM from different perspectives

Perspective	Definitions
The patient	Healthcare I've used for years and don't dare tell my doctor about
The doctor	Type of medicine many of my patients use (without telling me) and I know nothing about
The CAM provider	Healthcare that is universally appreciated by patients but suppressed by 'the establishment'
The regulator	Type of medicine which is outside our control
The manufacturer	Supplements which sell very well, even without investment into research
The scientist	Implausible treatments which can help patients through a powerful placebo effect
The politician	Private medicine which is popular and can win votes – should not be researched seriously; however, this might show efficacy (in which case the government ought to pay for it)

Table 16.2 Some commonly used modalities in CAM

Name	Description
Acupuncture	Insertion of a needle into the skin and underlying tissues in special sites, known as points, for therapeutic or preventive purposes
Aromatherapy	The controlled use of plant essences for therapeutic purposes
Bach flower remedies	A therapeutic system that uses specially prepared plant infusions to balance physical and emotional disturbances
Biofeedback	The use of apparatus to monitor, amplify, and feed back information on physiological responses so that a patient can learn to regulate these responses. It is a form of psychophysiological self-regulation
Chelation therapy	A method for removing toxins, minerals, and metabolic wastes from the bloodstream and vessel walls using intravenous EDTA (ethylenediaminetetra-acetic acid) infusions
Chiropractic	A system of healthcare which is based on the belief that the nervous system is the most important determinant of health and that most diseases are caused by spinal subluxations which respond to spinal manipulation
Craniosacral therapy	A proprietary form of therapeutic manipulation which is tissue-, fluid-, membrane-, and energy-orientated and more subtle than any other type of cranial work
Herbalism	The medical use of preparations that contain exclusively plant material
Homeopathy	A therapeutic method using preparations of substances whose effects when administered to healthy subjects correspond to the manifestations of the disorder (symptoms, clinical signs, and pathological states) in the unwell patient
Hypnotherapy	The induction of a trance-like state to facilitate the relaxation of the conscious mind and make use of enhanced suggestibility to treat psychological and medical conditions and effect behavioral changes
Massage	A method of manipulating the soft tissue of whole body areas using pressure and traction

(Continued)

Table 16.2 (Continued)	
Name	**Description**
Naturopathy	An eclectic system of healthcare, which integrates elements of complementary and conventional medicine to support and enhance self-healing processes
Osteopathy	A form of manual therapy involving massage, mobilization, and spinal manipulation
Reflexology	A therapeutic method that uses manual pressure applied to specific areas, or zones, of the feet (and sometimes the hands or ears) that are believed to correspond to areas of the body, in order to relieve stress and prevent and treat physical disorders
Relaxation therapy	Techniques for eliciting the 'relaxation response' of the autonomic nervous system
Spiritual healing	The direct interaction between one individual (the healer) and a second (sick) individual with the intention of bringing about an improvement or cure of the illness
Yoga	A practice of gentle stretching, exercises for breath control, and meditation as a mind-body intervention

Table 16.3 Positive and negative motivations for trying CAM

Positive motivations
- Hope for increased well-being and other positive outcomes
- Philosophical congruence:
  - spiritual dimension
  - emphasis on holism
  - active role of patient
  - explanation intuitively acceptable
  - natural treatments
- Personal control over treatment
- Good relationship with therapist:
  - on equal terms
  - time for discussion
  - allows for emotional factors
- Accessibility

- **Negative motivations**
- Dissatisfaction with certain aspects of conventional medicine:
  - ineffective
  - adverse effects
  - poor communication with healthcare practitioner
  - insufficient time with healthcare practitioner
- Total rejection of conventional medicine:
  - antiscience or antiestablishment attitude
- Desperation

Much of the popularity of CAM amounts to a criticism of conventional healthcare. This can be seen as a backlash from the spirit of the mid-20th century when science was expected to solve most problems. Reality turned out to be different. Many consumers now feel disappointed that many medical conditions (including PMDD) cannot be cured or adequately alleviated (i.e. without side effects); CAM, on the other hand, is 'free' of safety problems – at least this is what proponents incessantly claim.

THE EVIDENCE FOR OR AGAINST CAM

Even though sometimes denied by proponents of CAM, most therapies can be tested for efficacy/effectiveness in randomized clinical trials (RCTs). Occasionally, the standard RCT design requires adaptation to fit the demands of CAM,[7] but there are no compelling reasons why CAM should defy scientific testing in principle. The following discussion regarding the effectiveness of CAM to treat PMDD will therefore be based on evidence from clinical trials and (where available) systematic reviews of such studies.

Acupuncture/acupressure

A systematic review included four controlled clinical trials (CCTs) of acupuncture or acupressure for dysmenorrhea (not PMDD).[8] Even though they all generated results suggesting that acupuncture does in fact reduce symptoms, methodological limitations currently prevent definitive conclusions.

Biofeedback

Vaginal temperature feedback (12 weekly sessions) was compared with no treatment in two RCTs with 30 women.[9] Biofeedback alleviated both physiological and affective symptoms. However, methodological short-comings of these studies cast doubt on the validity of their findings.

Herbal medicine

Chaste tree

Chaste tree (*Vitex agnus-castus*) extracts have been tested in several uncontrolled studies. The results were invariably positive. In a large (*n* = 1634) study, for instance, 81% of all patients rated themselves 'much better'.[10] The results of double-blind RCTs (Table 16.4) are, however, not uniform.[11-13] One placebo-controlled RCT[11] failed to demonstrate efficacy whereas the other such study[13] suggested that chaste tree extract does alleviate symptoms. One RCT[12] compared the herbal extract to vitamin B_6. The results suggested equivalence, but it is unclear whether this indicates that both are similarly effective or ineffective. The value of chaste tree extracts has thus not been proven beyond reasonable doubt.

Evening primrose

A systematic review of evening primrose (*Oenothera biennis*) oil included seven uncontrolled studies as well as four randomized and placebo-controlled RCTs.[14] None of these investigations had large samples and most trials had other serious methodological weaknesses. The three most rigorous RCTs were all negative. The conclusion drawn from this evidence was that evening primrose oil seems to be of little value for PMDD. Evening primrose oil has been marketed extensively for PMS, PMDD, and for cyclical mastalgia and, although the evidence was limited, it was licensed for cyclical breast symptoms.

Ginkgo

Ginkgo (*Ginkgo biloba*) was investigated in a double-blind RCT with 163 women suffering from PMDD.[15] Patients were given either placebo or 160 mg ginkgo extract daily for 2 months. The results suggested that regular ginkgo intake may be helpful for breast pain, but not for other symptoms of PMDD.

Homeopathy

Two double-blind, placebo-controlled RCTs of classical homeopathy have been published. In the first one, stringent exclusion criteria led to the sample being too small (*n* = 10) for generating meaningful results.[16]

Table 16.4 Double-blind RCTs of chaste tree for premenstrual syndrome

Reference	Sample size	Interventions [dosage]	Result	Comment
Turner and Mills[11]	217	(A) Chaste tree [1800 mg/day] (B) Placebo	No difference	Postal study; other treatments not excluded
Lauritzen et al[12]	127	(A) Chaste tree [3.5–4.2 mg/day] (B) Vitamin B_6 [200 mg/day]	A was no different to B	Sample size lacked statistical power; efficacy of control intervention (B_6) was unclear
Schellenberg[13]	170	(A) Chaste tree [1 tab/day] (B) Placebo	A was superior to B	Responder rates were 52% (A) and 24% (B)

The other study comprised 105 patients treated over 3 months.[17] By the end of this treatment, symptom scores were lower in the homeopathically treated group compared with the placebo group. There was also less use of tranquillizers and analgesics and fewer work days lost than in the placebo group. Vis-à-vis these contradictory findings, no definitive conclusions about the value of homeopathy for PMDD are possible.

Massage

An RCT of massage therapy for 24 women with PMDD reported some improvements in symptoms immediately after massage sessions and after 1 month of treatment. However, the mood symptoms that are central to PMDD were not lowered at 1 month. Relaxation was used as a control, but intergroup analyses were not conducted.[18] The effectiveness of massage for PMDD therefore remains speculative.

Reflexology

An RCT ($n = 35$) of reflexology applied once weekly for 2 months reduced both somatic and psychological PMDD symptoms significantly more than sham reflexology, which involved treating points unrelated to premenstrual symptoms.[19] This study needs independent replication before recommendations can be made.

Relaxation

Progressive muscle relaxation training (twice weekly for 3 months) alleviated physical symptoms of PMDD in an RCT ($n = 46$) compared with the control interventions of reading and charting symptoms.[20] For women with severe complaints, there were also improvements in emotional symptoms. Independent replications of these data are required.

Spinal manipulation

A cross-over RCT of chiropractic manipulation included 25 PMDD patients. Superior results were noted for spinal manipulation compared with a sham treatment.[21] However, improvements were greatest with whichever intervention was received first. Therefore the perceived benefits may not be due to specific effects of spinal manipulation.

Dietary supplements

Calcium

Calcium supplementation has been demonstrated to be superior to placebo for most types of PMDD symptoms in two double-blind RCTs (Table 16.5).[22,23] The second of these trials is impressive in terms of size ($n = 466$) and methodological rigor and provides promising evidence in favor of calcium.

Magnesium

Two small double-blind RCTs of magnesium supplements have indicated some benefits over placebo.[24,25] However, the type of symptoms that improved was different in each study. The data are therefore not compelling and require independent replication.

Neptune Krill

Neptune Krill Oil has been compared to fish oil in an RCT with 70 women.[26] The results suggest that both have similar effects on dysmenorrhea and symptoms of

---

Table 16.5 Double-blind RCTs of calcium for premenstrual syndrome

Reference	Sample size	Interventions [dosage]	Result	Comment
Thys-Jacobs et al[22]	33	(A) Calcium [1000 mg/day for 3 months] (B) Placebo	A was superior in 3 of 4 symptoms	Cross-over trial; high drop-out rate; non-compliance
Thys-Jacobs et al[23]	466	(A) Calcium [1200 mg/day for 3 months] (B) Placebo	A was superior in all symptoms	Trial was rigorous but not all other treatments were excluded

PMDD. However, one cannot be sure that both were equally effective or ineffective.

Potassium

Potassium was investigated as a therapy in a non-randomized, placebo-controlled trial.[27] The results showed no effect on PMDD symptoms or premenstrual weight gain.

Vitamin B6

Vitamin B6 is a cofactor in the synthesis of serotonin from dietary tryptophan. It is self-prescribed extensively. The RCT evidence for vitamin B6 has been subjected to systematic review. A meta-analysis pooled the data of nine double-blind, placebo-controlled RCTs. Greater effect than placebo for overall symptoms and premenstrual depression were noted. The authors cautioned, however, that conclusions must remain limited due to the low quality of most trials. The authors also advised that doses in excess of 100 mg/day were not justified due to neurological adverse effects.[28] Combining vitamin B6 and magnesium reduces anxiety-related symptoms of PMDD.[29]

Table 16.6 Examples of risks associated with CAM

Obvious risks

Toxicity
- Toxic herbal remedies
- Toxic contaminants in oral remedies
- Adulteration of oral remedies with prescription drugs

Trauma
- Stroke after upper spinal manipulation
- Pneumothorax after acupuncture needle puncturing the lungs

Infection
- Hepatitis or other infections after improper use of acupuncture

Less obvious risks

- Use of CAM as a true alternative to effective healthcare
- Reliance on unreliable diagnostic techniques used by CAM providers
- Cost of ineffective treatments

Vitamin E

Vitamin E has been investigated in two double-blind, placebo-controlled RCTs.[30,31] Although both show positive results for some PMDD symptoms, the overall evidence is ambiguous and more research is required.

Other therapies

Aerobic exercise

A relatively large body of evidence from questionnaire studies, non-randomized trials, and case–control studies suggests that aerobic exercise training may help prevent or alleviate premenstrual symptoms (e.g. References 32–35).

Qi-therapy

Qi-therapy has generated encouraging results in two RCTs from the same research group.[36,37]

SAFETY ISSUES

Patients are continually being misled into believing (e.g. by the media or by the ~40 million websites promoting CAM) that CAM is natural and therefore safe. This misinformation can be dangerous, as none of the treatments is totally devoid of risks (Table 16.6). This is clearly not the place to review this complex area; the reader is referred to comprehensive overviews published elsewhere.[2,38]

CONCLUSIONS

Many CAM treatments are being promoted and used for PMDD: only some of them have been submitted to clinical trials. Frequently, the methodological rigor of these studies is wanting and, for each modality, trial data remain scarce. The most promising results so far suggest that acupuncture, calcium supplements, or vitamin B6 might alleviate some of the symptoms of PMDD.

REFERENCES

1. Ernst E, Resch KL, Mills S et al. Complementary medicine – a definition. Br J Gen Pract 1995; 45:506.
2. Ernst E. Prevalence of use of complementary/alternative medicine: a systematic review. Bull World Health Organ 2000; 78:252–7.
3. Barnes PM, Powell-Griner E, McFann K, Nahin RL. Complementary and alternative medicine use among adults: United States,

2002. Advance Data from Vital and Health Statistics. Hyattsville, Maryland: National Center for Health Statistics; 2004; 343:1.

4. Singh B, Berman B, Simpson R, Annechild A. Incidence of premenstrual syndrome and remedy usage: a national probability sample study. Altern Ther Health Med 1998; 4:75–9.

5. Corney RH, Stanton R. A survey of 658 women who report symptoms of premenstrual syndrome. J Psychosom Res 1991; 65:471–82.

6. Ernst E, Pittler MH, Wider B, Boddy K. The Desk Top Guide to Complementary and Alternative Medicine, 2nd edn. Edinburgh: Mosby/Elsevier; 2006.

7. Ernst E. Randomised clinical trials: unusual designs. Perfusion 2004; 17:416–21.

8. White AR. A review of controlled trials of acupuncture for women's reproductive healthcare. J Fam Plann Reprod Health Care 2003; 29:233–6.

9. Van Zak DB. Biofeedback treatments for premenstrual and premenstrual affective syndromes. Int J Psychosom 1994; 41:53–60.

10. Loch EG, Selle H, Boblitz N. Treatment of premenstrual syndrome with a phytopharmaceutical formulation containing Vitex agnus castus. J Womens Health Gend Based Med 2000; 9:315–20.

11. Turner S, Mills S. A double-blind clinical trial on a herbal remedy for premenstrual syndrome: a case study. Complement Ther Med 1993; 1:73–7.

12. Lauritzen C, Reuter HD, Repges R et al. Treatment of premenstrual tension syndrome with Vitex agnus castus: controlled, double-blind study versus pyridoxine. Phytomedicine 1997; 4:183–9.

13. Schellenberg R. Treatment for the premenstrual syndrome with agnus castus fruit extract: prospective, randomised, placebo controlled study. BMJ 2001; 322:134–7.

14. Budeiri D, Li Wan PA, Dornan JC. Is evening primrose oil of value in the treatment of premenstrual syndrome? Control Clin Trials 1996; 17:60–8.

15. Tamborini A, Taurelle R. Value of standardized Ginkgo biloba extract (EGb 761) in the management of congestive symptoms of premenstrual syndrome. [French]. Rev Fr Gynecol Obstet 1993; 88:447–57.

16. Chapman EH, Angelica J, Spitalny G, Strauss M. Results of a study of the homeopathic treatment of PMS. J Am Inst Homeopath 1994; 87:14–21.

17. Yakir M, Kreitler S, Brzezinski A, Vithoulkas G. Homeopathic treatment of premenstrual syndrome – repeated study. Proceedings of the Annual Conference of the International Homoeopathic League, Budapest, Hungary, May 2000.

18. Hernandez-Reif M, Martinez A, Field T et al. Premenstrual symptoms are relieved by massage therapy. J Psychosom Obstet Gynaecol 2000; 21:9–15.

19. Oleson T, Flocco W. Randomized controlled study of premenstrual symptoms treated with ear, hand and foot reflexology. Obstet Gynecol 1993; 82:906–11.

20. Goodale IL, Domar AD, Benson H. Alleviation of premenstrual syndrome symptoms with the relaxation response. Obstet Gynecol 1990; 75:649–55.

21. Walsh MJ, Polus BI. A randomized, placebo-controlled clinical trial on the efficacy of chiropractic therapy on premenstrual syndrome. J Manipulative Physiol Ther 1999; 22:582–5.

22. Thys-Jacobs S, Ceccarelli S, Bierman A et al. Calcium supplementation in premenstrual syndrome: a randomized crossover trial. J Gen Intern Med 1989; 4:183–9.

23. Thys-Jacobs S, Starkey P, Bernstein D, Tian J. Calcium carbonate and the premenstrual syndrome: effects on premenstrual and menstrual symptoms. Premenstrual Syndrome Study Group. Am J Obstet Gynecol 1998; 179:444–52.

24. Facchinetti F, Borella P, Sances G et al. Oral magnesium successfully relieves premenstrual mood changes. Obstet Gynecol 1991; 78:177–81.

25. Walker AF, De Souza MC, Vickers MF et al. Magnesium supplementation alleviates premenstrual symptoms of fluid retention. J Womens Health 1998; 7:1157–65.

26. Sampalis F, Bunea R, Pelland MF et al. Evaluation of the effects of Neptune Krill Oil on the management of premenstrual syndrome and dysmenorrhea. Altern Med Rev 2003; 8:171–9.

27. Reeves BD, Garvin JE, McElin TW. Premenstrual tension: symptoms and weight changes related to potassium therapy. Am J Obstet Gynecol 1971; 109:1036–41.

28. Wyatt KM, Dimmock PW, Jones PW, O'Brien PMS. Efficacy of vitamin B-6 in the treatment of premenstrual syndrome: systematic review. BMJ 1999; 318:1375–81.

29. De Souza MC, Walker AF, Robinson PA, Bolland K. A synergistic effect of a daily supplement for 1 month of 200 mg magnesium plus 50 mg vitamin B_6 for the relief of anxiety-related premenstrual symptoms: a randomized, double-blind, crossover study. J Womens Health Gend Based Med 2000; 9:131–9.

30. London RS, Sundaram GS, Murphy L, Goldstein PJ. The effect of alpha-tocopherol on premenstrual symptomatology: a double-blind study. J Am Coll Nutr 1983; 2:115–22.

31. London RS, Murphy L, Kitlowski KE, Reynolds MA. Efficacy of alpha-tocopherol in the treatment of the premenstrual syndrome. J Reprod Med 1987; 32:400–4.

32. Choi PY, Salmon P. Symptom changes across the menstrual cycle in competitive sportswomen, exercisers and sedentary women. Br J Clin Psychol 1995; 34:447–60.

33. Aganoff JA, Boyle GJ. Aerobic exercise, mood states and menstrual cycle symptoms. J Psychosom Res 1994; 38:183–92.

34. Steege JF, Blumenthal JA. The effects of aerobic exercise on premenstrual symptoms in middle-aged women: a preliminary study. J Psychosom Res 1993; 37:127–33.

35. Prior JC, Vigna Y, Sciarretta D, Alojado N, Schulzer M. Conditioning exercise decreases premenstrual symptoms: a prospective, controlled 6-month trial. Fertil Steril 1987; 47:402–8.

36. Jang HS, Lee MS. Effects of qi therapy (external qigong) on premenstrual syndrome: a randomized placebo-controlled study. J Altern Complement Med 2004; 10:456–62.

37. Jang HS, Lee MS, Kim MJ, Chong ES. Effects of Qi-therapy on premenstrual syndrome. Int J Neurosci 2004; 114:909–21.

38. Ernst E. Risks associated with complementary therapies. In: Dukes MNG, Aronson JK, eds. Meyler's Side Effects of Drugs, 14th edn. Amsterdam: Elsevier; 2000:1649–81.

17

Clinical evaluation and management

Andrea J Rapkin and Judy Mikacich

INTRODUCTION

The clinical approach to evaluation and management of premenstrual syndrome (PMS) or premenstrual dysphoric disorder (PMDD) involves taking an accurate history, prospective daily symptom monitoring to establish the diagnosis, patient-specific initial medical or psychological therapy, and adequate follow-up with appropriate alterations in the treatment plan. A typical patient can present with premenstrual irritability, mood swings, anxiety and/or depression, and physical symptoms that may include breast tenderness, bloating, fatigue, appetite, and sleep alterations, or difficulty concentrating; these conditions result in significant overall interference with daily activities or social interactions. As the symptoms are not unique in their nature but only in their timing, the diagnosis should be made only after the patient completes daily recording of bothersome symptoms for 2–3 consecutive months. However, a detailed psychiatric interview by an appropriately trained professional may rule out underlying affective disorder. This may be a useful compromise when only retrospective information is available.[1] Various medical and affective disorders included in the differential diagnosis must be excluded. Current management strategies include education and self-care, calcium supplementation, and the choice of a number of psychotropic agents that augment serotonin, administered either throughout the cycle or during the luteal phase alone. Pharmacological options include selective serotonin reuptake inhibitors (SSRIs), serotonin/norepinephrine reuptake inhibitors (SNRIs), serotonergic tricyclic antidepressants, or hormonal approaches that prevent ovulation, such as some oral contraceptives, gonadotropin-releasing hormone agonists (GnRH agonists), danazol, and high-dose estrogen. Psychological approaches, including cognitive/behavioral and relaxation therapy, may also be effective. The treatment plan should be designed according to the patient's specific symptoms, past pharmacological treatment experiences, and other current and past health and contraceptive needs.

CLINICAL EVALUATION

Diagnostic criteria

One of the limitations in establishing the diagnosis of a premenstrual disorder is the lack of universally accepted diagnostic criteria. Factors generic to the diagnosis of PMS and PMDD are that (1) the somatic, affective, and/or behavioral symptoms only occur in ovulatory women and that (2) the symptoms must recur cyclically in the luteal phase of the menstrual cycle and resolve by the end of menses, leaving a symptom-free interval in the late follicular phase, before ovulation.

The American College of Obstetricians and Gynecologists (ACOG) published a practice bulletin on PMS containing diagnostic criteria.[2] According to these criteria, the diagnosis of PMS requires that a woman must have one or more of the affective or somatic symptoms listed in Table 17.1.

The PMS criteria additionally specify that the symptoms must occur during the 5 days before menses in each of three prior menstrual cycles, with relief by day 4 of menses. This cyclic pattern must be confirmed in at least two consecutive months of prospective symptom charting. The symptoms must be bothersome, with the woman experiencing dysfunction in social and/or occupational spheres. These recurring symptoms must be present in the absence of pharmacological therapy, including hormones, or use of alcohol or drugs. Other psychiatric and medical disorders must have been excluded as a potential cause of the symptoms.[3,4]

Table 17.1 ACOG diagnostic criteria for premenstrual syndrome (PMS)

Affective symptoms	Somatic symptoms
Depression	Breast tenderness
Anger	Abdominal bloating
Irritability	Headache
Anxiety	Swelling of extremities
Confusion	
Social withdrawal	

PMS can be diagnosed after the patient prospectively documents at least one of the affective or somatic symptoms during the 5 days prior to menses for three menstrual cycles. Symptoms should be of such severity as to impact social or economic performance. Symptoms should abate during the first 4 days of the menstrual cycle and not recur until at least cycle day 13. There should be no concomitant pharmacological therapy, hormone ingestion, or drug or alcohol abuse.
Adapted from ACOG.[2]

Diagnostic criteria for PMDD, found in the Diagnostic and Statistical Manual of Mental Disorders, fourth edition, text revision (DSM-IV-TR), are more specific and include endorsement of five or more of the symptoms listed in Table 17.2, with at least one being a core symptom.[5]

Further PMS criteria are that the symptoms must be present during the last week of the luteal phase in most of the woman's menstrual cycles in the previous year, be relieved within the first few days of the follicular phase of the cycle, and must not have recurred during the week that follows menses. The criteria must be confirmed by prospective daily ratings for at least two consecutive symptomatic cycles. The symptoms must not represent an exacerbation of another disorder, such as a depressive or anxiety disorder, substance abuse, a personality disorder, perimenopause, or thyroid disease, although they can be superimposed on such a disorder. A diagnosis of PMDD requires that the symptoms be severe enough to interfere with the woman's work, social interactions, or usual activities. The National Institute of Mental Health also defines premenstrual changes as showing at least a 30% increase in symptom intensity during the late luteal phase of the cycle (6 days

Table 17.2 DSM-IV criteria for premenstrual dysphoric disorder (PMDD)

1. Experience five or more symptoms, including at least one core symptom:
   - Markedly depressed mood, hopelessness, self-deprecating thoughts[a]
   - Marked anxiety, tension[a]
   - Marked affective lability[a]
   - Persistent and marked anger or irritability[a]
   - Decreased interest in usual activities
   - Subjective sense of difficulty in concentrating
   - Subjective sense of being out of control
   - Lethargy, easy fatigability
   - Marked change in appetite
   - Hypersomnia or insomnia
   - Other physical symptoms, such as breast tenderness-headache.
2. Report symptoms during the last week of the luteal phase, with remission within a few days of the onset of menses
3. Document absence of symptoms during the week following menses
4. Demonstrate marked interference of symptoms with work, school, or social activities and relationships
5. Symptoms are not an exacerbation of another disorder
6. Prospective daily ratings confirm three of the above criteria during at least two consecutive symptomatic menstrual cycles.

[a]Core symptoms; PMDD can be diagnosed when, for most of the 12 cycles, the above criteria are met. Adapted from the Diagnostic and Statistical Manual of Mental Disorders, 4th edn (DSM-IV). Washington DC: American Psychiatric Association; 1994: 715–18.

prior to menses) compared with the follicular phase (days 5–10 of the cycle).[6]

The diagnostic process

There are no specific diagnostic tests for PMS or PMDD. Therefore, the diagnostic process is one of exclusion based on a clinical interview, physical examination, and prospective daily recordings. A comprehensive assessment is essential, exploring medical, gynecological, psychosocial, and psychosexual history, as well as substance abuse, domestic violence and life stressors, to determine the presence of past or current menstrual-related disorders, psychiatric disorders, or medical conditions (Table 17.3). It is very useful to perform assessment during the follicular phase to assess mood, cognition, and general level of functioning when premenstrual symptoms should be absent. An alteration in mental state during the follicular phase would suggest the necessity of a comprehensive psychiatric evaluation.[7,8] A thorough history, eliciting all bothersome premenstrual symptoms, is adequate, but a retrospective history or questionnaire, such as the Premenstrual Assessment Form (PAF), can be used.[9] The clinician must establish that the patient is ovulating, particularly if menses are not regular (ovulatory cycles are generally about 25–32 days in length.) Symptoms such as headache/migraine, fatigue, abdominal or breast pain, bloating, and vaginal spotting, presenting premenstrually, may be a result of other medical conditions. Symptoms of a depressive disorder, anxiety disorder, or personality disorder will not demonstrate a purely cyclic pattern, with a consistent asymptomatic phase before ovulation, although these disorders often worsen premenstrually.[10]

A thorough physical examination should be completed, including a breast and pelvic examination. Gynecological issues to be assessed include pregnancy, postpartum status, perimenopause, cycle irregularity, polycystic ovary syndrome, chronic pelvic pain, and endometriosis; fibrocystic disease, galactorrhea, and breast cancer should be evaluated in a woman who presents with breast symptoms. If a woman is using an oral contraceptive that suppresses ovulation, the symptoms experienced prior to the monthly bleeding are not PMS but could be attributed to hormone withdrawal associated with the hormone-free interval in the pill regimen.[11] Over age 40 years old, symptoms such as dysphoria, breast tenderness, headache, and sleep disturbances occurring during the premenopausal period should be differentiated from those of the perimenopause. The history and physical examination might prompt specific blood or radiological tests, such as complete blood count, thyroid- or follicle-stimulating

Table 17.3 Differential diagnosis of premenstrual disorders[3]

Psychiatric
Major depressive disorder
Dysthymic disorder
Anxiety disorder
Panic disorder
Bipolar disorder
Borderline personality disorder
Other

Medical disorders
Anemia
Autoimmune disorders
Chronic fatigue syndrome
Connective tissue diseases
Fibromyalgia
Diabetes
Thyroid disease
Liver or renal disease
Seizure disorders
Anorexia or bulimia
Endometriosis or chronic pelvic pain
Dysmenorrhea

Premenstrual exacerbation of:
Psychiatric diagnoses
Chronic pelvic pain
Migraine or other headache
Allergies
Irritable bowel syndrome
Any medical disorder noted above

Psychosocial
Sexual or physical abuse
Past or current domestic violence
Relationship or socioeconomic problems

Other
Perimenopause/climacteric symptoms
Alcohol or other substance abuse
Hormone withdrawal or other symptoms associated with hormonal contraceptive use

hormones, chemistry levels, and breast or pelvic imaging studies, although no specific tests are mandatory.

At the initial visit, educational information is imparted concerning lifestyle changes and treatment strategies to decrease premenstrual symptoms and reduce stress, as well as how to keep a prospective chart of symptoms for a period of 2 months. Some type of severity rating must be a part of these charts, such as using a scale ranging from '0' for no symptoms to '4' for severe symptoms, for example, and noting those that interfere with functioning. Various validated diaries will be discussed below.

The woman should then evaluate the impact of various lifestyle approaches during the recording of her symptoms. In order to minimize the her disappointment with the prospect of leaving the office without specific therapy, the following points should be made:

1. The diagnosis usually requires prospective monitoring to rule out affective disorders that would require daily, not luteal, therapy with specific psychotropics, as opposed to hormonal agents.
2. Treatment options will be better tailored to her symptom type and timing and to her other gynecological needs, such as treatment of dysmenorrhea or contraception.
3. Lifestyle change, stress reduction, and daily charting may be effective treatment.
4. Treatment is usually necessary for most of the reproductive years and thus the approach using the lowest dose of a pharmacological agent specific for the natural symptom duration and severity, and providing the best side-effect profile is preferable.

The second visit consists primarily of reviewing the symptom diary, establishing a diagnosis of a premenstrual disorder and choosing the optimal treatment approach. Dividing a woman's symptom ratings into the premenstrual, menstrual, and postmenstrual phases will determine if a temporal relationship exists between symptoms and menses.

Daily Rating Forms

There is a lack of agreement on the practicality of daily prospective symptom rating due to the amount of time required and delay in therapeutic interventions while symptoms are recorded. Some consider that an interview by an appropriately trained psychiatrist could suffice to exclude an underlying psychiatric disorder and could replace daily symptom recording. However, this is not universally accepted (particularly for research) and is contrary to the guidance in DSM-IV. Daily symptom diaries can also be therapeutic, increasing patient involvement and adherence to management strategies and allowing for the individualization of treatment. When the woman is unable to provide prospective data, the spouse/partner can keep a calendar of premenstrual observations to establish the type, severity, and pattern of symptoms. One must recognize

the limitations of self-reported retrospective measures. Biases include sociocultural, environmental, and patient and family expectations. Patients may forget to fill out the calendar daily and use recall to complete the missed days. The use of an electronic, voice-activated device that allows the patient to record daily while blinding prior entries may assist in obtaining more accurate information.[12]

Some clinicians may prefer to use a visually graphic evaluative tool. A visual analog scale (VAS) requires the patient to rate specific symptoms on a line, 100 mm in length. The anchor lines at the left- and right-hand ends of the scale represent '0,' or no symptoms, and '100,' extreme symptoms. The VAS was recently revised to more nearly reflect the DSM-IV-TR criteria for PMDD; it includes the four core symptoms (irritability, tension, depressed mood, and mood lability) and seven symptom clusters (decreased interest in usual activities, difficulty concentrating, lack of energy, appetite change, change in sleep, feeling out of control, and somatic symptoms).[1] The days most appropriate for calculating the follicular and luteal score in a clinical setting are cycle days 7 through 11 for the follicular score and days 16 through 22 for the late luteal score.[13]

The Calendar of Premenstrual Experiences (COPE) is a daily diary that includes 22 symptoms commonly reported by women with PMS.[14] The symptoms are rated on a four-point scale, ranging from '0' for no symptoms to '3,' which indicates that the symptoms are severe and the woman is unable to perform normal activities. PMS is diagnosed when the total of the points for the luteal phase (i.e. the last 7 days of the cycle) is at least 30% greater than the sum of points for the follicular phase of the cycle (i.e. days 3 through 9 of the cycle).

The Daily Record of Severity of Problems (DRSP) is a daily diary that has been developed for use in the diagnosis of PMDD.[15] The 11 symptoms included in the DSM-IV-TR diagnostic criteria for PMDD are described in 21 separate items. In addition, the DRSP includes three symptom-related areas of functional impairment that are necessary for the diagnosis of PMDD. Women are also instructed to list the days of bleeding. Symptoms are rated on a scale ranging from 1 = not at all to 6 = extreme. The individual and summary scores in the DRSP have high reliability and tend to be sensitive to treatment differences.

Severe PMS and PMDD can be difficult to differentiate from the premenstrual exacerbation of a medical or psychiatric disorder. At present, a diagnosis of PMDD specifically requires the exclusion of any psychiatric disorder that might explain the symptoms.[5] In screening for psychiatric disorders, it is especially important to determine any past or current episodes of depressive, anxiety, or bipolar disorders, postpartum illness, eating disorders, substance abuse, or personality disorders. Women with PMDD commonly have past episodes, postpartum episodes, or a family history of depressive and/or anxiety disorders.[10] Several studies have reported that women with severe premenstrual symptoms have a greater possibility for psychopathology and other significant difficulties.[16–19]

PMDD and psychiatric disorders may also be coexisting conditions. There is a high comorbidity of PMS and PMDD with anxiety, depressive, and other psychiatric disorders,[17] although PMDD is a distinct diagnostic entity separate from other affective disorders. The patient may have a history of mood disorder with current PMDD or the patient may have no mood disorder outside of PMDD. Symptoms of major depressive disorder, anxiety disorder, or personality disorder will not demonstrate a cyclic pattern with a constant symptom-free interval prior to ovulation.

Therapeutic approaches

Non-pharmacological or over-the-counter medical approaches are recommended during the 2-month prospective rating period. There is level A and B evidence for each of several modalities, including exercise, dietary supplements, and psychological interventions. Even daily recording can be therapeutic for the patient and her family.

Initiation of or increase in exercise, particularly the aerobic variety, can reduce premenstrual mood and physical symptoms and has other obvious potential health advantages. At least 3 days per week, 20–30 minutes of aerobic exercise should be performed.[20,21]

Dietary changes or calcium supplementation can be initiated. Calcium carbonate, 1200 mg/day in divided doses, has also shown efficacy in at least one randomized controlled trial for PMS.[22] Furthermore, in 105 women meeting DSM-IV criteria for PMDD, there was a statistically significant negative relationship between milk consumption and the following premenstrual complaints: abdominal bloating, cramps, craving for some foods, and increased appetite.[23] Vitamin supplementation with pharmacological doses of vitamin B_6 can also be initiated if the patient is not already taking a vitamin supplement. Vitamin B_6 intake in excess of 100 mg/day is not recommended and can be neurotoxic.[24] A review of published and unpublished randomized placebo trials of the use of vitamin B_6 in PMS concluded that doses up to 100 mg/day are likely to be helpful in the treatment of premenstrual symptoms, including depression.[25] Limited data indicate a possible benefit of a complex and simple carbohydrate-containing beverage taken twice per day premenstrually, allowing

for greater absorption of L-tryptophan, the amino acid precursor of serotonin.[26,27] However, the availability of this product is limited and each serving contains at least 200 calories.

For women with premenstrual mastalgia, abdominal discomfort, and headache, non-steroidal anti-inflammatory medication is helpful, but limited data investigating small groups of women given mefenamic acid or naproxen sodium suggest the psychological symptoms of PMS may also improve.[28,29]

Cognitive behavioral therapy (CBT) can also be initiated during the initial treatment or daily recording months. At least three studies have demonstrated reduction in PMS symptom severity with CBT.[30–32] Additionally, CBT added to the SSRI fluoxetine demonstrated longer maintenance of treatment effects than fluoxetine alone, but combining CBT and fluoxetine did not confer added benefit in terms of degree of response or rate of response.[30] The disadvantage of CBT is cost, but some practitioners offer CBT groups which are more affordable than individual therapy, and the skills acquired in CBT can also represent an important investment in one's own psychological well-being, as the approach is non-pharmacological and is useful for general stress reduction and coping with future adverse life events.

PHARMACOLOGICAL MANAGEMENT

Combined oral contraceptives

Many reproductive women request contraception, and hormonal contraception is the most commonly used reversible method worldwide. Other potential non-contraceptive benefits of oral contraceptives (OCs) are significant and include cycle regulation, reduction development of anemia and functional ovarian cysts, control of acne, decreased dysmenorrhea and pelvic pain for those with early endometriosis, and risk reduction for ovarian and endometrial carcinoma. For those women who also desire hormonal contraception, there is now evidence that OCs can be beneficial for PMS and PMDD; however, progestin-only methods have not been reliably studied for this indication and currently cannot be recommended.

Historically, OCs were not uniformly beneficial for women with PMS, despite the elimination of ovulation, but the higher doses of sex steroids in most of the earlier generations of OCs may provoke more symptoms.[33] The 7 days off active pills can also allow for follicular development and a minicycle of exposure to and withdrawal from endogenous steroids and residual PMS-like symptoms in susceptible women.

A newer OC, containing 20 or 30 μg of ethinyl estradiol + 3 mg of the progestin drospirenone, has demonstrated efficacy in the treatment of PMS and PMDD in a number of recent studies.[34–38] The antiandrogenic and antimineralocorticoid effects of drospirenone, a spironolactone derivative, combined with the ovulation inhibition of an OC, may contribute to efficacy. The drospirenone-containing 20 μg formulation provides a 24-day active/4-day placebo pill cycle, ensuring more complete hormonal suppression.[34,39,40] Shortening the hormone-free interval from 7 to 4 or fewer days serves to maintain sufficient circulating levels of exogenous estrogen and progestin to inhibit follicular development and suppress ovarian steroid synthesis. In the randomized controlled trials, nausea, headache, and break-through bleeding are more prevalent in OC users than in those assigned to placebo.

Psychopharmacology

Selective serotonin and serotonin/norepinephrine reuptake inhibitors

For women with a formal diagnosis of severe PMS or PMDD, but who do not desire hormonal therapy, have residual symptoms on OCs, or have contraindications for OCs, SSRIs are the treatment of choice. Many placebo-controlled trials have demonstrated a 50–70% response rate at standard daily SSRI doses, with significant improvement compared to placebo with all currently available SSRIs, including fluoxetine,[41] sertraline,[42] paroxetine,[1] and citalopram,[43] and the SNRI venlafaxine.[44] The only three pharmacological agents currently receiving a US Food and Drug Administration (FDA) indication for PMDD are fluoxetine hydrochloride (Sarafem), sertraline hydrochloride (Zoloft), and paroxetine hydrochloride (Paxil CR).

Before initiating SSRIs, prospective recording of symptoms to ensure a symptom-free postmenstrual phase is crucial (if the treating physician is not a psychiatrist) for many reasons. First, PMS necessitates long-term treatment, potentially until menopause, since it does not appear to go into remission as do depressive disorders. A retrospective analysis of two previous clinical trials of fluoxetine in PMDD demonstrated that symptoms recur within the first cycle after discontinuation. Secondly, it is important to rule out an underlying affective disorder, in particular bipolar disorder, as SSRIs can trigger a manic episode if prescribed without a mood-stabilizing agent. Thirdly, luteal phase therapy is effective for PMDD but not for depression. Finally, there are parallels with the treatment of depression in pregnancy but this is a separate and specific consideration

and is individualized; reference to other texts is appropriate.[45] Once the diagnosis of PMDD is well established and non-pharmacological approaches have failed, any of the SSRIs can be tried.[46] Fluoxetine has a recommended dose of 10–20 mg/day; in clinical studies, significantly more side effects without increased efficacy were seen with 60 mg daily.[40] Sertraline is initiated at a dose of 25–50 mg/day and can be increased up to 150 mg/day for daily dosing; the average effective dose is 100 mg/day. Paroxetine CR is initiated at a dose of 12.5 mg/day and can be increased to 25 mg/day. Citalopram is dosed at 20 mg/day.

Unlike the treatment of affective disorders, in which a clinical response requires 3–6 weeks of exposure to an SSRI, the response in PMS/PMDD patients occurs within the first days of exposure. The shorter response interval (1–2 days) in premenstrual disorders is the basis of intermittent treatment with SSRIs during the luteal phase, which has also proven effective in many studies and is the preferred mode of SSRI administration for PMDD or severe PMS without comorbid affective or anxiety disorders.[43,47,48] In severe PMS/PMDD patients, a randomized controlled trial of continuous vs intermittent dosing with sertraline at 50–100 mg/day for three cycles showed significant improvement in mood and physical symptoms in both groups of treated patients during the first month of treatment.[49] Luteal phase dosing begins on about day 14 or just after presumed time of ovulation, and continues until the onset of menses. Fluoxetine 20 mg/day, sertraline 50–100 mg/day, paroxetine CR 12.5–25 mg/day, and citalopram 20 mg/day can be initiated in this fashion More recently, intermittent, weekly luteal phase dosing of enteric-coated fluoxetine in 90 mg doses (two doses) was shown to be efficacious and well-tolerated.[50] Symptom-onset dosing with a newer SSRI, escitalopram (Lexapro), has been compared to luteal phase dosing with the same drug in PMDD patients. Although both dosing strategies resulted in significantly improved daily symptom reporting scores, women with more severe PMDD were less likely to improve with symptom-onset dosing.[51] Aside from equal, if not improved, effectiveness and compliance in luteal phase dosing, another clear advantage is the lack of discontinuation symptoms with the intermittent dosing[52] and possibly fewer side effects such as weight gain and sexual dysfunction.

In addition to improvement in mood, other aspects of PMS and PMDD are often relieved by treatment with SSRIs. At the higher dosing interval, SSRIs reduce the most common physical symptoms, such as bloating and breast tenderness, associated with PMDD.[40] However, intermittent luteal phase dosing of sertraline failed to demonstrate significant improvement in physical symptoms, but did effectively reduce complaints of premenstrual cognitive disturbance, increased appetite, increased sleep, and lethargy.[48] Paroxetine CR resulted in significant improvement compared to placebo in mood symptoms at 12.5 mg daily dosing, but physical symptom reduction required 25 mg daily dosing.[53] Fluoxetine reduced symptoms that negatively impact work capacity within the first cycle of treatment.[54]

If initial exposure to one of the SSRIs proves problematic due to side effects or lack of efficacy, another SSRI should be utilized. Common side effects can be found in Table 17.4.[55,56] Switching to another SSRI involves discontinuing the first drug quickly while the newer drug is titrated to an effective dose. If withdrawal effects from the first medication result, its discontinuation should be done more gradually. In the case of luteal dosing, the new drug can be started with the next menstrual cycle.

SSRIs should be taken in the morning, unless sedation results, in which case the dose can be taken in the late afternoon, generally before 4 pm to prevent insomnia. Gastrointestinal side effects and headache are usually transient; weight gain can also occur.[57] All SSRIs can be associated with lowered libido and delayed orgasm or anorgasmia.[58] Besides lowering dose or duration of therapy, antidotes include dopaminergic agents, such as bupropion; adrenergic agents such as Ritalin (methylphenidate); buspirone; and phosphodiesterase inhibitors like sildenafil.[58]

When the possibility of becoming pregnant exists, certain SSRIs might be preferred to others. As the PMDD will disappear with pregnancy, therapy will not be required. If the woman has underlying depression and requires treatment, known risks of SSRI therapy[59] warrant individualized care.

Discontinuation symptoms should also be considered in the choice of continuous, non-luteal dosing of SSRI, as symptoms vary considerably depending upon the drug and dosing schedule. Paroxetine has the most

significant withdrawal effects and is therefore weaned slowly, tapering by half the dose every several days until discontinued completely. The taper can be lengthened if symptoms occur. Sertraline should also be weaned slowly. Because of its long half-life, fluoxetine at 20 mg daily can be stopped without a taper. Escitalopram and citalopram should be tapered, but this can be done fairly rapidly.

If a woman conceives while using an SSRI and continues treatment, there are risks[60] of neonatal syndrome at birth. Hence, treatment should be discontinued or a psychiatric opinion should be sought if it is thought that her condition is so severe that further psychotropic therapy is required.

Anxiolytics

Other classes of psychotropic medications with some efficacy for luteal phase dosing only include buspirone ($5HT_{1A}$ agonist), 10 mg 2–3 times per day, and alprazolam ($GABA_A$ agonist), 0.25–0.5 mg taken 2–3 times per day. Although these agents have shown only minimal or modest usefulness for PMS/PMDD compared to SSRIs, their intake results in fewer sexual side effects.[52,61] These agents or other anxiolytics can also be added (in the luteal phase only, in order to preclude development of tolerance and addiction) to SSRIs if anxiety persists while taking an SSRI.

Diuretics

Specific physical symptoms that are most troubling to the patient may need to be addressed separately. For example, in women with severe mastalgia and bloating, use of spironolactone, an aldosterone receptor antagonist, may be a helpful adjunct. A dose of 100 mg from day 12 of the cycle to the onset of menses relieved PMS symptoms in a placebo-controlled trial, and by cycle three, with significant improvement in abdominal bloating, swelling of extremities, breast discomfort, and even mood symptoms of irritability, depression, anxiety, and tension.[62–64]

Gonadotropin-releasing hormone agonists

The use of a GnRH agonist to suppress ovarian sex steroids provides symptomatic relief in the majority of women with PMS;[65–68] however, long-term studies are lacking. Bone density, and cardiovascular and vaginal health can theoretically be maintained and vasomotor symptoms prevented with a menopausal dose of continuous estrogen/progestin or tibilone as hormone add-back therapy.[69] A GnRH analogue, even with hormone add-back therapy, remains a third-line therapy if

Table 17.4 Common side effects of daily SSRIs with an FDA indication for PMDD[55]

Side effect	Fluoxetine	Sertraline	Paroxetine
Anxiety	+++	+	+
Sedation	+	++	++++
Insomnia	++++	++++	++++
Nausea	++++	++++	++++
Decreased libido	+	+	+
Weight gain	0/+	+	++

psychotropics have failed or if there is a concurrent gynecological indication for its use, such as severe cyclic pelvic pain or endometriosis or prior to contemplating oophorectomy for severe symptoms. GnRH analogues can also be employed to help determine if severe premenstrual symptoms in women with an underlying mood disorder are related to PMDD or the primary mood disorder. Side effects of GnRH analogues include myalgias, arthralgias, headaches, and residual vasomotor symptoms if the doses of add-back hormone therapy are insufficient.

Danazol

Danazol is another option for women who also have endometriosis, or just bothersome dysmenorrhea, but who do not require contraception, or for whom estrogen is contraindicated. Danazol, however, is an androgen analogue and side effects can include weight gain, acne, hirsutism, and decreased breast size.[70,71] Many women will ovulate with the daily 400 mg dose; therefore, contraception is imperative in sexually active patients, as danazol can virilize the developing fetus.

Progesterone

Progesterone was evaluated in a systematic review of 319 women[72] and found to produce minimal improvement in PMS symptoms over that of placebo significantly eased PMS symptoms to a greater degree than placebo, but other individual studies have not demonstrated superior efficacy of suppositories or oral micronized progesterone, and side effects include nausea, breast pain and uterine bleeding irregularities.

Estradiol

Transdermal estradiol (200 μg) has demonstrated efficacy in controlling PMS symptoms if the dose is high enough to inhibit ovulation;[73] however, the endometrium must be protected with progestin. In the aforementioned study, norethindrone 5 mg/day from days 19 to 26 was administered.[73] As progestins can recreate PMS symptoms, an intrauterine device containing a 'progestin' is preferable. Skin patches are associated with skin irritation in some women. If estradiol subcutaneous implants are used, similar efficacy can be achieved and, while this avoids the use of the patch, it will require a simple insertion of the implant under local anesthetic.

The restimulation of symptoms by the oral progestagen can be avoided by using an intrauterine device containing levonorgestrel (levonorgestrel-releasing intrauterine system; LNG IUS). This protects the endometrium while keeping blood levels (and therefore CNS levels) or progestogen low. Although there is evidence that estradiol is effective in treating PMS symptoms and the LNG IUS prevents or even reverses endometrial hyperplasia, there are no published data to confirm the efficacy of the combination. There is a great deal of anecdotal evidence from UK clinical practice.

Tibolone

Tibolone is a synthetic steroid with estrogenic, androgenic, and progestogenic properties, with many studies demonstrating efficacy for menopausal symptoms but with some evidence for 2.5 mg daily (one small randomized placebo-controlled cross-over trial of 18 ovulatory women) for the treatment of PMS.[74] Significantly improved scores, as documented by the VAS, were noted in the 2nd and 3rd month of a 3-month trial. Recommendations concerning this compound await further confirmatory trials, although it is particularly useful as add-back therapy during the use of GnRH therapy.

COMPLEMENTARY AND ALTERNATIVE THERAPIES

Several complementary and alternative medicine approaches have demonstrated some efficacy, but also mixed results, in premenstrual disorders, and studies were small and some not well-controlled.[75] These include bright light therapy, certain herbal and nutritional supplements, the use of exercise, and various mind–body approaches.[21,76,77] L-Tryptophan, a serotonin precursor, given at a dose of 6 g/day, was significantly more effective than placebo in the control of extreme mood swings, dysphoria, irritability, and tension in patients with PMDD.[78] Vitamin B$_6$ was mentioned previously.[25] Chaste tree extracts (*Vitex agnus-castus*) are widely used to treat premenstrual symptoms, particularly mastalgia, with few reported side effects.[79,80]

SURGICAL OPTIONS

Hysterectomy with bilateral salpingo-oophrectomy is effective for severe PMS/PMDD[81,82] and can be proposed for women in their 40s who have completed childbearing and have failed other therapies or who are planning a hysterectomy for other gynecological indications. Oophorectomy before age 60 years old is theoretically associated with increased cardiovascular mortality,[83] and estrogen replacement should be administered. Hysterectomy alone is not effective for relief of

PMS, and bilateral oophorectomy alone requires both progestin and estrogen replacement with the risk of re-stimulating.

CONCLUSION

Premenstrual syndrome and premenstrual dysphoric disorder are common and often disabling conditions affecting reproductive-aged women. A formal diagnosis should be sought whenever premenstrual symptoms are described. Underlying medical, psychiatric, and psychosocial conditions should be excluded, and the premenstrual timing and postmenstrual relief of the symptoms documented prospectively by nightly recording for at least two cycles. Once a definitive diagnosis is made, initiation of various treatment strategies can be effective in alleviating symptoms. Education, lifestyle change, cognitive behavioral therapy, calcium supplementation, certain hormonal oral contraceptive preparations, and the diuretic spironolactone can be effective. The administration of a serotonergic antidepressant is likely to alleviate symptoms and improve significantly the quality of life and functional status. Luteal phase dosing is the preferred method of treatment with SSRIs in many cases, as discontinuation symptoms and overall side effects are minimized. The use of GnRH analogues and estradiol patches and implants should be reserved for the most severe cases.

REFERENCES

1. Steiner M, Hirschberg AL, Bergeron R et al. Luteal phase dosing with paroxetine controlled release (CR) in the treatment of premenstrual dysphoric disorder. Am J Obstet Gynecol 2005; 193(2):352–6.
2. American College of Obstetricians and Gynecologists. ACOG Practice Bulletin: Premenstrual Syndrome. Washington, DC: ACOG. Compendium of Selected Publications 2000; 15:1–9.
3. Rapkin AJ, Mikacich JA, Moatakef-Imani B et al. The clinical nature and formal diagnosis of premenstrual, postpartum, and perimenopausal affective disorders. Curr Psychiatry Rep 2002; 4:419–28.
4. Dell DL. Diagnostic challenges in women with premenstrual symptoms. Prim Psychiatry 2004; 1:41–6.
5. American Psychiatric Association. Diagnostic and Statistical Manual of Mental Disorders, 4th edn., Washington, DC: American Psychiatric Press; 1994.
6. Connolly M. Premenstrual syndrome: an update on definitions, diagnosis and management. Adv Psychiatr Treatment 2001; 7:469–77.
7. Ling FW. Recognizing and treating premenstrual dysphoric disorder in the obstetric, gynecologic, and primary care practices. J Clin Psychiatry 2000; 61:9–16.
8. Critchlow DG, Bond AJ, Wingrove J. Mood disorder history and personality assessment in premenstrual dysphoric disorder. J Clin Psychiatry 2001; 62:688–93.
9. Halbreich U, Endicott J, Schacht S et al. The diversity of premenstrual changes as reflected in the Premenstrual Assessment Form. Acta Psychiatr Scand 1982; 65:46–65.
10. Kim DR, Gyulai L, Freeman EW et al. Premenstrual dysphoric disorder and psychiatric co-morbidity. Arch Womens Ment Health 2004; 7:37–47.
11. Sulak PJ, Scow RD, Preece C et al. Hormone withdrawal symptoms in oral contraceptive users. Obstet Gynecol 2000; 95:261–6.
12. Wyatt KM, Dimmock PW, Hayes-Gill B et al. Menstrual symptometrics: a simple computer-aided method to quantify menstrual cycle disorders. Fertil Steril 2002; 78(1):96–101.
13. Steiner M, Streiner DL. Validation of a revised visual analog scale for premenstrual mood symptoms: results from prospective and retrospective trials. Can J Psychiatry 2205; 50:327–32.
14. Mortola JF, Girton L, Beck L et al. Diagnosis of premenstrual syndrome by a simple, prospective, and reliable instrument: the calendar of premenstrual experiences. Obstet Gynecol 1990; 76:302–7.
15. Endicott J, Nee J, Harrison W. Daily record of severity of problems (DRSP): reliability and validity. Arch Womens Ment Health 2006; 9:41–9.
16. Freeman EW, Schweizer E, Rickels K. Personality factors in women with premenstrual syndrome. Psychosom Med 1995; 57:453–9.
17. Pearlstein TB, Frank E, Rivera-Tovar A et al. Prevalence of axis I and axis II disorders in women with late luteal phase dysphoric disorder. J Affect Disord 1990; 20:129–34.
18. Wilson CA, Turner CW, Keye WR Jr. Firstborn adolescent daughters and mothers with and without premenstrual syndrome: a comparison. J Adolesc Health 1991; 12(2):130–7.
19. Perkonigg A, Yonkers KA, Pfister H et al. Risk factors for premenstrual dysphoric disorder in a community sample of young women: the role of traumatic events and posttraumatic stress disorder. J Clin Psychiatry 2004; 65(10):1314–22.
20. Prior JC, Vigna Y, Sciarretta D et al. Conditioning exercise decreases premenstrual symptoms: a prospective, controlled 6-month trial. Fertil Steril 1987; 47(3):402–8.
21. Girman A, Lee R, Kligler B. An integrative medicine approach to premenstrual syndrome. Am J Obstet Gynecol 2003; 188(Suppl 5):S56–65.
22. Thys-Jacobs S, Starkey P, Bernstein D et al. Calcium carbonate and the premenstrual syndrome: effects on premenstrual and menstrual symptoms. Premenstrual Study Group. Am J Obstet Gynecol 1998; 179:444–52.
23. Derman O, Kanbur NO, Tokur TE et al. Premenstrual syndrome and associated symptoms in adolescent girls. J Obstet Gynecol Reprod Biol 2004; 116(2):201–6.
24. Parry GJ. Sensory neuropathy with low dose pyridoxine. Neurology 1985; 35:166–8.
25. Wyatt KM, Dimmock PW, Jones PW et al. Efficacy of vitamin B-6 in the treatment of premenstrual syndrome: systematic review. BMJ 1999; 318(7195):1375–81.
26. Sayegh R, Schiff I, Wurtman J et al. The effect of a carbohydrate-rich beverage on mood, appetite, and cognitive function in women with premenstrual syndrome. Obstet Gynecol 1995; 86(4 pt 1):520–8.
27. Freeman EW, Stout AL, Endicott J et al. Treatment of premenstrual syndrome with a carbohydrate-rich beverage. Int J Gynaecol Obstet 2002; 77:253–4.
28. Jakubowicz DL, Godard E, Dewhurst J. The treatment of premenstrual tension with mefenamic acid: analysis of prostaglandin concentrations. Br J Obstet Gynaecol 1984; 91:78–84.
29. Mira M, McNeil D, Fraser IS et al. Mefenamic acid in the treatment of premenstrual syndrome. Obstet Gynecol 1986; 68:395–8.
30. Hunter MS, Ussher JM, Cariss M et al. Medical (fluoxetine) and psychological (cognitive-behavioural therapy) treatment for

premenstrual dysphoric disorder: a study of treatment processes. J Psychosom Res 2002; 53(3):811–17.

31. Christensen AP, Oei TPS. The efficacy of cognitive behavior therapy in treating premenstrual dysphoric changes. J Affect Disord 1995; 33:57–63.

32. Blake F, Salkovskis P, Gath D et al. Cognitive therapy for premenstrual syndrome: a controlled trial. J Psychosom Res 1998; 45(4):307–18.

33. Kurshan N, Epperson CN. Oral contraceptives and mood in women with and without premenstrual dysphoria: a theoretical model. Arch Womens Ment Health 2006; 9:1–14.

34. Freeman EW, Kroll R, Rapkin A et al; PMS/PMDD Research Group. Evaluation of a unique oral contraceptive in the treatment of premenstrual dysphoric disorder. J Womens Health Gend Based 2001; 20:561–96.

35. Apter D, Borsos A, Baumgartner W et al. Effect of an oral contraceptive containing drospirenone and ethinylestradiol on general well-being and fluid-related symptoms. Eur J Contracept Reprod Health Care 2003; 8:37–51.

36. Foidart JM, Wuttke W, Bouw GM et al. A comparative investigation of contraceptive reliability, cycle control and tolerance of two monophasic oral contraceptives containing either drospirenone or desogestrel. Eur J Contracept Reprod Health Care 2000; 5:124–34.

37. Sangthawan M, Taneepanichskul S. A comparative study of monophasic oral contraceptives containing either drospirenone 3 mg or levonorgestrel 150 µg on premenstrual symptoms. Contraception 2005; 71:1–7.

38. Borenstein J, Yu HT, Wade S et al. The effect of an oral contraceptive containing ethinyl estradiol and drospirenone (Yasmin) on premenstrual symptomatology and health-related quality of life. J Reprod Med 2003; 48(2):79–85.

39. Yonkers KA, Brown C, Pearlstein TB et al. Efficacy of a new low-dose oral contraceptive with drospirenone in premenstrual dysphoric disorder. Obstet Gynecol 2005; 106(3):492–501.

40. Pearlstein TB, Bachmann GA, Zacur HA et al. Treatment of premenstrual dysphoric disorder with a new drospirenone-containing oral contraceptive formulation. Contraception 2005; 72:414–21.

41. Steiner M, Steinberg S, Stewart D et al. Fluoxetine in the treatment of premenstrual dysphoria. N Engl J Med 1995; 332: 1529–34.

42. Freeman EW, Rickels K, Arredondo F et al. Full or half-cycle treatment of severe premenstrual syndrome with a serotonergic antidepressant. J Clin Psychopharmacol 1999; 19:3–8.

43. Wikander I, Sundblad C, Andersch B et al. Citalopram in premenstrual dysphoria: is intermittent treatment during luteal phases more effective than continuous medication throughout the menstrual cycle? J Clin Psychopharmacol 1998; 18:390–8.

44. Freeman EW, Rickels K, Yonkers KA et al. Venlafaxine in the treatment of premenstrual dysphoric disorder. Obstet Gynecol 2001; 98:737–44.

45. Pearlstein TB, Stone AB, Lund SA et al. Comparison of fluoxetine, bupropion, and placebo in the treatment of premenstrual dysphoric disorder. J Clin Psychopharmacol 1997; 17:261–6.

46. Wyatt KM, Dimmock PW, O'Brien PMS. Selective serotonin reuptake inhibitors for premenstrual syndrome. Cochrane Database Syst Rev 2002; (4):CD001396.

47. Halbreich U, Smoller JW. Intermittent luteal phase sertraline treatment of dysphoric premenstrual syndrome. J Clin Psychiatry 1997; 58:399–402.

48. Halbreich U, Bergeron R, Yonkers KA et al. Efficacy of intermittent, luteal phase sertraline treatment of premenstrual dysphoric disorder. Obstet Gynecol 2002; 100(6):1219–29.

49. Freeman EW, Rickels K, Sondheimer SJ et al. Continuous or intermittent dosing with sertraline for patients with severe premenstrual syndrome or premenstrual dysphoric disorder. Am J Psychiatry 2004; 161(2):343–51.

50. Miner C, Brown E, McCray S et al. Weekly luteal-phase dosing with enteric-coated fluoxetine 90 mg in premenstrual dysphoric disorder: a randomized, double-blind, placebo-controlled clinical trial. Clin Ther 2002; 24(3):417–33.

51. Freeman EW, Sondheimer SJ, Sammel MD et al. A preliminary study of luteal phase versus symptom-onset dosing with escitalopram for premenstrual dysphoric disorder. J Clin Psychiatry 2005; 66:769–73.

52. Freeman EW. Luteal phase administration of agents for the treatment of premenstrual dysphoric disorder. CNS Drugs 2004; 18(7):453–68.

53. Cohen LS, Soares CN, Yonkers KA et al. Paroxetine controlled release for premenstrual dysphoric disorder: a double-blind, placebo-controlled trial. Psychosom Med 2004; 66(5):707–13.

54. Steiner M, Brown P, Trzepacz J et al. Fluoxetine improves functional work capacity in women with premenstrual dysphoric disorder. Arch Womens Ment Health 2003; 6(1):71–7.

55. Ferguson JM. The effects of antidepressants on sexual functioning in depressed patients: a review. J Clin Psychiatry 2001; 62(Suppl 3): 22–34.

56. Sundstrom-Poromaa I, Bixo M, Bjorn I et al. Compliance to antidepressant drug therapy for treatment of premenstrual syndrome. J Psychosom Obstet Gynaecol 2000; 21:205–11.

57. Hirschfeld RM. Long-term side effects of SSRIs: sexual dysfunction and weight gain. J Clin Psychiatry 2003; 64(Suppl 18):20–4.

58. Zajecka J. Strategies for the treatment of antidepressant-related sexual dysfunction. J Clin Psychiatry 2001; 62(Suppl 3):35–43.

59. Dillon AJ, for GlaxoSmithKline, Inc., endorsed by Health Canada, new safety information regarding paroxetine. Findings suggest increased risk over other antidepressants, of congenital malformations, following first trimester exposure to paroxetine. Available: www.hc-sc.gc.ca/dhp-mps/medeff/advisories-avis/prof/paxil_3_hpc-cps_e.html.

60. Moses-Kolko EL, Bogen D, Perel J et al. Neonatal signs after late in utero exposure to serotonin reuptake inhibitors. JAMA 2005; 293:2372–83.

61. Landen M, Eriksson O, Sundblad C et al. Compounds with affinity or serotonergic receptors in the treatment of premenstrual dysphoria: a comparison of buspirone, nefazodone and placebo. Psychopharmacologia 2001; 155:292–8.

62. Ginsburg KA, Dinsay R. Premenstrual syndrome. In: Ransom SB, ed. Practical Strategies in Obstetrics and Gynecology. Philadelphia: WB Saunders; 2000:684–94.

63. Vellacott ID, Shroff NE, Pearce MY et al. A double-blind, placebo-controlled evaluation of spironolactone in the premenstrual syndrome. Curr Med Res Opin 1987; 10:450–6.

64. Wang M, Hammarback S, Lindhe BA et al. Treatment of premenstrual syndrome by spironolactone: a double-blind, placebo-controlled study. Acta Obstet Gynecol Scand 1995; 74:803–8.

65. Muse KN, Cetel NS, Futterman LA et al. The premenstrual syndrome – effects of 'medical ovariectomy.' N Engl J Med 1984; 311:1345–9.

66. Mortola JF, Girton L, Fischer U. Successful treatment of severe premenstrual syndrome by combined use of gonadotropin-releasing hormone agonist and estrogen/progestin. J Clin Endocrinol Metab 1991; 71:252a–f.

67. Mezrow G, Shoupe D, Spicer D et al. Depot leuprolide acetate with estrogen and progestin add-back for long-term treatment of premenstrual syndrome. Fertil Steril 1994; 62:932–7.

68. Wyatt KM, Dimmock PW, Ismail KM, Jones PW, O'Brien PM. The effectiveness of GnRHa with and without 'add-back' therapy in treating premenstrual syndrome: a meta analysis. BJOG 2004; 111(6):585–93.

69. Studd J, Leather AT. The need for add-back with gonadotrophin-releasing hormone agonist therapy. Br J Obstet Gynaecol 1996; 103(Suppl 14):1–4.

70. Hahn PM, Van Vugt DA, Reid RL. A randomized, placebo-controlled, crossover trial of danazol for the treatment of premenstrual syndrome. Psychoneuroendocrinology 1995; 20:193–209.

71. Deeny M, Hawthorn R, McKay HD. Low dose danazol in the treatment of the premenstrual syndrome. Postgrad Med J 1991; 67:450–4.

72. Wyatt K, Dimmock P, Jones P et al. Efficacy of progesterone and progestogens in management of premenstrual syndrome: systematic review. BMJ 2001; 323:776–80.

73. Watson NR, Studd JW, Savvas M et al. Treatment of severe premenstrual syndrome with oestradiol patches and cyclical oral norethisterone. Lancet 1989; 2:730–2.

74. Taskin O, Gokdeniz R, Yalcinoglu A et al. Placebo-controlled cross-over study of effects of tibolone on premenstrual symptoms and peripheral beta-endorphin concentrations in premenstrual syndrome. Hum Reprod 1998; 13:2402–5.

75. Stevinson C, Ernst E. Complementary/alternative therapies for premenstrual syndrome: a systematic review of randomized controlled trials. Am J Obstet Gynecol 2001; 185:227–35.

76. Lam RW, Carter D, Misri S et al. A controlled study of light therapy in women with late luteal phase dysphoric disorder. Psychiatry Res 1999; 86(3):185–92.

77. Krasnik C, Montori VM, Guyatt GH et al.; Medically Unexplained Syndromes Study Group. The effect of bright light therapy on depression associated with premenstrual dysphoric disorder. Am J Obstet Gynecol 2005; 193:658–61.

78. Steinberg S, Annable L, Young SN et al. A placebo-controlled clinical trial of L-tryptophan in premenstrual dysphoria. Biol Psychiatry 1999; 45:313–20.

79. Wuttke W, Jarry H, Christoffel V et al. Chaste tree (Vitex agnus-castus) – pharmacology and clinical indications. Phytomedicine 2003; 10(4):348–57.

80. Schellenberg R. Treatment for the premenstrual syndrome with agnus castus fruit extract: prospective, randomised, placebo controlled study. BMJ 2001; 322(7279):134–7.

81. Casper RF, Hearn MT. The effect of hysterectomy and bilateral oophorectomy in women with severe premenstrual syndrome. Am J Obstet Gynecol 1990; 162:105–9.

82. Casson P, Hahn PM, Van Vugt DA et al. Lasting response to ovariectomy in severe intractable premenstrual syndrome. Am J Obstet Gynecol 1990; 162:99–105.

83. Parker WH, Broder MS, Liu Z et al. Ovarian conservation at the time of hysterectomy for benign disease. Obstet Gynecol 2005; 106(2):219–26.

18

Genetics of premenstrual dysphoric disorder

Julia L Magnay and Khaled MK Ismail

INTRODUCTION

Males and females differ in their predisposition to certain clinical disorders. One of the most widely documented findings in psychiatric epidemiology is that women have higher rates of major depressive episodes than men, a phenomenon observed worldwide using a variety of diagnostic schemes and interview methods.[1,2] The prevalence of depression among women in these studies was reported to be between 1.5 and 3 times that of men. Although a genetic predisposition to major depression has been extensively postulated, the actual mechanisms involved in this disorder are still being investigated. Several authors have reported similarities and associations between the symptoms of affective disorders such as anxiety, panic disorder, major depression, and seasonal affective disorder, and premenstrual syndrome/premenstrual dysphoric disorder (PMS/ PMDD).[3–8] It has also been noted that the incidence of anxiety, mood disorders, and depression among women suffering with PMS is greater than that of the general population.[9–11]

Evidence supporting the view that a genetically determined vulnerability plays a major role in the expression of PMS/PMDD is derived from twin and family studies,[12–15] that showed a high correlation between mothers and daughters and also between mono- and dizygotic twins. Additionally, a similarity of PMS subtypes was noted between mothers and daughters. Thus, genetic factors have been implicated repeatedly in the pathogenesis of PMS/PMDD, although no specific susceptibility gene has been identified.

PMDD AND BRAIN NEUROTRANSMITTERS

We have seen in earlier chaperts (Chapter 10) that the definitive cause of PMS is unknown but it appears to be directly related to the ovarian cycle trigger. The concept of a hormonal imbalance has been popular, but there is no supportive evidence. The hormone status of PMS patients does not appear to differ from that of asymptomatic women.[16–21]

Several lines of evidence suggest that an underlying dysregulation of serotonergic neurotransmission plays a pivotal role in PMDD.[22–32] Data from both animal and clinical studies indicate that (serotonin; 5-hydroxytryptamine, 5-HT) exerts an *inhibitory* effect on symptoms such as irritability, affect lability, and depression, which are core features of premenstrual dysphoria.[33,34] Ovarian steroids have been shown to profoundly influence the activity of the serotonergic system.[35–37] In the central nervous system (CNS), there is evidence of region-specific effects on serotonin synthesis, turnover, uptake, and release, and on specific receptors by estradiol and progesterone.[38,39] Falling levels of ovarian hormones (e.g. in the late-luteal phase of the menstrual cycle) have been associated with decreased serotonergic activity.[40]

Low serotonin levels in red blood cells and platelets[27–29,41] have been demonstrated in PMS patients compared with controls. This serotonin deficiency has been proposed to enhance CNS sensitivity to normal progesterone following ovulation.[42] Further credence to the potential involvement of serotonin in the pathogenesis of premenstrual dysphoria is provided by the effectiveness of selective serotonin reuptake inhibitors (SSRIs) such as fluoxetine and sertraline[43] in the treatment of severe PMS/PMDD. Vitamin B_6 (pyridoxine) is a cofactor in the final step in the synthesis of serotonin and dopamine from tryptophan. No data have yet demonstrated consistent abnormalities of either brain amine synthesis or deficiency of cofactors such as vitamin B_6 in PMDD.[44]

There is also increasing support for the hypothesis that ovarian hormones modulate γ-aminobutyric acid (GABA) neuronal function. GABA is the primary inhibitory neurotransmitter in the CNS. Disorders in

GABAergic neurotransmission have been linked to epilepsy, anxiety disorders, schizophrenia, and PMDD.[45,46] Plasma and cortical GABA levels of women with PMDD have been demonstrated to be lower during the late-luteal phase of the menstrual cycle, compared with the mid-follicular phase.[45–48] Data from animal studies suggest that the GABAergic system is substantially modulated by menstrual cycle phase.[49] This raises the possibility of disturbances in cortical GABA neuronal function and modulation by neuroactive steroids as potentially important contributors to the pathogenesis of PMDD.[50,51]

Moreover, progesterone is converted to neuroactive steroids (5α-pregnane steroids) in the brain. Progesterone metabolites (allopregnanolone and pregnanolone) appear to have anxiolytic and hypnotic properties via GABA type A (GABA-A) agonistic activity. Therefore, dysfunction in the GABA-A/neurosteroid system has been implicated in the pathogenesis of mood disorders and premenstrual syndrome.[42,52] Diminished levels of luteal phase β-endorphin have been shown in women with PMS/PMDD compared with asymptomatic controls.[53–55] Symptoms such as anxiety, food craving, and physical discomfort have been associated with a significant premenstrual decline in β-endorphin levels.[56–58] Other neurotransmitters may have relevance to PMDD, for example dopamine and acetylcholine, although the evidence for these is less convincing.

If the above suppositions are substantiated, it would seem that PMDD is not caused by an endocrine imbalance per se, but rather from an increased sensitivity to normal circulating level of ovarian hormones, particularly progesterone, secondary to a neuroendocrine disturbance.

THE SEROTONERGIC PATHWAY

As a result of the impressive therapeutic effects of SSRIs in up to 60–70% of women with PMS/PMDD, dysregulation of serotonin neurotransmission is a popular hypothesis in the pathogenesis of premenstrual dysphoria. Serotonin is a monoamine neurotransmitter stored at several sites in the body. The majority (95%) is located in the enterochromaffin cells of the intestinal mucosa. Smaller amounts occur in platelets and in the CNS, where the highest concentrations are found in the raphe nuclei of the brainstem. Serotonergic neurons project from the raphe nuclei to various brain regions, and play a vital role in modulating emotion, motor function, and cognition, as well as circadian and neuroendocrine functions such as appetite, sleep, and sexual activity. Serotonin is synthesized from the amino acid tryptophan, a reaction catalyzed by tryptophan

hydroxylase (TPH), and is stored in presynaptic vesicles until required. Upon neuronal firing, serotonin is released extracellularly and binds to postsynaptic receptor proteins, thereby transmitting a signal from one cell to the next (Figure 18.1). It also binds to presynaptic autoreceptors (5-HT_{1A} and 5-$HT_{1B/D}$), which regulate further serotonin release. Synaptic serotonin concentration is directly controlled by its rapid reuptake into the presynaptic terminal by a specific transporter protein (5-hydroxytryptamine transporter, 5-HTT). Serotonin uptake in platelets occurs by a similar active transport process.[59] Furthermore, the amino acid sequences of the two transporter proteins are identical and are encoded by the same gene.[60,61] Monoamine oxidase A (MAOA) catalyzes the catabolism of serotonin to 5-hydroxyindoleacetic acid (5-HIAA) and is pivotal in the regulation of intracellular serotonin levels (Figure 18.2).

PMDD and psychiatric disorders share several key symptoms, such as anxiety, depression, tension, and affective lability.[3,6–8] In light of this association, and the myriad of publications linking serotonergic polymorphisms to depressive disorders, the lack of reported genetic studies in PMDD is surprising. Below, we describe potential candidate gene polymorphisms suitable for study in PMDD, and include relevant evidence from numerous psychiatric studies.

GENETICS OF THE SEROTONERGIC SYSTEM IN PMDD

The concept of genetic polymorphisms

The fundamental basis of genetic polymorphism in a population is variation of the nucleotide sequence of DNA at homologous locations in the genome. These differences in sequence can result from mutations involving a single nucleotide or from deletions or insertions of variable numbers of contiguous nucleotides. At many loci within the human genome, two or more alleles may occur with significant frequency in the same population. These loci are said to be polymorphic. Their existence allows for multiple combinations of alleles at different loci, and is responsible for both the incredible diversity in populations and the uniqueness of individuals. However, this very diversity is also thought to account for genetic susceptibility to many diseases. Thus, the study of polymorphisms in key candidate genes is a potentially powerful tool in the investigation of complex polygenic diseases, in which multiple genes (each of which may have a relatively minor effect) and environmental factors collaborate to cause disease. Applying this concept to PMDD, polymorphisms of genes controlling

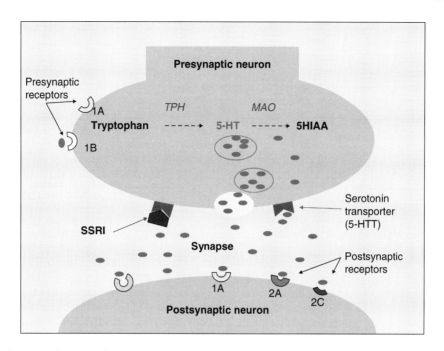

Figure 18.1 Schematic diagram of 5-HT metabolism.

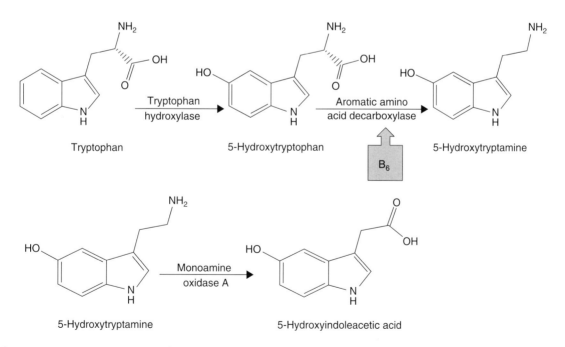

Figure 18.2 Serotonin (5-HT) synthesis and catabolism.

the serotonin or other neurotransmitter pathways may influence susceptibility, with cyclical ovarian hormone fluctuations providing the environmental trigger.

Allelic variants can occur anywhere in the genome: some are found within exons, which are the coding regions of genes, whereas others are located in introns, promoter regions, or sites that are not closely linked to any known expressed gene.[62]

Types of genetic polymorphisms

Single-nucleotide polymorphisms (SNPs) are allelic variants that have been generated as the result of conversion of one nucleotide to another at a homologous position. When present within a coding region (exon) of a gene, the expressed product may or may not have a single amino acid difference, depending on the resulting codon change. In some cases, the resulting codon stops the transcription process and results in the production of a truncated peptide. SNPs that are located in regulatory regions of an expressed gene can alter the transcription efficiency of that gene but not the protein sequence.[62] Some polymorphisms coincide with the target nucleotide sequences recognized by restriction enzymes. Polymorphisms that occur at restriction enzyme sites are known as restriction fragment length polymorphisms (RFLPs). RFLPs are extremely useful because they can be used to identify genetic markers.[63] Deletion or insertion mutants have also been found in functional genes. The consequence of a deletion depends on its precise location: whether it produces a mutation that results in an alteration in the reading frame of the gene and the function of the expressed product.

Other types of allelic variance in association with a particular gene are repetitive sequence elements which are arranged in tandem. Depending on the repeat unit length and the degree of repetition per locus, these repetitive sequence elements are known as satellite, minisatellite and microsatellite. Polymorphisms created by such elements are termed variable number of tandem repeats (VNTR) polymorphisms.[63]

Below, we describe potential candidate gene polymorphisms suitable for study in PMDD, and include relevant evidence from numerous psychiatric studies.

Candidate genes in the serotonergic pathway

Tryptophan hydroxylase

TPH catalyzes the rate-limiting step in serotonin synthesis, and is one of the most important regulators of the serotonergic system. In humans, two different TPH genes exist, which encode two enzymes (TPH1 and TPH2), with an overall sequence homology of 71%.[64] TPH1 is expressed in peripheral tissues and in the pineal body, whereas TPH2 appears to be responsible for serotonin synthesis in the rest of the brain. Since the existence of TPH2 is a relatively recent discovery (2003), most studies conducted to date have focused on TPH1 markers. Numerous TPH1 sequence variants have been reported.[65] Of these, the most commonly studied are the two promoter polymorphisms G-6526A and G-5806T, and the two markers A218C and A779C in intron 7. It has been suggested that sequence variations within the promoter region may modify TPH1 expression and affect serotonin synthesis, and this has been supported by successive deletion analysis of the promoter region, which led to a decrease in promoter activity.[66] The A218C marker has been studied extensively in psychiatric disorders.[67] The exact mechanism linking the A218C polymorphism to reduced expression of the gene product remains unknown; however, the functional relevance of this polymorphism has been demonstrated for a series of clinical syndromes (e.g. bipolar disorder, suicide attempts, and suicidal behavior).[68–74] The A allele has been associated with decreased serotonin synthesis[75] and slower response to SSRIs[76,77] in subjects with major depressive disorders. Numerous studies have attempted to link TPH1 polymorphisms with a variety of mood disorders, but have given conflicting data.[78–81] In a recent study, we found no significant associations between PMDD and the G-6526A, G-5806T, or the A218C polymorphisms of the TPH1 gene.[82] Until recently, TPH1 was believed to be the sole rate-limiting enzyme for neuronal serotonin synthesis, which occurs in the raphe nuclei of the brainstem. This lack of association is not surprising in the light of the discovery of a second tryptophan hydroxylase (TPH2) isoform,[64] which is expressed predominantly in the brainstem but not in peripheral tissues.[83,84] Initial reports of TPH2 polymorphisms indicate an association between several SNPs and major depression.[85–87] Thus, TPH2 may be a strong candidate gene for future study in PMDD.

The serotonin transporter

The serotonin transporter (5-HTT) protein is the primary mechanism for removing serotonin from the synaptic cleft. Three common 5-HTT polymorphisms have been studied in psychiatric disorders: 5-HTT LPR, VNTR-2, and 3′UTR G/T. The 5-HTT LPR is a 44 nucleotide insertion/deletion in the promoter region giving rise to long (L) or short (S) alleles.[88] This polymorphism has been evaluated in several studies. Infants with the short homozygous (S/S) 5-HTT LPR genotype had higher scores on negative emotionality and distress than infants with the L/S or L/L genotypes.[89] The 5-HTT LPR was also strongly associated with childhood aggression.[90] Homozygosity for the short variant of the 5-HTT LPR polymorphism was shown to be significantly more frequent in bipolar patients than in controls.[73] Courtet and associates[74] reported a significant association between the 5-HTT LPR S/S genotype and further suicide attempts among patients who had previously attempted suicide. The S allele was also more likely to have higher symptom counts for aggressivity, attention deficit, and conduct disorders in males. However, among females, the short variant (S/S, L/S) was associated with lower levels of such behavior.[91] The S variant has been shown in vitro to be less transcriptionally active than the L allele, resulting in decreased 5-HTT expression and uptake,[92] and a poorer response to SSRI therapy in Caucasian subjects with mood disorders.[93,94]

The 5-HTT VNTR-2 polymorphism comprises 9, 10, or 12 copies of a 17 base pair repeat element in intron 2.[95] This polymorphism has been suggested to regulate transcriptional activity of the 5-HTT gene, and the 12-repeat allele has been associated with increased 5-HTT expression, compared with the 9- and 10-repeat variants.[95,96] Using an ethnically homogeneous sample of highly aggressive Caucasian children and their matched controls, Beitchman and colleagues[97] reported an association of this polymorphism with aggression. It has also been suggested that 5-HTT VNTR-2 influences age of onset in patients with bipolar affective disorder.[72] Moreover, a recent meta-analysis of 12 population-based association studies consisting of 2177 cases and 2369 control subjects showed a highly significant association between the 5-HTT VNTR-2 polymorphism and schizophrenia.[98] The 3'UTR G/T is an SNP located in a putative polyadenylation site of the 3'untranslated region of the 5-HTT gene.[99] This polymorphism has been linked with bipolar and attention deficit hyperactivity disorders.[100,101]

To date, studies of these three 5-HTT polymorphisms in PMDD have found no significant differences in genotype distribution between healthy controls and PMDD subjects in any of the markers.[102,103]

Monoamine oxidase A

MAOA is a mitochondrial enzyme that catalyzes the oxidative deamination of neurotransmitters such as dopamine, norepinephrine, and serotonin. Increased MAOA activity might feasibly be expected to contribute to the pathogenesis of conditions associated with reduced serotonergic neurotransmission, such as PMDD. Several different polymorphisms in the MAOA gene have been identified: of these, the VNTR-1 and the *Fnu 4H1*

RFLP are of particular interest. Transcriptional activity of the human MAOA gene is modulated by the VNTR-1 polymorphism. Based on functional characterization, alleles with 3.5 or 4 copies of the repeat sequence are transcribed 2–10 times more efficiently than those with 3 or 5 copies of the repeat.[104,105] The presence of an *Fnu 4H1* restriction site in exon 8 (the G allele) has been associated with a high MAOA activity in healthy individuals.[106] MAOA gene polymorphisms have been linked to the pathogenesis of major depression, associated with insomnia in depressed individuals, attention deficit hyperactivity disorder, alcoholism and binge drinking.[106–109]

Our collaborative group has recently studied the association between the VNTR-1 and *Fnu 4H1* polymorphisms and PMDD.[103] We found no significant distribution pattern associated with the high-activity alleles 3.5 and 4, or the lower-activity alleles 4 and 5 in the VNTR-1 in our cases and controls. Although the G/T genotype in the *Fnu 4H1* RFLP was more common in the PMDD group than in the controls, this difference was not statistically significant, and the overall frequency of the G and T alleles was similar in both cohorts.[103]

Serotonin receptors

Over the past decade, more than 14 different serotonin receptors have been cloned through molecular biological techniques. There are seven classes of serotonin receptors. Some of these are divided into several subclasses based on structural and operational characteristics (e.g. $5HT_{1A}$, $5HT_{1B}$, $5HT_{1D}$, $5HT_{1E}$, $5HT_{1F}$, $5HT_{2A}$, $5HT_{2B}$, and $5HT_{2C}$).

The proposed mechanisms by which gonadal hormones influence neurotransmitters, in general, and serotonin, in particular, are not only achieved by affecting their rate of production and catabolism but also by modulating their individual receptor's function and responsivity. For example, it has been shown that estrogen increases serotonin (5-HT) postsynaptic responsivity, up-regulates 5-HT_1 receptors, and down-regulates 5-HT_2 receptors.[110,111] Research investigating vulnerability to anxiety and irritability indicated that agonists of 5-HT_{1A} receptor and antagonists of the activating 5-HT_2 receptor decrease anxiety.[112–114] Moreover, the 5-HT_{1A} receptor is expressed as a postsynaptic receptor, in addition to being the major presynaptic autoreceptor on serotonergic raphe neurons.[114] The electrophysiological activity of serotonergic neurons is regulated, at least in part, through a negative feedback mechanism triggered by the stimulation of presynaptic 5-HT_{1A} autoreceptors. This receptor activity has also been linked to responsiveness to SSRI therapy in some psychiatric disorders. An initial delayed response to SSRIs is thought to be secondary to activation of the $5-HT_{1A}$ autoreceptors, as a result of the immediate increase in extracellular serotonin at the somatodendritic level following treatment initiation.[114] Therefore, the associations between serotonergic receptor gene polymorphisms, PMDD, and response to SSRIs therapy are undoubtedly interesting areas for future research.

CONSIDERATIONS FOR GENETIC STUDIES IN PMDD

If genetic studies of PMDD are to be conducted, it is absolutely vital that participants are diagnosed correctly so that the description of the phenotype is precise. The importance of clinical categorization using strict inclusion and exclusion criteria cannot be overemphasized. Before completing any prospective rating, it is essential to ensure that potential participants are not taking any hormonal contraceptives or replacement therapy both during the monitored cycles and for a minimum of 2 months previously. Women should be excluded if they are pregnant, planning a pregnancy, have an existing or past history of psychiatric disorder, or are taking psychotropic medications. Diagnosis of PMDD can present significant challenges, owing to the subjective nature of symptom interpretation and reporting. Medical researchers and clinicians offer conflicting opinions about whether PMDD and its milder variant, PMS, are synonymous or separate diagnoses[115] (see Chapter 2).

Gonadal hormonal influences on the brain processes involved in regulation of mood, behavior, and cognitive functions are complex and are not limited to the serotonergic system, but also involve other major neurotransmitter pathways such as the noradrenergic, dopaminergic, acetyl cholinergic, and GABAergic systems. There is increasing support for the hypothesis that gonadal steroids involved in the regulation of the human menstrual cycle modulate GABA neuronal function. Moreover, several polymorphisms in genes controlling the GABAergic system have been linked to mental health and substance misuse problems.[116–120] Hence, genes regulating the GABAergic system are potentially strong candidates to be investigated for any association with PMDD.

The polygenic approach

At present, there are a significant number of genetic markers that can be used in genetic association studies of PMDD. Although each polymorphism can be studied in isolation, it is much more informative to analyze a panel of putative markers in a region of interest. The combination of marker alleles on a single chromosome is called a haplotype. For haplotypes which include markers tightly linked with each other (such as those within the same gene), alleles often display statistical dependence, a phenomenon called linkage dysequilibrium (LD), or allelic association. One major aspect of haplotype analysis is to identify LD patterns in different regions and different populations, since the very existence of LD among markers makes it possible to localize genetic variants underlying complex traits.[46] When multiple markers associated with a specific chromosomal region are studied to assess the association between this region and traits of interest, a statistical analysis based on haplotypes may be more meaningful than separate analyses of each individual marker. This has been demonstrated by both simulation and empirical studies.[46]

CONCLUSION

Individual hypersensitivity to physiological hormonal fluctuations that occur during periods of hormonal change such as the menstrual cycle, postpartum, and the perimenopause contributes to the vulnerability to PMS, PMDD, postpartum, and perimenopausal behavioral disorders. Family and twin studies have shown that this hypersensitivity has a genetically determined component. However, the assumption that PMS/PMDD results from an isolated neurotransmitter disorder is probably too simplistic, and an imbalance or disturbed feedback mechanisms between several transmitter systems or disturbed feedback between several components and stages within the same system is a more plausible hypothesis.

GLOSSARY OF TERMS

(Adapted from the National Human Genome Research Institute: www.genome.gov)

Allele: one of the variant forms of a gene at a particular locus.

Exon: a nucleotide sequence in DNA that carries the code for the final messenger RNA molecule and thus defines a protein's amino acid sequence.

Gene: the functional and physical unit of heredity passed from parent to offspring.

Genotype: the genetic identity of an individual that does not show as outward characteristics.

Intron: a non-coding region of DNA that is originally copied into RNA but is cut out of the final RNA transcript.

Derby Hospitals NHS Foundation Trust

Library and Knowledge Service

Linkage: the association of genes and/or markers that lie near each other on a chromosome. Linked genes and markers tend to be inherited together.

Locus: the place on a chromosome where a specific gene is located (plural: loci).

Nucleotide: one of the structural components of DNA and RNA, consisting of a base (guanine, thymine, adenine, or cytosine) plus a molecule of sugar and a molecule of phosphoric acid.

PCR (polymerase chain reaction): a fast, inexpensive technique for making an unlimited number of copies of any piece of DNA.

Phenotype: the observable traits or characteristics of an organism, such as hair color, weight, or presence or absence of disease.

Polymorphism: a common variant in the sequence of DNA among individuals.

Promoter: the part of a gene that contains the information to turn the gene on or off. The process of transcription is initiated at the promoter.

RFLP (restriction fragment length polymorphisms): genetic variations at a site where a restriction enzyme cuts a piece of DNA. Such variations affect the size of the resulting fragments.

SNP (single nucleotide polymorphism): common, single nucleotide variations that occur in human DNA at a frequency of one every 1000 bases.

Transcription: the process through which a DNA sequence is copied to produce a complementary RNA; i.e. the transfer of information from DNA to RNA.

VNTR: short repeated segments of identical DNA at a particular locus in the human genome. This number of repeated units varies between individuals.

REFERENCES

1. Weissman MM, Klerman GL. Depression: current understanding and changing trends. Annu Rev Public Health 1992; 13:319–39.
2. Weissman MM, Bland RC, Canino GJ et al. Cross-national epidemiology of major depression and bipolar disorder. JAMA 1996; 276(4):293–9.
3. De Ronchi D, Muro A, Marziani A, Rucci P. Personality disorders and depressive symptoms in late luteal phase dysphoric disorder. Psychother Psychosom 2000; 69(1):27–34.
4. De Ronchi D, Ujkaj M, Boaron F et al. Symptoms of depression in late luteal phase dysphoric disorder: a variant of mood disorder? J Affect Disord 2005; 86(2–3):169–74.
5. Harlow BL, Cohen LS, Otto MW, Spiegelman D, Cramer DW. Early life menstrual characteristics and pregnancy experiences among women with and without major depression: the Harvard study of moods and cycles. J Affect Disord 2004; 79(1–3):167–76.
6. Harlow BL, Cohen LS, Otto MW, Spiegelman D, Cramer DW. Prevalence and predictors of depressive symptoms in older premenopausal women: the Harvard Study of Moods and Cycles. Arch Gen Psychiatry 1999; 56(5):418–24.
7. Maskall DD, Lam RW, Misri S et al. Seasonality of symptoms in women with late luteal phase dysphoric disorder. Am J Psychiatry 1997; 154(10):1436–41.
8. Hendrick V, Altshuler LL. Recurrent mood shifts of premenstrual dysphoric disorder can be mistaken for rapid-cycling bipolar II disorder. J Clin Psychiatry 1998; 59(9):479–80.
9. Barnhart KT, Freeman EW, Sondheimer SJ. A clinician's guide to the premenstrual syndrome. Med Clin North Am 1995; 79(6):1457–72.
10. Halbreich U, Endicott J. Relationship of dysphoric premenstrual changes to depressive disorders. Acta Psychiatr Scand 1985; 71(4):331–8.
11. Roca CA, Schmidt PJ, Rubinow DR. A follow-up study of premenstrual syndrome. J Clin Psychiatry 1999; 60(11):763–6.
12. Dalton K, Dalton ME, Guthrie K. Incidence of the premenstrual syndrome in twins. Br Med J (Clin Res Ed) 1987; 295(6605):1027–8.
13. Condon JT. The premenstrual syndrome: a twin study. Br J Psychiatry 1993; 162:481–6.
14. Kendler KS, Karkowski LM, Corey LA, Neale MC. Longitudinal population-based twin study of retrospectively reported premenstrual symptoms and lifetime major depression. Am J Psychiatry 1998; 155(9):1234–40.
15. Widholm O, Kantero RL. A statistical analysis of the menstrual patterns of 8,000 Finnish girls and their mothers. Acta Obstet Gynecol Scand Suppl 1971; 14(Suppl 14):1–36.
16. Dennerstein L, Brown JB, Gotts G et al. Menstrual cycle hormonal profiles of women with and without premenstrual syndrome. J Psychosom Obstet Gynaecol 1993; 14(4):259–68.
17. Cerin A, Collins A, Landgren BM, Eneroth P. Hormonal and biochemical profiles of premenstrual syndrome. Treatment with essential fatty acids. Acta Obstet Gynecol Scand 1993; 72(5):337–43.
18. Bloch M, Schmidt PJ, Su TP, Tobin MB, Rubinow DR. Pituitary–adrenal hormones and testosterone across the menstrual cycle in women with premenstrual syndrome and controls. Biol Psychiatry 1998; 43(12):897–903.
19. O'Brien PM, Selby C, Symonds EM. Progesterone, fluid, and electrolytes in premenstrual syndrome. Br Med J 1980; 280(6224):1161–3.
20. Hammarback S, Damber JE, Backstrom T. Relationship between symptom severity and hormone changes in women with premenstrual syndrome. J Clin Endocrinol Metab 1989; 68(1):125–30.
21. van Leusden HA. Premenstrual syndrome no progesterone; premenstrual dysphoric disorder no serotonin deficiency. Lancet 1995; 346(8988):1443–4.
22. Ashby CR Jr, Carr LA, Cook CL, Steptoe MM, Franks DD. Inhibition of serotonin uptake in rat brain synaptosomes by plasma from patients with premenstrual syndrome. Biol Psychiatry 1992; 31(11):1169–71.
23. Ashby CR Jr, Carr LA, Cook C, Steptoe MM, Franks DD. Effect of plasma from premenstrual syndrome and control patients on human platelet and rat brain synaptosome monoamine oxidase B activity. Neuropsychobiology 1992; 25(3):121–5.
24. Ashby CR Jr, Carr LA, Cook CL, Steptoe MM, Franks DD. Alteration of 5-HT uptake by plasma fractions in the premenstrual syndrome. J Neural Transm Gen Sect 1990; 79(1–2):41–50.
25. Ashby CR Jr, Carr LA, Cook CL, Steptoe MM, Franks DD. Alteration of platelet serotonergic mechanisms and monoamine oxidase activity in premenstrual syndrome. Biol Psychiatry 1988; 24(2):225–33.
26. Halbreich U, Tworek H. Altered serotonergic activity in women with dysphoric premenstrual syndromes. Int J Psychiatry Med 1993; 23(1):1–27.
27. Rapkin AJ. The role of serotonin in premenstrual syndrome. Clin Obstet Gynecol 1992; 35(3):629–36.

28. Rapkin AJ, Edelmuth E, Chang LC et al. Whole-blood serotonin in premenstrual syndrome. Obstet Gynecol 1987; 70(4):533–7.

29. Rapkin AJ, Buckman TD, Sutphin MS, Chang LC, Reading AE. Platelet monoamine oxidase B activity in women with premenstrual syndrome. Am J Obstet Gynecol 1988; 159(6):1536–40.

30. Rojansky N, Halbreich U, Zander K, Barkai A, Goldstein S. Imipramine receptor binding and serotonin uptake in platelets of women with premenstrual changes. Gynecol Obstet Invest 1991; 31(3):146–52.

31. Parry BL. The role of central serotonergic dysfunction in the aetiology of premenstrual dysphoric disorder: therapeutic implications. CNS Drugs 2001; 15(4):277–85.

32. Eriksson O, Wall A, Marteinsdottir I et al. Mood changes correlate to changes in brain serotonin precursor trapping in women with premenstrual dysphoria. Psychiatry Res 2006; 146(2):107–16.

33. Ho HP, Olsson M, Westberg L, Melke J, Eriksson E. The serotonin reuptake inhibitor fluoxetine reduces sex steroid-related aggression in female rats: an animal model of premenstrual irritability? Neuropsychopharmacology 2001; 24(5):502–10.

34. Eriksson E, Humble M. Serotonin in psychiatric pathophysiology. A review of data from experimental and clinical research. In: Gershon S, Pohl R, eds. Progress in Basic Clinical Pharmacology. Basel: Karger; 1990:66–119.

35. Rubinow DR, Schmidt PJ, Roca CA. Estrogen–serotonin interactions: implications for affective regulation. Biol Psychiatry 1998; 44(9):839–50.

36. Joffe H, Cohen LS. Estrogen, serotonin, and mood disturbance: where is the therapeutic bridge? Biol Psychiatry 1998; 44(9): 798–811.

37. Eriksson E, Alling C, Andersch B, Andersson K, Berggren U. Cerebrospinal fluid levels of monoamine metabolites. A preliminary study of their relation to menstrual cycle phase, sex steroids, and pituitary hormones in healthy women and in women with premenstrual syndrome. Neuropsychopharmacology 1994; 11(3):201–13.

38. Leibenluft E, Fiero PL, Rubinow DR. Effects of the menstrual cycle on dependent variables in mood disorder research. Arch Gen Psychiatry 1994; 51(10):761–81.

39. Bethea CL, Pecins-Thompson M, Schutzer WE, Gundlah C, Lu ZN. Ovarian steroids and serotonin neural function. Mol Neurobiol 1998; 18(2):87–123.

40. FitzGerald M, Malone KM, Li S et al. Blunted serotonin response to fenfluramine challenge in premenstrual dysphoric disorder. Am J Psychiatry 1997; 154(4):556–8.

41. Rapkin AJ, Reading AE, Woo S, Goldman LM. Tryptophan and neutral amino acids in premenstrual syndrome. Am J Obstet Gynecol 1991; 165(6 Pt 1):1830–3.

42. Rapkin AJ, Morgan M, Goldman L et al. Progesterone metabolite allopregnanolone in women with premenstrual syndrome. Obstet Gynecol 1997; 90(5):709–14.

43. Dimmock PW, Wyatt KM, Jones PW, O'Brien PM. Efficacy of selective serotonin-reuptake inhibitors in premenstrual syndrome: a systematic review. Lancet 2000; 356(9236):1131–6.

44. van den Berg H, Louwerse ES, Bruinse HW, Thissen JT, Schrijver J. Vitamin B$_6$ status of women suffering from premenstrual syndrome. Hum Nutr Clin Nutr 1986; 40(6):441–50.

45. Stromberg J, Haage D, Taube M, Backstrom T, Lundgren P. Neurosteroid modulation of allopregnanolone and GABA effect on the GABA-A receptor. Neuroscience 2006; 143(1):78–81.

46. Wong CG, Bottiglieri T, Snead OC 3rd. GABA, gamma-hydroxybutyric acid, and neurological disease. Ann Neurol 2003; 54(Suppl 6):S3–12.

47. Epperson CN, Haga K, Mason GF et al. Cortical gamma-aminobutyric acid levels across the menstrual cycle in healthy women and those with premenstrual dysphoric disorder: a proton magnetic resonance spectroscopy study. Arch Gen Psychiatry 2002; 59(9):851–8.

48. Halbreich U, Petty F, Yonkers K et al. Low plasma gamma-aminobutyric acid levels during the late luteal phase of women with premenstrual dysphoric disorder. Am J Psychiatry 1996; 153(5):718–20.

49. Gulinello M, Gong QH, Smith SS. Progesterone withdrawal increases the anxiolytic actions of gaboxadol: role of alpha4betadelta GABA(A) receptors. Neuroreport 2003; 14(1): 43–6.

50. Lovick TA. Plasticity of GABAA receptor subunit expression during the oestrous cycle of the rat: implications for premenstrual syndrome in women. Exp Physiol 2006; 91(4):655–60.

51. Maguire JL, Stell BM, Rafizadeh M, Mody I. Ovarian cycle-linked changes in GABA(A) receptors mediating tonic inhibition alter seizure susceptibility and anxiety. Nat Neurosci 2005; 8(6):797–804.

52. Romeo E, Strohle A, Spalletta G et al. Effects of antidepressant treatment on neuroactive steroids in major depression. Am J Psychiatry 1998; 155(7):910–13.

53. Rapkin AJ, Shoupe D, Reading A et al. Decreased central opioid activity in premenstrual syndrome: luteinizing hormone response to naloxone. J Soc Gynecol Investig 1996; 3(2):93–8.

54. Chuong CJ, Coulam CB, Kao PC, Bergstralh EJ, Go VL. Neuropeptide levels in premenstrual syndrome. Fertil Steril 1985; 44(6):760–5.

55. Chuong CJ, Hsi BP, Gibbons WE. Periovulatory beta-endorphin levels in premenstrual syndrome. Obstet Gynecol 1994; 83(5 Pt 1):755–60.

56. Giannini AJ, Melemis SM, Martin DM, Folts DJ. Symptoms of premenstrual syndrome as a function of beta-endorphin: two subtypes. Prog Neuropsychopharmacol Biol Psychiatry 1994; 18(2):321–7.

57. Giannini AJ, Martin DM, Turner CE. Beta-endorphin decline in late luteal phase dysphoric disorder. Int J Psychiatry Med 1990; 20(3):279–84.

58. Giannini AJ, Price WA, Loiselle RH. Beta-endorphin withdrawal: a possible cause of premenstrual tension syndrome. Int J Psychophysiol 1984; 1(4):341–3.

59. Marcusson JO, Ross SB. Binding of some antidepressants to the 5-hydroxytryptamine transporter in brain and platelets. Psychopharmacology (Berl) 1990; 102(2):145–55.

60. Lesch KP, Wolozin BL, Murphy DL, Riederer P. Primary structure of the human platelet serotonin uptake site: identity with the brain serotonin transporter. J Neurochem 1993; 60(6): 2319–22.

61. Lesch KP, Wolozin BL, Estler HC, Murphy DL, Riederer P. Isolation of a cDNA encoding the human brain serotonin transporter. J Neural Transm Gen Sect 1993; 91(1):67–72.

62. Milford EL, Carpenter CB. Immunogenetics of Disease: Genetic Polymorphism. Dale DC, Federman DD, eds. http://www.medscape.com/viewarticle/534976 6. 2000. WebMD Inc.

63. Winter PC, Hickey GI, Fletcher HL. Instant Notes in Genetics. 2nd edn. Oxford: BIOS Scientific Publishers; 2000.

64. Walther DJ, Peter JU, Bashammakh S et al. Synthesis of serotonin by a second tryptophan hydroxylase isoform. Science 2003; 299(5603):76.

65. Paoloni-Giacobino A, Mouthon D, Lambercy C et al. Identification and analysis of new sequence variants in the human tryptophan hydroxylase (TpH) gene. Mol Psychiatry 2000; 5(1):49–55.

66. Teerawatanasuk N, Carr LG. CBF/NF-Y activates transcription of the human tryptophan hydroxylase gene through an inverted CCAAT box. Brain Res Mol Brain Res 1998; 55(1):61–70.

67. Rotondo A, Schuebel K, Bergen A et al. Identification of four variants in the tryptophan hydroxylase promoter and association to behavior. Mol Psychiatry 1999; 4(4):360–8.

68. Nielsen DA, Goldman D, Virkkunen M et al. Suicidality and 5-hydroxyindoleacetic acid concentration associated with a tryptophan hydroxylase polymorphism. Arch Gen Psychiatry 1994; 51(1):34–8.

69. Bennett PJ, McMahon WM, Watabe J et al. Tryptophan hydroxylase polymorphisms in suicide victims. Psychiatr Genet 2000; 10(1):13–17.

70. Geijer T, Frisch A, Persson ML et al. Search for association between suicide attempt and serotonergic polymorphisms. Psychiatr Genet 2000; 10(1):19–26.

71. Abbar M, Courtet P, Bellivier F et al. Suicide attempts and the tryptophan hydroxylase gene. Mol Psychiatry 2001; 6(3):268–73.

72. Bellivier F, Leroux M, Henry C et al. Serotonin transporter gene polymorphism influences age at onset in patients with bipolar affective disorder. Neurosci Lett 2002; 334(1):17–20.

73. Bellivier F, Henry C, Szoke A et al. Serotonin transporter gene polymorphisms in patients with unipolar or bipolar depression. Neurosci Lett 1998; 255(3):143–6.

74. Courtet P, Picot MC, Bellivier F et al. Serotonin transporter gene may be involved in short-term risk of subsequent suicide attempts. Biol Psychiatry 2004; 55(1):46–51.

75. Jonsson EG, Goldman D, Spurlock G et al. Tryptophan hydroxylase and catechol-O-methyltransferase gene polymorphisms: relationships to monoamine metabolite concentrations in CSF of healthy volunteers. Eur Arch Psychiatry Clin Neurosci 1997; 247(6):297–302.

76. Serretti A, Zanardi R, Cusin C et al. Tryptophan hydroxylase gene associated with paroxetine antidepressant activity. Eur Neuropsychopharmacol 2001; 11(5):375–80.

77. Serretti A, Zanardi R, Rossini D et al. Influence of tryptophan hydroxylase and serotonin transporter genes on fluvoxamine antidepressant activity. Mol Psychiatry 2001; 6(5):586–92.

78. Serretti A, Cristina S, Lilli R et al. Family-based association study of 5-HTTLPR, TPH, MAO-A, and DRD4 polymorphisms in mood disorders. Am J Med Genet 2002; 114(4):361–9.

79. Bellivier F, Chaste P, Malafosse A. Association between the TPH gene A218C polymorphism and suicidal behavior: a meta-analysis. Am J Med Genet B Neuropsychiatr Genet 2004; 124(1):87–91.

80. Manuck SB, Flory JD, Ferrell RE et al. Aggression and anger-related traits associated with a polymorphism of the tryptophan hydroxylase gene. Biol Psychiatry 1999; 45(5):603–14.

81. Lalovic A, Turecki G. Meta-analysis of the association between tryptophan hydroxylase and suicidal behavior. Am J Med Genet 2002; 114(5):533–40.

82. Magnay JL, Ismail KM, Chapman G et al. Serotonin transporter, tryptophan hydroxylase, and monoamine oxidase A gene polymorphisms in premenstrual dysphoric disorder. Am J Obstet Gynecol 2006; 195(5):1254–9.

83. Zill P, Buttner A, Eisenmenger W, Bondy B, Ackenheil M. Regional mRNA expression of a second tryptophan hydroxylase isoform in postmortem tissue samples of two human brains. Eur Neuropsychopharmacol 2004; 14(4):282–4.

84. Zhang X, Beaulieu JM, Gainetdinov RR, Caron MG. Functional polymorphisms of the brain serotonin synthesizing enzyme tryptophan hydroxylase-2. Cell Mol Life Sci 2006; 63(1):6–11.

85. Zill P, Buttner A, Eisenmenger W et al. Single nucleotide polymorphism and haplotype analysis of a novel tryptophan hydroxylase isoform (TPH2) gene in suicide victims. Biol Psychiatry 2004; 56(8):581–6.

86. Zill P, Baghai TC, Zwanzger P et al. SNP and haplotype analysis of a novel tryptophan hydroxylase isoform (TPH2) gene provide evidence for association with major depression. Mol Psychiatry 2004; 9(11):1030–6.

87. Zhang X, Gainetdinov RR, Beaulieu JM et al. Loss-of-function mutation in tryptophan hydroxylase-2 identified in unipolar major depression. Neuron 2005; 45(1):11–16.

88. Heils A, Teufel A, Petri S et al. Allelic variation of human serotonin transporter gene expression. J Neurochem 1996; 66(6):2621–4.

89. Auerbach J, Geller V, Lezer S et al. Dopamine D4 receptor (D4DR) and serotonin transporter promoter (5-HTTLPR) polymorphisms in the determination of temperament in 2-month-old infants. Mol Psychiatry 1999; 4(4):369–73.

90. Beitchman JH, Baldassarra L, Mik H et al. Serotonin transporter polymorphisms and persistent, pervasive childhood aggression. Am J Psychiatry 2006; 163(6):1103–5.

91. Cadoret RJ, Langbehn D, Caspers K et al. Associations of the serotonin transporter promoter polymorphism with aggressivity, attention deficit, and conduct disorder in an adoptee population. Compr Psychiatry 2003; 44(2):88–101.

92. Lesch KP, Bengel D, Heils A et al. Association of anxiety-related traits with a polymorphism in the serotonin transporter gene regulatory region. Science 1996; 274(5292):1527–31.

93. Serretti A, Benedetti F, Zanardi R, Smeraldi E. The influence of Serotonin Transporter Promoter Polymorphism (SERTPR) and other polymorphisms of the serotonin pathway on the efficacy of antidepressant treatments. Prog Neuropsychopharmacol Biol Psychiatry 2005; 29(6):1074–84.

94. Smith GS, Lotrich FE, Malhotra AK et al. Effects of serotonin transporter promoter polymorphisms on serotonin function. Neuropsychopharmacology 2004; 29(12):2226–34.

95. Lesch KP, Balling U, Gross J et al. Organization of the human serotonin transporter gene. J Neural Transm Gen Sect 1994; 95(1):157–62.

96. MacKenzie A, Quinn J. A serotonin transporter gene intron 2 polymorphic region, correlated with affective disorders, has allele-dependent differential enhancer-like properties in the mouse embryo. Proc Natl Acad Sci USA 1999; 96(26):15251–5.

97. Beitchman JH, Davidge KM, Kennedy JL et al. The serotonin transporter gene in aggressive children with and without ADHD and nonaggressive matched controls. Ann NY Acad Sci 2003; 1008:248–51.

98. Fan JB, Sklar P. Meta-analysis reveals association between serotonin transporter gene STin2 VNTR polymorphism and schizophrenia. Mol Psychiatry 2005; 10(10):928–38, 891.

99. Battersby S, Ogilvie AD, Blackwood DH et al. Presence of multiple functional polyadenylation signals and a single nucleotide polymorphism in the 3′ untranslated region of the human serotonin transporter gene. J Neurochem 1999; 72(4):1384–8.

100. Kent L, Doerry U, Hardy E et al. Evidence that variation at the serotonin transporter gene influences susceptibility to attention deficit hyperactivity disorder (ADHD): analysis and pooled analysis. Mol Psychiatry 2002; 7(8):908–12.

101. Mynett-Johnson L, Kealey C, Claffey E et al. Multimarker haplotypes within the serotonin transporter gene suggest evidence of an association with bipolar disorder. Am J Med Genet 2000; 96(6):845–9.

102. Melke J, Westberg L, Landen M et al. Serotonin transporter gene polymorphisms and platelet [³H] paroxetine binding in premenstrual dysphoria. Psychoneuroendocrinology 2003; 28(3):446–58.

103. Magnay JL, Ismail KM, Chapman G et al. Serotonin transporter, tryptophan hydroxylase, and monoamine oxidase A gene polymorphisms in premenstrual dysphoric disorder. Am J Obstet Gynecol 2006; 195(5):1254–9.

104. Sabol SZ, Hu S, Hamer D. A functional polymorphism in the monoamine oxidase A gene promoter. Hum Genet 1998; 103(3):273–9.

105. Denney RM, Koch H, Craig IW. Association between monoamine oxidase A activity in human male skin fibroblasts and genotype of the MAOA promoter-associated variable number tandem repeat. Hum Genet 1999; 105(6):542–51.

106. Hotamisligil GS, Breakefield XO. Human monoamine oxidase A gene determines levels of enzyme activity. Am J Hum Genet 1991; 49(2):383–92.

107. Contini V, Marques FZ, Garcia CE, Hutz MH, Bau CH. MAOA-uVNTR polymorphism in a Brazilian sample: further support for the association with impulsive behaviors and alcohol dependence. Am J Med Genet B Neuropsychiatr Genet 2006; 141(3):305–8.

108. Du L, Bakish D, Ravindran A, Hrdina PD. MAO-A gene polymorphisms are associated with major depression and sleep disturbance in males. Neuroreport 2004; 15(13):2097–101.

109. Herman AI, Kaiss KM, Ma R et al. Serotonin transporter promoter polymorphism and monoamine oxidase type A VNTR allelic variants together influence alcohol binge drinking risk in young women. Am J Med Genet B Neuropsychiatr Genet 2005; 133(1):74–8.

110. Chakravorty SG, Halbreich U. The influence of estrogen on monoamine oxidase activity. Psychopharmacol Bull 1997; 33(2):229–33.

111. Halbreich U, Rojansky N, Palter S et al. Estrogen augments serotonergic activity in postmenopausal women. Biol Psychiatry 1995; 37(7):434–41.

112. Katz RJ, Landau PS, Lott M et al. Serotonergic (5-HT2) mediation of anxiety–therapeutic effects of serazepine in generalized anxiety disorder. Biol Psychiatry 1993; 34(1–2):41–4.

113. Dubovsky SL, Thomas M. Serotonergic mechanisms and current and future psychiatric practice. J Clin Psychiatry 1995; 56(Suppl 2):38–48.

114. Brawman-Mintzer O, Lydiard RB. Biological basis of generalized anxiety disorder. J Clin Psychiatry 1997; 58(Suppl 3):16–25.

115. Endicott J, Amsterdam J, Eriksson E et al. Is premenstrual dysphoric disorder a distinct clinical entity? J Womens Health Gend Based Med 1999; 8(5):663–79.

116. Kim SA, Kim JH, Park M, Cho IH, Yoo HJ. Association of GABRB3 polymorphisms with autism spectrum disorders in Korean trios. Neuropsychobiology 2007; 54(3):160–5.

117. Soyka M, Preuss UW, Hesselbrock V et al. GABA-A2 receptor subunit gene (GABRA2) polymorphisms and risk for alcohol dependence. J Psychiatr Res 2007; Jan 4 (Epub ahead of print).

118. Lou XY, Ma JZ, Sun D, Payne TJ, Li MD. Fine mapping of a linkage region on chromosome 17p13 reveals that GABARAP and DLG4 are associated with vulnerability to nicotine dependence in European-Americans. Hum Mol Genet 2007; 16(2):142–53.

119. Lo WS, Harano M, Gawlik M et al. GABRB2 association with schizophrenia: commonalities and differences between ethnic groups and clinical subtypes. Biol Psychiatry 2007; 61(5):653–60.

120. Dick DM, Plunkett J, Wetherill LF et al. Association between GABRA1 and drinking behaviors in the collaborative study on the genetics of alcoholism sample. Alcohol Clin Exp Res 2006; 30(7):1101–10.

19

Future directions in the pathophysiology of premenstrual dysphoric disorder: steps to future treatments

Peter J Schmidt and David R Rubinow

INTRODUCTION

Premenstrual dysphoric disorder (PMDD) represents an affective syndrome, the symptoms of which are confined to the luteal phase of the menstrual cycle and are of sufficient severity to interfere with normal life activities. PMDD causes substantial suffering to the approximately 5–10% of women of reproductive age with this disorder. The degree of functional impairment is at least equivalent to that seen with dysthymia (i.e. chronic depression) and, in some aspects (e.g. social/leisure and parental impairment) is equivalent to chronic or recurrent major depression. Given the prevalence of PMDD (almost four million women), the years at risk, and an average of 6 days of severe symptoms per cycle, the World Health Organization's model calculates the burden of PMDD in the United States alone as 14.5 million disability adjusted life years. Two forms of treatment have demonstrated efficacy in PMDD (i.e. selective serotonin reuptake inhibitors [SSRI] and ovarian suppression); however, neither treatment is effective in all women with PMDD, and predictors of response to either treatment are not known, nor are the mechanisms of their therapeutic actions.

The timing of symptoms of PMDD both distinguishes this condition and leads to speculation about its underlying pathophysiology. Since the menstrual cycle is a series of hormonal events involving endocrine activity at the hypothalamus, pituitary, and ovary, it was presumed that the symptoms of PMDD must result from abnormal levels of some ovarian or menstrual cycle-dependent factor, much in the way that depression may result from other endocrinopathies involving thyroid or adrenal dysfunction. Studies reviewed in previous chapters in this textbook, however, have overwhelmingly, refuted the presumption that circulating gonadal steroid levels are abnormal in women with PMDD. Thus, traditional hormone deficiency-based models of behavioral regulation do not provide adequate explanations for PMDD. Speculation about the pathophysiology of PMDD may be informed by those characteristics of women with this disorder that are consistently demonstrated in the literature: evidence of altered serotonergic system function in women with PMDD compared with controls, the therapeutic efficacy of SSRIs but not other antidepressants, and the provocation of PMDD symptoms by physiological levels of ovarian steroids. Nonetheless, to propose that PMDD simply reflects an interaction between a hormonal signal and an abnormality of neurotransmitters (e.g. serotonergic dysfunction) is not adequate, since neither the nature of the signal nor the nature of the neurotransmitter abnormality is understood. Moreover, there are several characteristics of PMDD that need to be included in efforts to develop a disease model for PMDD. First, PMDD involves symptoms of both affective dysregulation and cognitive disturbance and, therefore, it is in large part a brain disease. Thus, in addition to understanding the nature of the hormonal signal, the brain regions targeted by this signal and the relevant neurocircuitry of PMDD need to be identified. Finally, an appropriate disease model for PMDD must not only account for the timing of the symptoms during the luteal phase but also their emergence with time (appearing commonly in the late 20s or 30s) and their minimal expression in most women (only 5–10% of women have PMDD). An attempt to model these characteristics not only results in a reconceptualization of PMDD that will generate new hypotheses to be examined but also permits the development of theoretically derived and evidence-based treatment strategies for this condition.

In this chapter we first provide a brief summary of the data that we believe provide directions for the design of future investigations into the pathophysiology of this condition. Next, we discuss several hormonal mechanisms and physiological substrates that potentially are involved in the development of PMDD. Specifically, we focus on the nature of the hormonal signal or trigger for symptom occurrence, the substrates that are implicated in the symptoms of PMDD (i.e. brain regions and connections, hypothalamic–pituitary–adrenal [HPA] axis), and finally, the mechanisms whereby a hormonal signal could be differentially modulated to alter stress responsivity and produce affective, cognitive, and behavioral symptoms in a subgroup of women.

BACKGROUND

Once investigators had agreed on the appropriate methods for sample selection in studies of PMDD, they were then able to reasonably attempt to test hypotheses about physiological disturbances accompanying PMDD. Several studies documented that there were no differences in plasma levels of gonadotropins or gonadal steroids in women with prospectively confirmed PMDD compared with controls in whom the absence of premenstrual symptoms were prospectively confirmed (see Chapter 10). These data, therefore, failed to support hypotheses of excesses or deficiencies of circulating gonadal steroids (either progesterone or estradiol) in PMDD. Indeed, both observational and controlled studies also demonstrated that the symptoms of PMDD could be dissociated from the endocrine events of the luteal phase. Specifically, PMDD symptoms were observed despite blinded luteal phase function, including during luteal phase truncation with high doses of the progesterone receptor antagonist RU-486[1] as well as during luteal phase administration of low doses of RU-486.[2] Thus, the symptoms of PMDD could occur in the absence of the endocrine events of a normal luteal phase.

These data then raised the next question of whether reproductive-endocrine events occurring prior to the luteal phase might nonetheless be influencing subsequent symptom development. To test this possibility, several studies examined the effects on PMDD of either ovarian suppression with gonadotropin-releasing hormone (GnRH) agonists (under placebo-controlled conditions) or oophorectomy (during unblinded observational follow-up) in women with prospectively confirmed PMDD. The findings of these studies consistently documented that the elimination of cyclic ovarian activity reduced both symptom severity and cyclicity in the majority of women with PMDD (see Chapter 10).

Two studies pursued these observations further and examined the effects of administering physiological doses of ovarian steroids to those women whose PMDD was in remission during ovarian suppression[3] or postoophorectomy,[4] respectively. In the approximately 60% of women whose PMDD symptoms were significantly attenuated or eliminated by ovarian suppression, symptoms returned within 2 weeks of initiating replacement of estradiol or progesterone to physiological levels, and remitted by the fourth week of administration. In contrast, in the study by Schmidt et al,[3] in the group of control women lacking a history of PMDD, neither the hypogonadal nor the hormone replacement conditions were associated with any perturbation of mood. Consistent with the findings from basal hormone studies, then, it appears that PMDD represents an abnormal response to normal hormone changes or levels rather than a 'normal' response to a hormonal abnormality.

Ovarian suppression is effective in approximately 60% of women with PMDD, and in these women physiological levels of estradiol and/or progesterone trigger a recurrence of PMDD symptoms; nonetheless, we cannot infer a simple relationship between PMDD and ovarian hormone secretion. For example, in these same studies many women with otherwise identical forms of PMDD continued to experience cyclic symptoms despite hormonal evidence of adequate ovarian suppression. Thus, a considerable proportion (i.e. 20–40%) of women with PMDD show a 'hormone-independent' condition, since PMDD symptoms did not improve with ovarian suppression. Additionally, GnRH agonists also suppress ovarian androgen production, which contributes approximately 50% of circulating androgens in women. Thus, the ability of GnRH agonists (with or without estradiol and progesterone) to regulate symptom expression must be interpreted in the context of accompanying relative hypoandrogenism.

These caveats notwithstanding, in the women with PMDD whose symptoms are eliminated by ovarian suppression, changes in estradiol or progesterone secretion 'trigger' the onset of symptoms. Our studies, then, raised several questions:

1. Why do similar changes in, or levels of, gonadal steroids trigger mood deterioration in women with PMDD while showing no apparent effect on mood in women lacking this history?
2. Is it the rate of change in the hormone level or the exceeding of a critical threshold that results in the triggering effect?
3. Will continued exposure to stable levels of gonadal steroids be associated with the continuation, disappearance, or episodic recurrence of mood symptoms?

NATURE OF HORMONAL TRIGGER

The ability of ovarian steroids to precipitate mood symptoms in women with PMDD could reflect either a change in gonadal steroid levels or the exceeding of a critical threshold of hormone secretion above which cyclic symptoms are manifest. We initiated a study in which we continuously administer hormone replacement for 3 months in women with PMDD in whom we document that ovarian suppression eliminates symptom severity and cyclicity. Women with PMDD receive Lupron (leuprolide; 3.75 mg IM every month) for 6 months. After month 2, those women showing elimination of PMDD symptoms receive placebo for 1 month (to identify placebo-related symptom induction). Those women not showing symptoms on placebo during the third month then receive estradiol (Estraderm patch 100 μg every day) and progesterone (200 mg suppository twice a day) for the next 3 months. We reasoned that if the symptoms recurred monthly, it would suggest that the change in steroid levels is of no consequence (as no change occurs after the first month) and it is the level of gonadal steroids that is relevant and necessary but not sufficient (i.e. there must occur some other cyclical process [e.g. an infradian rhythm that is ovarian steroid-dependent] that allows for the precipitation and remission of symptoms while constant gonadal steroid levels are maintained). If subjects were symptomatic during the first month and then experienced no recurrence of symptoms during the next 2 months, it would rule out the importance of the level of gonadal steroids per se (even in the presence of an infradian factor) as the precipitant of symptoms. To date, preliminary data suggest that the change in gonadal steroids triggers mood destabilization, with no further symptomatic episodes recurring over the subsequent 3 months.[5] These data do not permit us to identify whether it is the change in progesterone or the change in estradiol that is the triggering stimulus. Future studies employing either selective estrogen and progesterone receptor antagonists or the selective withdrawal of estrogen and progesterone could dissect out the roles of estrogen and/or progesterone as the steroid signal in PMDD. Finally, these preliminary data suggest that continuously (rather than sequentially) administered oral contraceptives might successfully treat PMDD, a significant potential advance in the available therapeutic options.[6,7]

NATURE OF SUBSTRATE

While the obvious candidate for mediating PMDD symptoms is the 'central nervous system', most studies to date regard PMDD as an array of negative affects and behavioral symptoms without further consideration of how changes in the brain could mediate these symptoms other than through vague reference to 'disturbances of neurotransmitters'. Such a conception both ignores the phenomenology of the symptomatic state in women with PMDD[8,9] and fails to incorporate recent discoveries in affective neuroscience. Clinical observations in women with PMDD suggest that the neurocircuitry targeted by ovarian steroids comprises those brain regions implicated in the regulation of affective state and the stress response, abnormalities of which are also described in depression. Indeed, PMDD shares many common features with traditional affective disorders. First, the symptoms of PMDD are similar to those of an atypical depression, e.g. sadness, anxiety, carbohydrate craving, and hypersomnia. Additionally, as part of this dysphoric state, women with PMDD demonstrate negative affective bias and report anhedonia (inability to enjoy otherwise pleasurable events), social avoidance, and emotional overreaction to stressful situations along with other symptoms of affective maladaptation. Secondly, the prevalence of a past history of major depression is substantially increased in women with PMDD compared with the normal population. Thirdly, some of the efficacious (e.g. SSRIs) or putatively efficacious (sleep deprivation, phototherapy) treatments for PMDD are also employed in the treatment of depression. Fourthly, some of the biological systems that are 'dysregulated' with increased frequency in women with PMDD are the same systems that have shown increased frequency of dysregulation in depression: e.g. blunted or exaggerated adrenocorticotropic hormone (ACTH) response to corticotropin-releasing hormone (CRH), blunted or exaggerated thyroid-stimulating hormone (TSH) response to thyrotropin-releasing hormone (TRH), decreased serotonin peripheral binding and uptake, and phase-shifted circadian rhythms.

Additionally, as suggested by Rubinow and Schmidt,[10] PMDD comprises several other disturbances during the luteal phase indicative of dysfunctions in specific brain regions:

- changes in valuation of or valence assignment to experiences
- increase in negative information processing bias
- inability to access/recall positive mood states or maintain positive mood state
- disturbances in arousal/reactivity
- inability to suppress negative responses
- inability to change affective state[11,12] (Rubinow et al, personal communication).

Many of these processes are regulated by and reflect the input of several interconnected brain regions (circuits), including the prefrontal cortex (PFC), orbitofrontal cortex (OFC), anterior cingulate cortex (ACC), amygdala, striatum, and ventral tegmentum/nucleus accumbens. Excessive activation (e.g. amygdala activation) or deficient activation (i.e. loss of inhibition from PFC or OFC) of specific brain regions is associated with dysphoric states. For example, increased amygdala activation (or inappropriate amygdala activation) is associated with prolonged negative mood states and with trait vulnerability to experience depression.[13,14] The findings of many investigators[15–20] emphasize that symptoms of affective dysregulation can be understood by studying the activation patterns of interconnected and reciprocal inhibitory brain regions (e.g. OFC and amygdala) rather than in the activity of one specific brain region acting in isolation. Deficient PFC activation, for example, may result in unrestrained amygdala activation,[17] with aforementioned negative impact on mood, and in unrestrained stress-related dorsal raphe activation,[21] with consequent amplification of the adverse biological and behavioral effects of stress. Similarly, interconnecting neurocircuits have been described between the PFC and the locus coeruleus that could be important for the regulation of arousal, focused attention, and performance during conflict or stress.[22,23] While stimulated PFC and amygdala function have not been examined in PMDD, deficits in the recognition of facial emotion during the luteal phase in women with PMDD[12] is suggestive of abnormal amygdala function, similar to observations in depressed subjects, of both altered amygdala activation in response to masked faces[24] as well as deficits in facial emotion recognition.[25] Women with PMDD but not controls showed menstrual cycle-related variation in performance on the Facial Discrimination Task (FDT), with both impaired performance and prominent negative bias (e.g. identifying neutral faces as sad) seen during the luteal phase. No menstrual cycle phase effect nor diagnostic effect was seen on a control task. The bias in affective processing in women with PMDD is state-related (although not correlated with symptom ratings) and suggests that events related to the luteal phase may trigger functional dysregulation in those brain regions mediating the recognition of emotional facial expression (e.g. amygdala, OFC, fusiform gyrus, superior temporal sulcus), brain regions that have also been implicated in depression. Additionally, the bias in affect assessment (the experience of stimuli as both more emotional and more negative) in the luteal phase in women with PMDD may contribute to the generation and perpetuation of negative affective states. For example, Hooker et al[26] show that an inability to perform reversal learning with emotionally charged faces is associated with an oversensitivity to negative

social cues, cognitive inflexibility, and a differential pattern of brain regional activation on functional magnetic resonance imaging (fMRI). Disturbances observed in women with PMDD during the luteal phase may also implicate other elements of the affective neurocircuitry. The negative bias/affective misperception could reflect the mis-assessment of emotional information seen with dysfunction of the normal balance between dorsal and ventral anterior cingulate cortical activity.[27] The failure to access positive mood states and to update frontal representations, and the consequent maladaptive behavioral response selection, may suggest dysfunctional reward circuitry, with impaired phasic mid-brain dopaminergic modulation of prefrontal cortical activity.[28] This possibility is enhanced by our observation of decreased capacity for emotional reappraisal and recovery in women with PMDD (Dancer et al, personal communication). Studies by Schultz and colleagues[29] demonstrate that a reward that is smaller than that expected will actually inhibit the firing of dopamine neurons associated with the expectation of the reward. Thus, an affective misperception may contribute to as well as reflect the experience of anhedonia or dysphoria.

If the actual physiological substrates (i.e. neurocircuits, neurotransmitters, and stress axis) implicated in PMDD can be identified, then a critical question is whether the functions of these systems are regulated by ovarian steroids. Two strategies are employed to answer this question: comparison of outcome measures in the follicular and luteal phases of the menstrual cycle; and comparison during GnRH agonist-induced hypogonadism and hormone replacement.

Recent brain imaging studies in asymptomatic women (i.e. women without PMDD) confirm for the first time in humans that physiological levels of ovarian steroids have the capacity to modulate the neurocircuitry thought to be involved in both normal and pathological affective states. First, Berman et al performed cognition-activated ^{15}O PET (positron emission tomography) scans in women during conditions of GnRH agonist-induced hypogonadism and gonadal steroid replacement. They observed the elimination of Wisconsin Card Sort-activated regional cerebral blood flow (rCBF) in the dorsolateral prefrontal cortex as well as an attenuation of cortical activation in the inferior parietal lobule and posterior inferior temporal cortex (bilaterally) during GnRH agonist-induced hypogonadism.[30] The characteristic pattern of cortical activation re-emerged during both estradiol and progesterone add-back. Additionally, they observed a differential pattern of hippocampal activation, with estradiol increasing and progesterone decreasing activation relative to hypogonadism. This was the first demonstration that ovarian steroids have activational effects on rCBF

Derby Hospitals NHS Foundation
Trust
Library and Knowledge Service

during cognitive stimulation in the brain regions (i.e. PFC) implicated in disorders of affect and cognition. Secondly, Goldstein et al[31] observed an increase in amygdala activity and arousal (as measured by fMRI and skin conductance, respectively) during the late follicular phase of the menstrual cycle (higher estradiol levels) compared with the early follicular phase (characterized by relatively low estradiol levels). Thirdly, Protopopescu et al[32] employed an affective pictures task in an fMRI study and observed increased OFC activity (a region that in some studies exerts inhibitory control over amygdala functioning) during the luteal compared with the follicular phase. Moreover, preliminary data from these same investigators in women with PMDD (DC Silbersweig, pers comm) suggest a relative loss of OFC activity (decreased inhibition) in women with PMDD during the luteal phase. Notwithstanding the caveat that decreased cortical 'activity' could also reflect more efficient or optimal function, these data suggest that a reduction in OFC inhibition of amygdala function during the luteal phase is associated with PMDD symptoms. Finally, Dreher et al[33] performed an event-related fMRI study of reward processing across the menstrual cycle in women with PMDD and controls. The paradigm employed disentangles transient reward error prediction (PFC) from sustained response to reward uncertainty (ventral striatum). Preliminary data in the controls demonstrate, for the first time in humans, that ovarian steroids modulate reward system function, with increased follicular phase activation of the OFC and amygdala during reward anticipation and of the midbrain, striatum, and left ventrolateral PFC during reward delivery. New analytical approaches will allow for testing the hypothesis that the hormonally induced alteration in function includes changes in interregional neural interactions. These findings then suggest that cognitive and affective information processes may serve as probes to identify candidate circuits for the mediation of gonadal steroid-dependent affective dysregulation. Additionally, neuroimaging studies in women suggest that ovarian steroids can influence many neural processes and systems relevant to PMDD, including arousal, stress responsivity, and reward processing.

The description of altered stress reactivity[34–36] during the luteal phase in women with PMDD suggest that the HPA axis might also be an important target for ovarian steroids in women with PMDD. Although we[37,38] were unable to confirm reported (albeit inconsistent) differences between patients and controls in *basal* plasma β-endorphin, ACTH, or cortisol, we did find significant differences in *stimulated* HPA axis activity.[39,40] Consequently, we examined exercise stress-stimulated levels of arginine vasopressin (AVP), ACTH, and cortisol in PMDD patients and controls during both the follicular and luteal phases of the menstrual cycle. Women with PMDD failed to demonstrate the luteal phase-enhanced HPA axis activation seen in the controls.[41] These data are of interest for several reasons. First, the luteal phase-related enhancement of stimulated HPA axis activity seen in the controls complements the observation that the HPA axis response is significantly increased in the presence of progesterone during GnRH agonist-induced ovarian suppression (comparable to the luteal phase).[41] Thus, not only is it progesterone rather than estradiol that has the greater impact on HPA axis activation in humans (unlike in rodents) but also the HPA axis response to progesterone appears to differ in women with PMDD and controls.

Thus, several physiological substrates that control both affective and stress adaptation are also regulated by gonadal steroids and, therefore, could be sites of the differential response to the hormone signal in PMDD. Future studies employing probes of these systems combined with multimodal brain imaging techniques will better characterize and, possibly, confirm the relevance of these substrates in PMDD.

GONADAL STEROID SIGNAL MODULATION: ROLE OF CONTEXT

As more is learned about steroid–steroid receptor signaling, the possible sources of altered steroid signaling in PMDD grow exponentially. Several observations in women with PMDD must be incorporated into the search for the contextual variables that differentially modulate steroid signaling in PMDD. First, the actions of ovarian steroids at non-CNS sites appear to be normal in women with PMDD and, therefore, the differential steroid signal is substrate/tissue specific. Thus, women with PMDD could have a differential metabolism of steroids, resulting in locally (i.e. within specific regions of the CNS) increased or decreased tissue levels of steroids or their metabolites. Secondly, PMDD demonstrates a high rate of heritability, suggesting genotypic variation may contribute to altered (and tissue-specific) steroid signaling. Finally, symptoms develop over the course of reproductive life in those women with PMDD, suggesting either behavioral sensitization or possible epigenetic modification of steroid signaling pathways, perhaps by interaction with other contextual variables such as early-life trauma, reproductive aging, or the occurrence of episodes of major/minor depressions (both reproductive and non-reproductive-related). Whereas mood disorders may be seen in association with the pathological function of certain endocrine organs (e.g. adrenal, thyroid), mood disturbances precipitated by gonadal steroids in PMDD appear in the context of normal ovarian function. Thus, although substrates such as OFC/PFC–anterior cingulate–amygdala neurocircuits, the serotonergic system, and HPA axis can be identified as potential targets for the ovarian steroid signal, studies must examine means by which otherwise normal steroid signals elicit a change in behavioral state.

The neurosteroid metabolites of progesterone (and androgens) are of considerable interest as possible mediators of the behavioral effects of gonadal steroids in PMDD (see Chapter 10). Whereas reports of altered allopregnanolone levels in PMDD are inconsistent, several findings suggest the relevance of neurosteroids in PMDD, including the following:

- allopregnanolone plasma levels have been correlated with PMDD symptoms
- altered sensitivity to benzodiazepines/neurosteroids has been found in women with PMDD
- women with PMDD fail to show the normal luteal phase-related blunting of cortical activation presumed to be due to allopregnanolone.[42]

Although we previously reported no differences in luteal phase allopregnanolone and pregnanolone levels in women with PMDD compared with controls,[43] studies during GnRH agonist-induced ovarian suppression enabled us to examine the metabolism of progesterone during constant daily dosing and without the confound of variable ovarian progesterone production. In preliminary data, women with PMDD differed from controls, showing a greater decrease for peak allopregnanolone and 5α-dihydroprogesterone (DHP) levels (PMDD). Further, in women with PMDD, evidence of decreased 5α-reductase activity (decreased DHP) and 3α-hydroxysteroid oxidoreductase (3α-HSD) activity (decreased allopregnanolone) correlated with symptom ratings. These findings suggest that differences in the activity of the synthetic (or metabolic) enzymes for neurosteroids (or differences in metabolite conversion, sequestration, or clearance) might translate into phenotypic differences. This possibility is strengthened by observations that different metabolites of progesterone have opposite central neuromodulatory effects (e.g. 3α-metabolites are $GABA_A$ receptor agonists, whereas 3β-metabolites are $GABA_A$ antagonists)[44] and changes in reproductive hormones are known to modulate 5α-reductase activity in the amygdala of non-human primates.[45]

In collaboration with Dr Synthia Mellon, we have been measuring the activity of one of the two major enzymes responsible for the production of allopregnanolone (3α-HSD) in women with PMDD to determine whether lower activity of this enzyme might account for both gonadal steroid-triggered symptoms (due to low allopregnanolone levels and elevated dihydrotestosterone (DHT) levels) and responsivity to SSRIs (which stimulate the activity of the enzyme). While initial efforts have been primarily directed at determining the effect of menstrual cycle phase on enzyme activity in controls, preliminary data suggest that women with PMDD may have (paradoxically) increased conversion of DHP to allopregnanolone compared with controls (Rubinow et al, pers comm). Additionally, women with PMDD have increased levels of lymphocyte 3α-HSD mRNA but no differences in 5α-reductase mRNA levels.

Allopregnanolone is also a positive modulator of the $GABA_A$ receptor. Animal study data from several laboratories[46–48] demonstrate that both chronic (3–5 days) exposure to and subsequent withdrawal from progesterone or allopregnanolone alter the expression of $GABA_A$ subunits (and the composition of the receptor) in such a way as to greatly diminish both the sensitivity to benzodiazepine potentiation and the agonist response of the $GABA_A$ receptor/chloride ion channel. Blockade of the formation of allopregnanolone with either 5α-reductase inhibitors (finasteride) or 3α-HSD inhibitors (indomethacin) prevented the adverse behavioral effects (irritability and withdrawal-like symptoms) seen following progesterone exposure in rats.[49,50] Thus, the blockade of allopregnanolone-induced alterations in $GABA_A$ receptor activity might similarly prevent progesterone/luteal phase-related symptom appearance in women with PMDD. Given the toxicity of indomethacin and the lack of efficacy of finasteride against type I 5α-reductase (the isoform present in the brain), this hypothesis could be tested only recently with the development of dutasteride, which antagonizes type I 5α-reductase.

Finally, as metabolomic techniques develop, investigators will have the ability to more directly examine the products of cellular metabolism. The advantages of metabolic profiling are compelling and described elsewhere.[65] The estimated number of human cellular metabolites is several orders of magnitude smaller than the numbers of genes, transcripts, or proteins. Further, metabolomic technology permits inferences about disturbances in metabolic pathways. For example, if 5α-reductase activity is altered in women with PMDD, as suggested to be the case in polycystic ovary syndrome (increased),[51] one would expect an array of changes in metabolic profile, including changes in allopregnanolone, 5α-dihydroprogesterone, dihydrotestosterone, and progesterone concentrations. Thus, potential alterations in neurosteroid metabolism should be more comprehensively demonstrated with this technique, because the extended metabolic pathway of a substance/enzyme is being measured. These studies may enable investigators to determine both the metabolic consequences of ovarian steroid exposure, as well as the identity of candidate mediators of the differential behavioral response (i.e. altered pattern of metabolites) observed in women with PMDD.

A second possible site of differential steroid signal modification is at the level of the steroid receptor. Steroid receptor function is modified by an array of tissue-specific factors including the relative concentration of co-regulator proteins, the presence and activity of receptors for other members of the steroid family or receptor subtypes, and concurrent action of the steroid at the cell membrane. In human disease one of the best characterized sources of variation in steroid receptor function is genomic. Polymorphisms in gonadal steroid receptors have been shown to alter receptor transcriptional efficacy (e.g. CAG repeat in exon 1 of the androgen receptor; progins insertion in intron 7 of the progesterone receptor; T1057G in exon 5 of β-estrogen receptor) and to be associated with differential illness risk (i.e. prostate cancer, breast cancer).[52–55] Additionally, the susceptibility to the disruptive effects of estradiol on reproductive development differs enormously (up to 100-fold) between mouse strains, with the genotype contributing more to the variance than the dose of estradiol employed.[56] Finally, a single nucleotide polymorphism enables progesterone to activate a receptor, the mineralocorticoid receptor, at which it normally functions only as a competitive inhibitor, thus providing a means by which normal steroid levels create a different phenotype (hypertension).[57] There is precedent, then, for expecting that polymorphisms in the gonadal steroid signaling pathway or in gonadal steroid-regulated genes could alter the nature or strength of the steroid signal as well as phenotype. Alternatively, non-steroid-related genes could be implicated in the vulnerability to develop the differential behavioral response to ovarian steroids in PMDD. For example, Caspi et al[58] demonstrated that the risk of developing depression is predicted by the experience of stressful life events in combination with a specific genetic background but is not predicted by either the genetic or environmental factors when considered separately. Thus gene–environment interactions represent a promising explanation for the differential behavioral sensitivity to gonadal steroids seen in women with PMDD. Analogous to the suggestion by Caspi et al, PMDD symptoms could develop after a hormonal stimulus (i.e. the environmental event) against the background of a specific genetic context.

Whereas some earlier candidate gene studies did not find significant associations with PMDD,[59] we have recently identified a region of the ESR1 gene containing multiple polymorphic alleles that associate with PMDD, thus lending support to the idea that the effects of multiple genes may interact in creating a dysphoric behavioral response to normal gonadal steroid levels.[64]

The contributions of genotypic variation to PMDD phenotype could be modified by several other factors, including both epigenetic processes as well as gene–environment or gene–steroid interactions. For example, Meaney et al[60,61] have demonstrated that the behavioral phenotype can be determined by environment-induced alterations in the expression of the genome. Thus, early-life trauma or past episodes of depression, both frequent accompaniments of PMDD,[62] could potentially modify the substrate response to the gonadal steroid trigger. As more is learned about both the nature of gonadal steroid signaling in the brain and the complexities of gonadal steroid-regulated behaviors, the sources of the differential response to gonadal steroids in PMDD will be clarified. In summary, women with PMDD could have excessive or deficient gonadal steroid signaling that might alter the processing of stressors and lead to a dysregulated affective response[63] or altered learning that could favor the development of behavioral sensitization or steroid-dependent interoceptive cueing of behavioral states.

CONCLUSIONS

In PMDD there is a well-defined endocrine stimulus that for many women with this condition is critical in the precipitation of affective state disturbances. This affords a unique opportunity to identify neural substrates involved in the regulation of the affective state that could be targeted in the development of novel treatment strategies. Our pursuits of several testable hypotheses in PMDD will advance our understanding of this disorder, illuminate mechanisms by which reproductive steroids may regulate the affective state, and help identify the locus of the differential sensitivity that permits reproductive steroids to destabilize mood in some but not all women. A better understanding of the pathophysiology of this complex disorder will permit the development of theoretically driven treatment strategies and, hopefully, predictors of therapeutic response for the considerable number of women with PMDD who are not responsive to either ovarian suppression strategies or SSRIs.

ACKNOWLEDGMENT

The research was supported by the Intramural Research Programs of the NIMH.

REFERENCES

1. Schmidt PJ, Nieman LK, Grover GN et al. Lack of effect of induced menses on symptoms in women with premenstrual syndrome. N Engl J Med 1991; 324:1174–9.
2. Chan AF, Mortola JF, Wood SH et al. Persistence of premenstrual syndrome during low-dose administration of the progesterone antagonist RU 486. Obstet Gynecol 1994; 84:1001–5.
3. Schmidt PJ, Nieman LK, Danaceau MA et al. Differential behavioral effects of gonadal steroids in women with and in those without premenstrual syndrome. N Engl J Med 1998; 338: 209–16.
4. Henshaw C, Foreman D, Belcher J, Cox J, O'Brien S. Can one induce premenstrual symptomatology in women with prior hysterectomy and bilateral oophorectomy? J Psychosom Obstet Gynaecol 1996; 17:21–8.
5. Schmidt PJ, Nieman LK, Rubinow DR. Kinetics of hormone replacement and symptoms recurrence in MRMD. Abstr 33rd Annu Meeting Soc Neurosci, 2003.
6. Yonkers KA, Brown C, Pearlstein TB et al. Efficacy of a new low-dose oral contraceptive with drospirenone in premenstrual dysphoric disorder. Obstet Gynecol 2005; 106:492–501.
7. Sulak PJ, Carl J, Gopalakrishnan I et al. Outcomes of extended oral contraceptive regimens with a shortened hormone-free interval to manage breakthrough bleeding. Contraception 2004; 70: 281–7.
8. Smith MJ, Schmidt PJ, Rubinow DR. Operationalizing DSM-IV criteria for PMDD: selecting symptomatic and asymptomatic cycles for research. J Psychiatr Res 2003; 37:75–83.
9. Bloch M, Schmidt PJ, Rubinow DR. Premenstrual syndrome – evidence for symptom stability across cycles. Am J Psychiatry 1997; 154:1741–6.
10. Rubinow DR, Schmidt PJ. Gonadal steroid regulation of mood: the lessons of premenstrual syndrome. Front Neuroendocrinol 2006; 27:210–16.
11. Schmidt PJ, Grover GN, Hoban MC et al. State-dependent alterations in the perception of life events in menstrual-related mood disorders. Am J Psychiatry 1990; 147:230–4.
12. Rubinow DR, Smith MJ, Schenkel LA et al. Facial emotion discrimination across the menstrual cycle in women with premenstrual dysphoric disorder (PMDD) and controls. J Affective Discord 2007, in press.
13. Gotlib IH, Joormann J, Minor KL et al. Cognitive and biological functioning in children at risk for depression. In: Canli T, ed. Biology of Personality and Individual Differences. New York: Guilford Press; 2005.
14. Siegle GJ, Steinhauer SR, Thase ME et al. Can't shake that feeling: event-related fMRI assessment of sustained amygdala activity in response to emotional information in depressed individuals. Biol Psychiatry 2002; 51:693–707.
15. Drevets WC. Neuroplasticity in mood disorders. Dial Clin Neurosci 2004; 6:199–216.
16. Mayberg HS, Liotti M, Brannan SK et al. Reciprocal limbic-cortical function and negative mood: converging PET findings in depression and normal sadness. Am J Psychiatry 1999; 156:675–82.
17. Davidson RJ. Anxiety and affective style: role of prefrontal cortex and amygdala. Biol Psychiatry 2002; 51:68–80.
18. Haldane M, Frangou S. New insights help define the pathophysiology of bipolar affective disorder: neuroimaging and neuropathology findings. Prog Neuropsychopharmacol Biol Psychiat 2004; 28:943–60.
19. Holland PC, Gallagher M. Amygdala–frontal interactions and reward expectancy. Curr Opin Neurobiol 2004; 14:148–55.
20. Tunbridge E, Harrison P, Weinberger D. Catechol-o-methyltransferase, cognition and psychosis: Val^{158}Met and beyond. Biol Psychiatry 2006; 60:141–51.
21. Amat J, Baratta MV, Paul E et al. Medial prefrontal cortex determines how stressor controllability affects behavior and dorsal raphe nucleus. Nat Neurosci 2005; 8:365–71.
22. Aston-Jones G, Cohen JD. Adaptive gain and the role of the locus coeruleus–norepinephrine system in optimal performance. J Comp Neurol 2005; 493:99–110.
23. Cohen JD, Ashton-Jones G. Decision amid uncertainty. Nature 2005; 436:471–2.
24. Sheline YI, Barch DM, Donnelly JM et al. Increased amygdala response to masked emotional faces in depressed subjects resolves with antidepressant treatment: an fMRI study. Biol Psychiatry 2001; 50:651–8.
25. Gur RC, Erwin RJ, Gur RE et al. Facial emotion discrimination: II. Behavioral findings in depression. Psychiatry Res 1992; 42:241–51.
26. Hooker CI, Germine LT, Owen E et al. Neural mechanisms involved in learning from happy and fearful facial expressions. Abstr 34th Annu Meeting Soc Neurosci 2004; 203.6.
27. Bush TL. Preserving cardiovascular benefits of hormone replacement therapy. J Reprod Med 2000; 45:259–72.
28. Montague PR, Hyman SE, Cohen JD. Computational roles for dopamine in behavioural control. Nature 2004; 431:760–7.
29. Schultz W. Neural coding of basic reward terms of animal learning theory, game theory, microeconomics and behavioural ecology. Curr Opin Neurobiol 2004; 14:139–47.
30. Berman KF, Schmidt PJ, Rubinow DR et al. Modulation of cognition-specific cortical activity by gonadal steroids: a positron-emission tomography study in women. Proc Natl Acad Sci USA 1997; 94:8836–41.
31. Goldstein JM, Jerram M, Poldrack R et al. Hormonal cycle modulates arousal circuitry in women using functional magnetic resonance imaging. J Neurosci 2005; 25:9309–16.
32. Protopopescu X, Pan H, Altemus M et al. Orbitofrontal cortex activity related to emotional processing changes across the menstrual cycle. Proc Natl Acad Sci USA 2005; 102:16060–5.
33. Dreher J, Schmidt P, Kohn P et al. Menstrual cycle phase modulates the reward-related neural function in women. Proc Natl Acad Sci USA 2007; 104: 2465–70.
34. Girdler SS, Pedersen CA, Straneva PA et al. Dysregulation of cardiovascular and neuroendocrine responses to stress in premenstrual dysphoric disorder. Psychiatry Res 1998; 81:163–78.
35. Girdler SS, Sherwood A, Hinderliter AL et al. Biological correlates of abuse in women with premenstrual dysphoric disorder and healthy controls. Psychosom Med 2003; 65:849–56.
36. Van Goozen SHM, Frijda NH, Wiegant VM et al. The premenstrual phase and reactions to aversive events: a study of hormonal influences on emotionality. Psychoneuroendocrinology 1996; 21:479–97.
37. Rosenstein DL, Kalogeras KT, Kalafut M et al. Peripheral measures of arginine vasopressin, atrial natriuretic peptide and adrenocorticotropic hormone in premenstrual syndrome. Psychoneuroendocrinology 1996; 21:347–59.
38. Bloch M, Schmidt PJ, Su T-P et al. Pituitary–adrenal hormones and testosterone across the menstrual cycle in women with premenstrual syndrome and controls. Biol Psychiatry 1998; 43:897–903.
39. Su T-P, Schmidt PJ, Danaceau M et al. Effect of menstrual cycle phase on neuroendocrine and behavioral responses to the serotonin agonist m-chlorophenylpiperazine in women with premenstrual syndrome and controls. J Clin Endocrinol Metab 1997; 82:1220–8.
40. Rabin DS, Schmidt PJ, Campbell G et al. Hypothalamic–pituitary–adrenal function in patients with the premenstrual syndrome. J Clin Endocrinol Metab 1990; 71:1158–62.
41. Roca CA, Schmidt PJ, Altemus M et al. Differential menstrual cycle regulation of hypothalamic–pituitary–adrenal axis in

women with premenstrual syndrome and controls. J Clin Endocrinol Metab 2003; 88:3057–63.

42. Smith MJ, Adams LF, Schmidt PJ et al. Abnormal luteal phase excitability of the motor cortex in women with premenstrual syndrome. Biol Psychiatry 2003; 54:757–62.

43. Schmidt PJ, Purdy RH, Moore PH Jr et al. Circulating levels of anxiolytic steroids in the luteal phase in women with premenstrual syndrome and in control subjects. J Clin Endocrinol Metab 1994; 79:1256–60.

44. Lundgren P, Stromberg J, Backstrom T et al. Allopregnanolone-stimulated GABA-mediated chloride ion flux is inhibited by 3β-hydroxy-5α-pregnan-20-one (isoallopregnanolone). Brain Res 2003; 982:45–53.

45. Roselli CE, Stadelman H, Horton LE et al. Regulation of androgen metabolism and luteinizing hormone-releasing hormone content in discrete hypothalamic and limbic areas of male rhesus macaques. Endocrinology 1987; 120:97–106.

46. Smith MJ, Adams LF, Schmidt PJ et al. Effects of ovarian hormone on human cortical excitability. Ann Neurol 2002; 51:599–603.

47. Smith SS, Ruderman Y, Frye C, Homanics G, Yuan M. Steroid withdrawal in the mouse results in anxiogenic effects of 3α,5β-THP: a possible model of premenstrual dysphoric disorder. Psychopharmacology (Berl) 2006; 186:323–33.

48. Maguire JL, Stell BM, Rafizadeh M et al. Ovarian cycle-linked changes in GABAA receptors mediating tonic inhibition after seizure susceptibility and anxiety. Nat Neurosci 2005; 8: 797–804.

49. Gallo MA, Smith SS. Progesterone withdrawal decreases latency to and increases duration of electrified prod burial: a possible rat model of PMS anxiety. Pharmacol Biochem Behav 1993; 46:897–904.

50. Frye CA, Walf AA. Changes in progesterone metabolites in the hippocampus can modulate open field and forced swim test behavior of proestrous rats. Horm Behav 2002; 41:306–15.

51. Fassnacht M, Schlenz N, Schneider SB et al. Beyond adrenal and ovarian androgen generation: increased peripheral 5α-reductase activity in women with polycystic ovary syndrome. J Clin Endocrinol Metab 2003; 88:2760–6.

52. Zhao X-Y, Boyle B, Krishnan AV et al. Two mutations identified in the androgen receptor of the new human prostate cancer cell line MDA PCA 2A. J Urol 1999; 162:2192–9.

53. Beilin J, Zajac JD. Function of the human androgen receptor varies according to CAG repeat number within the normal range. Abstr 81st Annu Meeting Endocr Soc 1999; 500.

54. Giovannucci E, Stampfer MJ, Krithivas K et al. The CAG repeat within the androgen receptor gene and its relationship to prostate cancer. Proc Natl Acad Sci USA 1997; 94:3320–23.

55. Wang-Gohrke S, Chang-Claude J, Becher H et al. Progesterone receptor gene polymorphism is associated with decreased risk for breast cancer by age 50. Cancer Res 2000; 60:2348–50.

56. Spearow JL, Doemeny P, Sera R et al. Genetic variation in susceptibility to endocrine disruption by estrogen in mice. Science 1999; 285:1259–61.

57. Geller DS, Farhi A, Pinkerton N et al. Activating mineralocorticoid receptor mutation in hypertension exacerbated by pregnancy. Science 2000; 289:119–23.

58. Caspi A, Sugden K, Moffitt TE et al. Influence of life stress on depression: moderation by a polymorphism in the 5-HTT gene. Science 2003; 301:291–3.

59. Melke J, Westberg L, Landen M et al. Serotonin transporter gene polymorphisms and platelet [³H]paroxetine binding in premenstrual dysphoria. Psychoneuroendocrinology 2003; 28:446–58.

60. Meaney MJ, Szyf M. Environmental programming of stress responses through DNA methylation: life at the interface between a dynamic environment and a fixed genome. Dial Clin Neurosci 2005; 7:103–23.

61. Weaver IC, Diorio J, Seckl JR et al. Early environmental regulation of hippocampal glucocorticoid receptor gene expression: characterization of intracellular mediators and potential genomic target sites. Ann NY Acad Sci 2004; 1024:182–212.

62. Girdler SS, Thompson KS, Light KC et al. Historical sexual abuse and current thyroid axis profiles in women with premenstrual dysphoric disorder. Psychosom Med 2004; 66:403–10.

63. Shansky RM, Glavis-Bloom C, Lerman D et al. Estrogen mediates sex differences in stress-induced prefrontal cortex dysfunction. Mol Psychiatry 2004; 9:531–8.

64. Huo L, Straub RE, Schmidt PJ et al. Risk for premenstrual dysphoric disorder is associated with genetic variation in ESRI, the estrogen receptor alpha gene. Biol Psychiatry 2006, in press.

65. Binder EB, Nemeroff CB, Implications for the practice of Psychiatry. Prog Brain Res 2006; 158: 275–93.

Index

Note to index: PMS is used for PMS/PMDD; italic page numbers denote illustrations/tables.

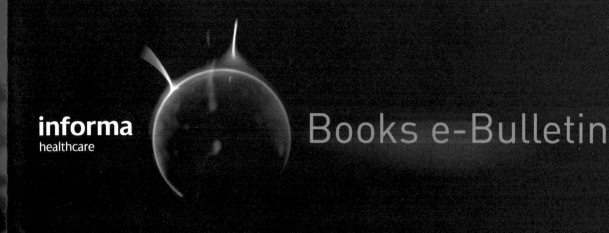

Books e-Bulletin

informa healthcare

Subscribe to the Informa Healthcare books e-Bulletin

Now you can keep your finger on the pulse with monthly highlights of all the latest and forthcoming publications from Informa Healthcare. You'll also receive special offers and promotions and a listing of all the key exhibitions Informa Healthcare are attending throughout the year.

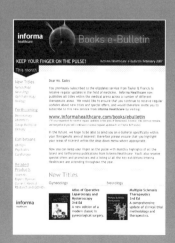

To Subscribe to the Books e-Bulletin please visit:
www.informahealthcare.com/books/ebulletin

OBSTETRICS AND GYNAECOLOGY/ REPRODUCTIVE MEDICINE

Informa Healthcare provides a wide range of Obstetrics and Gynaecology journals.

Journal of Obstetrics and Gynaecology

Journal of Obstetrics and Gynaecology represents an established forum for the entire field of obstetrics and gynaecology with an affiliation with the British Society for the Study of Vulval Disease (BSSVD). It publishes a broad range of high quality original, peer-reviewed papers, from scientific and clinical research to reviews relevant to practice and case reports.

www.informaworld.com/cjog

Editors in Chief: Harry Gordon, Alan MacLean

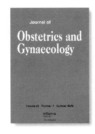

Climacteric

Climacteric is the official Journal of the International Menopause Society with a current Impact Factor of 2.299, ranking it in the top tier of all journals in obstetrics and gynaecology. It has an increased frequency of 6 issues per year.

www.informaworld.com/dcli

Editor in Chiefs: David Sturdee, Alastair MacLennan

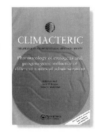
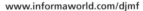

The Journal of Maternal-Fetal and Neonatal Medicine

This monthly publication is the official journal of the European Association of Perinatal Medicine, the Federation of Asia and Oceania Perinatal Societies, and the International Society of Perinatal Obstetricians. It publishes a wide range of peer-reviewed original research on the obstetric, medical, genetic, mental health and surgical complications of pregnancy and their effects on the mother, fetus and neonate.

www.informaworld.com/djmf

Editors in Chief: Gian Carlo Di Renzo, Dev Maulik

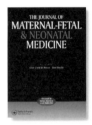

The European Journal of Contraception and Reproductive Health Care

For over 11 years, *The European Journal of Contraception and Reproductive Health Care* is the official journal of the European Society of Contraception. It has published published original peer-reviewed research papers, review papers and other appropriate educational material on all aspects of contraception and reproductive health care.

www.informaworld.com/dejc

Editor in Chief: Jean-Jacques Amy,

Editors: Medard Lech, Dan Apter, Dimitris Lazaris

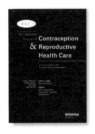
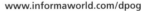

Journal of Psychosomatic Obstetrics and Gynecology

Journal of Psychosomatic Obstetrics and Gynecology is the official journal of the International Society of Psychosomatic Obstetrics and Gynecology. It provides a scientific forum for gynaecologists, psychiatrists and psychologists as well as for all those who are interested in the psychosocial and psychosomatic aspects of women's health.

www.informaworld.com/dpog

Editors in Chief: Willibrord C.M Weijmar Schultz, Harry B.M Van de Wiel

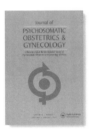

Gynecological Endocrinology

Gynecological Endocrinology, published monthly is the official journal of the International Society of Gynecological Endocrinology. It includes topics relating to the control and function of the different endocrine glands in females, the effects of reproductive events on the endocrine System and the consequences of endocrine disorders on reproduction.

www.informaworld.com/dgye

Editor in Chief: Andrea R. Genazzani

Human Fertility

Human Fertility is the official Journal of the British Fertility Society, the Association of Clinical Embryologists, the British Infertility Counselling Association, the Royal College of Nursing Fertility Nurses Group, and the British Andrology Society. Topics include molecular medicine and healthcare delivery.

www.informaworld.com/thuf

Editor in Chief: Henry Leese

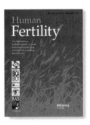

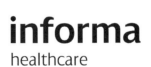

Only £45/AU$110

Pathology

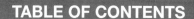

Special theme issue: Gynaecological pathology
Invited guest editor: Peter Russell

TABLE OF CONTENTS

HISTORY
- The rich history of gynaecological pathology: brief notes on some of its personalities and their contributions
  R. H. YOUNG

MOLECULAR STUDIES
- Molecular targets in gynaecological cancers
  A. N. Y. CHEUNG

- Molecular genetic changes in epithelial, stromal and mixed neoplasms of the endometrium
  S. F. LAX

- Uterine sarcomas
  F. MOINFAR, M. AZODI, AND F. A. TAVASSOLI

- Endometrial carcinoma: pathology and genetics
  J. PRAT, A. GALLARDO, M. CUATRECASAS AND L. CATASUS

- The pathology of gestational trophoblastic disease: recent advances
  M. WELLS

IMMUNOHISTOCHEMISTRY
- Immunohistochemistry as a diagnostic aid in cervical pathology
  W. G. McCLUGGAGE

DIAGNOSTIC PATHOLOGY
- Neoplasms of the fallopian tube and broad ligament: a selective survey including historical perspective and emphasising recent developments
  R. H. YOUNG

- Minimal uterine serous carcinoma: current concepts in diagnosis and prognosis
  J. T. RABBAN AND C. J. ZALOUDEK

- Undifferentiated carcinoma of the endometrium: a review
  E. SILVA, M. DEAVERS AND A. MALPICA

- The enigma of struma ovarii
  L. ROTH AND A. TALERMAN

INTERSEX
- Neoplasms and pathology of sexual developmental disorders (intersex)
  S. J. ROBBOY AND F. JAUBERT

This special theme issue on Gynaecological Pathology contains contributions from some of the finest international pathologists in the field. They provide an insight into common yet difficult aspects of surgical pathology of the female reproductive tract.

Visit **www.informaworld.com/pathology**
for general Journal information

To order the special issue, contact:
Louise Porter, Marketing Manager, Informa Healthcare,
69-77 Paul Street, London, EC2A 4LQ; **Email:** Louise.Porter@informa.com